NUTRACEUTICAL DELIVERY SYSTEMS

Promising Strategies for Overcoming Delivery Challenges

NUTRACEUTICAL DELIVERY SYSTEMS

Promising Strategies for Overcoming Delivery Challenges

Edited by
Pankaj V. Dangre, PhD
Debarshi Kar Mahapatra, PhD

A∧P APPLE
ACADEMIC
PRESS

First edition published 2023

Apple Academic Press Inc.
1265 Goldenrod Circle, NE,
Palm Bay, FL 32905 USA

4164 Lakeshore Road, Burlington,
ON, L7L 1A4 Canada

CRC Press
6000 Broken Sound Parkway NW,
Suite 300, Boca Raton, FL 33487-2742 USA

4 Park Square, Milton Park,
Abingdon, Oxon, OX14 4RN UK

© 2023 by Apple Academic Press, Inc.

Apple Academic Press exclusively co-publishes with CRC Press, an imprint of Taylor & Francis Group, LLC

Library and Archives Canada Cataloguing in Publication

Title: Nutraceutical delivery systems : promising strategies for overcoming delivery challenges / edited by
 Pankaj V. Dangre, PhD, Debarshi Kar Mahapatra, PhD.
Names: Dangre, Pankaj V., editor. | Mahapatra, Debarshi Kar, editor.
Description: First edition. | Includes bibliographical references and index.
Identifiers: Canadiana (print) 20220171335 | Canadiana (ebook) 20220171408 | ISBN 9781774637166 (hardcover) |
 ISBN 9781774637999 (softcover) | ISBN 9781003189671 (ebook)
Subjects: LCSH: Drug delivery systems. | LCSH: Functional foods.
Classification: LCC RS199.5 .N88 2023 | DDC 615/.6—dc23

Library of Congress Cataloging-in-Publication Data

....

CIP data on file with US Library of Congress

....

ISBN: 978-1-77463-716-6 (hbk)
ISBN: 978-1-77463-799-9 (pbk)
ISBN: 978-1-00318-967-1 (ebk)

About the Editors

Pankaj V. Dangre, PhD

Associate Professor and Vice-Dean (Research),
Department of Pharmaceutics, Datta Meghe College of Pharmacy,
DMIMS (DU), Wardha, Maharashtra, India

Pankaj V. Dangre, PhD, is currently an Associate Professor and Vice-Dean (Research), Department of Pharmaceutics, Datta Meghe College Of Pharmacy, DMIMS (DU), Maharashtra, India. He was formerly Assistant Professor in the Department of Pharmaceutics at the R. C. Patel Institute of Pharmaceutical Education and Research at North Maharashtra University, Nagpur, India. He is an academician dedicated to teaching, a passionate researcher, and an administrator. He taught modern pharmaceutics and novel drug delivery systems (NDDS) at undergraduate and postgraduate levels and has mentored students in various research projects at both levels. His area of interest includes drug delivery, formulation development, and nutraceutical innovations. He has published a number of research papers on bioavailability enhancement and controlled-release formulations along with book chapters and laboratory manuals on basic pharmaceutical formulations and physical pharmaceutics. He is an active reviewer for several international journals and a member of a number of professional bodies.

Debarshi Kar Mahapatra, PhD

Assistant Professor, Department of Pharmaceutical Chemistry,
Dadasaheb Balpande College of Pharmacy,
Rashtrasant Tukadoji Maharaj Nagpur University, Maharashtra, India

Debarshi Kar Mahapatra, PhD, is currently an Assistant Professor in the Department of Pharmaceutical Chemistry at Dadasaheb Balpande College of Pharmacy at RTM Nagpur University, Nagpur, India. He has taught medicinal chemistry and computational chemistry at both undergraduate and postgraduate levels and has mentored a number of students in various research projects. His area of interest includes computer-assisted rational designing, synthesis of low molecular weight ligands against druggable targets, development of drug delivery systems, and optimization of unconventional formulations. He has published several research papers, review articles, and imperative case studies in various reputed international journals and has presented his original contributions at several international platforms, for which he received several awards by a number of scientific and professional bodies. He has contributed several edited books, syllabus-based textbooks, lab manuals, book chapters, magazine articles, and guidebooks on pharmaceutical chemistry, natural products, pharmacology, and pharmaceutics. Presently, he is as an active reviewer and serves as an editorial board member for several journals of national and international repute. He is an active member of a number of professional and international scientific societies. He held the positions of Chief Advisor and Chief Executive Manager in the Indian Pharma Educational Society (IPES) and presently holds the position of Chief Advisor in the Health Society of Global Pharmacovigilance Professionals.

Contents

Contributors

Sumit Arora
Department of Pharmacognosy, Gurunanak College of Pharmacy, Rashtrasant Tukadoji Maharaj Nagpur University, Nari, Nagpur, Maharashtra, India

Shashikant Bagade
NMIMS, School of Pharmacy and Technology Management, Shirpur, Maharashtra, India

Sanjaykumar B. Bari
H.R Patel Institute of Pharmaceutical Education and Research, Shirpur, Dhule, Maharashtra, India

Veena S. Belgamwar
Department of Pharmaceutical Sciences, RTM Nagpur University, Nagpur, Maharashtra, India

Sachin Borikar
Department of Pharmacology, Rajarshi Shahu College of Pharmacy, Buldhana, Maharashtra. India

Shailesh S. Chalikwar
Department of Pharmaceutical Quality Assurance, R.C. Patel Institute of Pharmaceutical Education and Research, Shirpur, Dhule, Maharashtra, India

Kaushalendra Chaturvedi
Lachman Institute for Pharmaceutical Analysis Laboratory at Long Island University, New York, USA

Kanhaiya M. Dadure
Department of Chemistry, J. B. College of Science, Wardha – 442001, Maharashtra, India

Pankaj V. Dangre
Department of Pharmaceutics, Data Meghe College of Pharmacy, Wardha 442004, Maharashtra, India

Manik Das
Department of Pharmaceutical Chemistry, Gokaraju Rangaraju College of Pharmacy, Hyderabad, Telangana, India

Vivek S. Dave
St. John Fisher College, Wegmans School of Pharmacy, Rochester, New York, USA

Prashant K. Deshmukh
Department of Pharmaceutics, H.R. Patel Institute of Pharmaceutical Education and Research, Shirpur, Maharashtra–425405, India

Poorva P. Dusad
Department of Pharmaceutical Quality Assurance, R.C. Patel Institute of Pharmaceutical Education and Research, Shirpur, Dhule, Maharashtra, India

Bhavin Gajera
Formulation Scientist, Impel NeuroPharma, Washington, USA

Surendra G. Gattani
School of Pharmacy, S.R.T.M. University, Vishnupuri, Nanded–431606, Maharashtra, India

Ankita A. Gorhe
Department of Pharmaceutical Quality Assurance, SRES's Sanjivani College of Pharmaceutical
Education and Research, Kopargaon, Maharashtra, India

Vishal S. Gulecha
School of Pharmaceutical Sciences, Sandip University, Nashik, Maharashtra, India

Vishal C. Gurumukhi
Department of Pharmaceutics and Quality Assurance, R. C. Patel Institute of Pharmaceutical Education
and Research, Shirpur, Dhule, Maharashtra–425405, India, E-mail: vishalgurumukhi1584@gmail.com

Abhay Ittadwar
Gurunanak College of Pharmacy, Rashtrasant Tukadoji Maharaj Nagpur University, Nagpur,
Maharashtra, India

Snehal S. Jagtap
Department of Pharmaceutical Quality Assurance, SRES's Sanjivani College of Pharmaceutical
Education and Research, Kopargaon, Maharashtra, India

Shirish P. Jain
Department of Pharmaceutics, Rajarshri Shahu College of Pharmacy, Buldhana, Maharashtra, India

Tomy Muringayil Joseph
Chemical Faculty, Polymers Technology Department, Gdansk University of Technology,
Gdansk–80233, Poland

Prajakta Joshi
Private Practitioner, VIBGYOR Pediatric and Family Dental Clinic, Mumbai–400024, Maharashtra, India

Pallavi S. Kandalkar
Department of Pharmaceutical Quality Assurance, SRES's Sanjivani College of Pharmaceutical
Education and Research, Kopargaon, Maharashtra, India

Asmita K. Kedar
Department of Pharmaceutical Quality Assurance, SRES's Sanjivani College of Pharmaceutical
Education and Research, Kopargaon, Maharashtra, India

Vaishali Kilor
Department of Pharmaceutics, Gurunanak College of Pharmacy, Rashtrasant Tukadoji Maharaj Nagpur
University, Nagpur, Maharashtra, India, E-mail: v_kilor@yahoo.com

Abhijeet D. Kulkarni
Pharmaceutical Quality Assurance Department, SRES's Sanjivani College of Pharmaceutical Education
and Research, Shinganapur, Kopargaon, Ahmednagar, Maharashtra–423603, India,
Tel.: (02423)222862; 223362, 226947, Mobile: +91 9021038338; 7875038969, Fax: (02423)222682,
E-mail: kulkarniabhijeet11@gmail.com

Parag A. Kulkarni
SVKM's NMIMS, School of Pharmacy and Technology Management, Shirpur Campus, Shirpur, Dhule,
Maharashtra, India

Dileep Kumar
Department of Pharmaceutical Chemistry, Poona College of Pharmacy, Bharati Vidyapeeth
(A Deemed to be University), Pune, Maharashtra, India

Pranesh Kumar
Department of Pharmacology, Aryakul College of Pharmacy & Research, Lucknow, Uttar Pradesh,
India

Vaibhav A. Mahale
Department of Pharmaceutical Quality Assurance, SRES's Sanjivani College of Pharmaceutical Education and Research, Kopargaon, Maharashtra, India

Debarshi Kar Mahapatra
Department of Pharmaceutical Chemistry, Dadasaheb Balpande College of Pharmacy, Nagpur–440037, Maharashtra, India, E-mail: mahapatradebarshi@gmail.com

Mahesh P. More
Department of Pharmaceutics, SVKM's Institute of Pharmacy, Dhule, Maharashtra–424001, India; Department of Pharmaceutics, H.R. Patel Institute of Pharmaceutical Education and Research, Shirpur, Maharashtra–425405, India

Pankaj Padmakar Nerkar
Associate Professor, Department of Quality Assurance, R.C. Patel Institute of Pharmaceutical Education and Research, Shirpur, Maharashtra, India, Mobile: +919420151343, E-mail: nerkarpankaj@rediffmail.com

Amit B. Page
SVKM's NMIMS, School of Pharmacy and Technology Management, Shirpur Campus, Shirpur, Dhule, Maharashtra, India

Chandrakantsing V. Pardeshi
R. C. Patel Institute of Pharmaceutical Education and Research, Shirpur, Maharashtra, India, Tel.: +91-9881414752, E-mail: chandrakantpardeshi11@gmail.com

Unnati M. Patel
Department of Pharmaceutical Quality Assurance, SRES's Sanjivani College of Pharmaceutical Education and Research, Kopargaon, Maharashtra, India

Kiran Patil
NMIMS, School of Pharmacy and Technology Management, Shirpur, Maharashtra, India

Swapnil G. Patil
School of Pharmacy, S.R.T.M. University, Vishnupuri, Nanded–431606, Maharashtra, India

Anil M. Pethe
Department of Pharmaceutics, Datta Meghe College of Pharmacy, Wardha, Maharashtra. India.

Prasad A. Pofali
National Institute of Immunohematology, Mumbai, Maharashtra, India, E-mail: prasad.pofali@gmail.com

Manisha Puranik
Institute of Pharmaceutical Education and Research, Borgaon (Meghe), Wardha, Maharashtra, India, E-mail: manisha68_12@yahoo.com

Jyotiranjan Roul
Institute of Pharmaceutical Education and Research, Rashtrasant Tukadoji Maharaj Nagpur University, Borgaon (Meghe), Wardha, Maharashtra, India

Anjali S. Sabale
Department of Pharmaceutical Quality Assurance, SRES's Sanjivani College of Pharmaceutical Education and Research, Kopargaon, Maharashtra, India

Nidhi Sapkal
Gurunanak College of Pharmacy, Rashtrasant Tukadoji Maharaj Nagpur University, Nagpur, Maharashtra, India

Harsh Shah
Lachman Institute for Pharmaceutical Analysis Laboratory at Long Island University, New York, USA

Sanjay J. Surana
Department of Pharmaceutical Quality Assurance, R.C. Patel Institute of Pharmaceutical Education and Research, Shirpur, Dhule, Maharashtra, India

Mohamad Taleuzzaman
Department of Pharmaceutical Chemistry, Faculty of Pharmacy, Maulana Azad University, Jodhpur, Rajasthan, India

Darshan R. Telange
Department of Pharmaceutics, Data Meghe College of Pharmacy, Wardha 442004, Maharashtra, India

Alok Ubgade
Department of Pharmacognosy, Gurunanak College of Pharmacy, Rashtrasant Tukadoji Maharaj Nagpur University, Nari, Nagpur, Maharashtra, India

Shobha Ubgade
Department of Pharmacognosy, Gurunanak College of Pharmacy, Rashtrasant Tukadoji Maharaj Nagpur University, Nari, Nagpur, Maharashtra, India

Pramod Yeole
Institute of Pharmaceutical Education and Research, Rashtrasant Tukadoji Maharaj Nagpur University, Borgaon (Meghe), Wardha, Maharashtra, India

Amar G. Zalte
School of Pharmaceutical Sciences, Sandip University, Nashik, Maharashtra, India

Abbreviations

AD	Alzheimer's disease
AFM	atomic force microscopy
API	active pharmaceutical ingredient
ASE	accelerated solvent extraction
ATP	adenosine triphosphate
AUC	area under the curve
BCRP	breast cancer-resistant proteins
BCS	biopharmaceutical classification system
CAA	consumer affairs agency
CD	cyclodextrin
CFSAN	center for food safety and applied nutrition
CHT	chitosan
CMC	critical micelle concentration
CMP	carboxymethylpachyman
CMT	continuous multipurpose melt
CO_2	carbon dioxide
CoQ10	co-enzyme Q10
COS	chitooligosaccharides derivatives
CQAs	critical quality attributes
CRSD	controlled release solid dispersion
Cur	curcumin
CVD	cardiovascular disease
CYP 450	cytochrome p450
DCM	dichloromethane
DF	dietary fiber
DHA	docosahexaenoic acid
DI	deionized
DLS	dynamic light scattering
DMF	5,7-dimethoxyflavone
DNA	deoxyribonucleic acid
DoE	design of experiment
DS	dietary supplements
DSC	differential scanning calorimetry
DSHEA	Dietary Supplement Health and Education Act

DTPA	diethylenetriaminepentaacetic acid
EC	European Council
EE	entrapment efficiency
EFSA	European Food and Safety Authority
EPA	eicosapentaenoic acid
EPA	Environmental Protection Agency
FDA	Food and Drug Administration
FDAMA	FDA Modernization Act
FDP	freeze drying process
FF	functional fiber
FIM	foundation for innovation in medicine
FMCG	fast-moving consumer goods
FMEA	failure mode effect analysis
FNFC	foods with nutrient function claims
FOSHU	foods for specified health use
FPLC	flavonoids-phospholipids complexes
FSSAI	Food Safety and Standards Authority of India
FT-IR	Fourier transform infrared
GCP	good clinical practice
Gd	gadolinium
GI	gastrointestinal
GIT	gastrointestinal tract
GMP	good manufacturing practice
GMS	glyceryl monostearate
GPCR	g-protein-coupled receptors
GRAS	generally recognized as safe
HHS	health and human services
HLB	hydrophilic-lipophilic balance
Hot HPH	hot high-pressure homogenization
HPH	high-pressure homogenization
HPLC	high-performance liquid chromatography
HPMC	hydroxypropyl methylcellulose
ICH	International Council for Harmonization
IDF	insoluble dietary fiber
KP	Kaempferia parviflora
Lac	lactose
LC	liquid crystalline
LD	laser diffraction
LFCS	lipid formulation classification system

LUV	large unilamellar vesicles
MAE	microwave-assisted extraction
MePEGCA-HDCA	methoxy-polyethyleneglycol cyanoacrylate-co-hexadecylcyanoacrylate
MEs	microemulsions
METAC	methacryloxyethyl trimethylammonium
MHLW	ministry of health, labor, and welfare
MLV	multilamellar vesicles
MPS	mononuclear phagocyte system
MYR	myricetin
N_2O	nitrous oxide
NCDs	non-communicable diseases
NCEs	new chemical entities
NIH	National Institutes of Health
NLCs	nanostructured lipid carriers
NLEA	nutrition labeling and education act
nm	nanometer
NM	nutrient material
NMR	nuclear magnetic resonance
NPs	nanoparticles
NRG	naringenin
NSS	national sample survey
NuBACS	nutraceutical bioavailability classification scheme
O/W	oil-in-water
O/W/O	oil/water/oil
OTC	over the counter
P	pressure
PAC	poly(acrylic acid)
PBS	phosphate buffer saline
P_c	critical pressure
PC	phosphatidyl choline
PCA	poly(cyanoacrylate)
PDADMAC	poly(diallyldimethylammonium chloride)
PDI	polydispersity index
PE	phosphatidylethanolamine
PEG	polyethylene oxide
PEI	poly(ethyleneimine)
PEO	poly(ethylene oxide)
PF	propolis flavonoid

P-gp	p-glycoproteins
PIP	piperine
PLA	poly(lactic acid)
PLG	poly(D, L-glycolide)
PLGA	poly(D,L-lactide-co-glycolide)
PMCA	polymethylcyanoacrylate
PMF	3,5,7,3′,4′-pentamethoxyflavone
PMMA	poly methyl methacrylate
PS	phytosterols
P-SNP	phytosomal soft nanoparticles
PSS	poly(styrenesulfonate)
PUFA	polyunsaturated fatty acids
PVA	polyvinylalcohol
PXRD	powder x-ray diffraction
PZA	piezoelectric actuator
QbD	quality by design
QC	quality control
RES	reticulo-endothelial system
RESS	rapid expansion of supercritical solution
RH	relative humidity
RPM	rotation per min
RPN	risk priority number
SAS	supercritical antisolvent
$ScCo_2$	supercritical carbon dioxide
SCF	supercritical fluid
SD	Sprague Dawley
SDF	soluble dietary fiber
SDs	solid dispersions
SEM	scanning electron microscopy
SFE	supercritical fluid extraction
SLNs	solid lipid nanoparticle
SLS	sodium lauryl sulfate
SMEDDS	self-micro-emulsifying drug delivery system
SP	soya phospholipids
SPs	sulfated polysaccharides
SSA	significant scientific agreement
S-SEDDS	supersaturable self-emulsifying drug delivery system
SUV	small unilamellar vesicles
T	temperature

T2D	type-2 diabetes
T_c	critical temperature
TEM	transmission electron microscopy
TMC	N-trimethyl chitosan
TMF	5,7,4′-trimethoxy flavone
TPGS	tocopherol polyethylene glycol succinate
UAE	ultrasound-assisted extraction
USFDA	United States Food and Drug Administration
W/O	water-in-oil
WSA	wet spherical agglomeration
XRD	X-ray diffraction

Foreword

It is an extremely pleasurable moment in my life to write a foreword for the reference book entitled *Nutraceutical Delivery Systems: Promising Strategies for Overcoming Delivery Challenges*, edited by Pankaj V. Dangre, PhD, and Debarshi Kar Mahapatra, PhD, which is of great interest to academic members, medical practitioners, industry personnel, clinical dieticians, nutraceutical experts and a wide, range of biological researchers. This book provides new insights for PhD scholars involved in drug delivery fields, postdoctoral researchers, allied multidisciplinary students (medical, dental, nursing, physiotherapy, etc.), independent nutraceutical researchers, students enrolled in several scientific courses, and those with professional degrees like BS, BSc, BTech, BPharm, MS, MSc, MTech, MPharm, MBBS, etc. This book focuses on the current research aspects of interest to nutraceutical companies, pharmaceutical organizations, private producers, and innovation-oriented small- to large-scale companies.

This book highlights the recent work in nutraceutical delivery systems encompassing various strategies and approaches to get maximum health benefits to the patients. The book focuses the recent research-oriented work in nutraceutical delivery, including recent facts, global perspectives, isolation techniques, various strategies, and approaches such as phytosomes, solid dispersions (SDs), micelles, self-emulsifying drug delivery system (SEDDS), microemulsions (MEs), solid lipid nanoparticles (SLN), oral delivery, and polymeric nanoparticles to get maximum health benefits to the patients with various ailments like cancer, diabetes, etc. This book has includes adequate illustrations of instruments, small diagrams, high-resolution graphical representations, and other varied figures, which will positively guide readers in grasping the modern concepts and improving the theoretical knowledge and practical techniques several-folds.

I personally recommend this book to global readers and students. I also wish good luck to the editors and all the contributing authors for their enormous efforts.

—**Prof. (Dr.) R. S. Gaud**

Director, SVKM's Pharma Institutions (Mumbai, Shirpur, Dhule, Hyderabad)
and Mukesh Patel Technology Park, Shirpur Campus, Shirpur,
Dhule, Maharashtra, India

Preface

Nutraceutical is a hybrid term that originated from "nutrition" and "pharmaceuticals." The term is applied to products that are food or part of food that have numerous medical and health benefits, including the protection and treatment of chronic diseases. It encompasses a wide range of products from herbs, functional food, dietary supplements (DS), isolated nutrients, and genetically discovered foods. These components have been systematically categorized based on the source, mechanism of action, and chemical nature into various groups such as polyphenols, polyunsaturated fatty acids (PUFAs), antioxidant vitamins, dietary fibers (DFs), probiotics, bioactive peptides, etc. These nutraceuticals have shown promising results in various complications such as diabetes, cancer, cardiovascular diseases (CVDs), obesity, arthritis, and osteoporosis, leading to a new era of investigation on natural products. The consumption of nutraceuticals for health-related benefits has ascended drastically in recent years; the global nutraceutical market is anticipated to rise to US$ 279 billion by 2021, with a cumulative annual growth rate of 7.3%. With the versatility in pharmacological action as well as a strong presence in a global market, it is imperative to optimize the formulations to gain maximum health-related benefits.

This innovative edited book highlights the recent work in nutraceutical delivery, encompassing various strategies and approaches to get maximum health benefits to the patients. The book highlights the recent research-oriented work in the nutraceutical delivery with recent facts, global perspectives, isolation techniques, various strategies, and approaches such as phytosomes, liposomes, solid dispersions, micelles, self-emulsifying drug delivery system (SEDDS), microemulsions (MEs), solid lipid nanoparticles (SLN), polyelectrolyte complexes, oral delivery, and polymeric nanoparticles to get maximum health benefits to the patients in treating various ailments. The book also focuses on facts, global perspectives, and isolation techniques on nutraceutical components and/or products.

—**Pankaj V. Dangre, PhD**
Debarshi Kar Mahapatra, PhD

PART I

Basics Concepts and Global Progress in Nutraceutical Sciences

CHAPTER 1

Recent Facts and Global Perspectives of Nutraceuticals in Medicine

MANISHA PURANIK, JYOTIRANJAN ROUL, and PRAMOD YEOLE

Institute of Pharmaceutical Education and Research, Borgaon (Meghe), Wardha, Maharashtra, India, E-mail: manisha68_12@yahoo.com (M. Puranik)

ABSTRACT

This book chapter comprehensively describes the fundamentals of nutraceuticals, translated concepts, plausible benefits, developed new products (vitamin, minerals, herbal, polyphenols, dietary fiber (DF), etc.), paradigms, challenges, global economy, worldwide demands, global scenario, and regulatory aspects (USA, Europe, Japan, and India).

1.1 INTRODUCTION

Globalization of the economy is linked with the globalization of the western diet. Wealth and financial development resulted in a superior intake of total, saturated, and trans-fat; people consume more ready-prepared refined foods, beverages, snacks, and meals with an increased glycemic index. These foods are deficient in micronutrients, amino acids, antioxidants, and omega-3 fatty acids. They are rich in refined carbohydrates, fat, vitamins, and salt. Increased consumption of Junk foods is linked with increased risk of non-communicable diseases (NCDs), hypertension, angina, type-2 diabetes (T2D), cancer, liver diseases, gastrointestinal (GI) diseases, joint disorders, degenerative bone diseases, and depression-like psychological diseases. These diseases are related to dietary habits, which will continue to expand gradually. So, it is recommended for the intake of plant-related food to overcome these diseases and to improve quality of life [1–5].

Food security and food self-sufficiency are significant challenges for developed and underdeveloped countries. One of the most influential groups that bear the brunt of nutritional problems are lactating mothers and school-going children; many of them suffer from under-nutrition and malnutrition. The world still ignores seasonal diversity, food diversity, and the adequacy of nutrients. The nutrient adequacy is abundant in the Indian diet because of food consumption patterns. The new sedentary lifestyle adopted by the population has altered the essential food habits, use of junk foods has increased manifold, leading to the increased prevalence of lifestyle-related diseases. Obesity is a global health issue. Heart diseases report many deaths, followed by osteoporosis, arthritis, cancers, and many others. Excessive industrialization has caused air as well as water pollution, leading to soil and food contamination. It leads to increased occurrences of physiological, psychological, and degenerative diseases leading to severe immune dysfunction. Consumers are frustrated with expensive, high-tech, side effect prone, disease-treatment, and management approach and are seeking a complementary, manageable, low-cost, customer-friendly, and alternative approach. Moreover, customers are consuming food items of minimal nutritive value and pretend that they do not have sufficient time for preparing a healthy balanced meal. For compensation of these frustrations and losses, dietary supplements (DS) should be included in today's lifestyle [6–11].

1.2 NUTRACEUTICALS

Dr. Stephen L. DeFelice, the Founder and Chairman of Foundation for Innovation in Medicine (FIM), Cranford, NJ, coined the term 'Nutritive Pharmaceuticals.' According to him, the amalgamated commercial term, 'Nutraceuticals,' means foods or food products that might help to prevent and treat diseases. These are usually natural substances derived from food sources with more health benefits in addition to the fundamental nutritional value found in foods and, unlike drugs, are not synthesized for a specific purpose and include isolated nutrients, diets, and genetically prepared foods, herbal products, and processed foods. Nutraceuticals are non-specific biological therapies used to control several symptoms, encourage general health well-being, and avert destructive progressions [2]. Health Canada defines nutraceuticals as "an innovative component prepared from foods, sold in the form of pills, or powder (potions) or in other medicinal formulations, not typically linked with foods." The art and science behind nutraceuticals are to focus on the health value of our diet and improve the medical condition at an economically affordable cost, according to Greek Physician, Hippocrates, *"let food be thy medicine."*

The nutraceutical market is growing and diversifying rapidly, and in the global market, nutraceuticals have become a multibillion-dollar industry. Nutraceuticals are over food but less than pharmaceuticals. Unfortunately, even after two decades, there is still no globally acknowledged description of these products, and therefore, the regulations vary country by country. However, in most countries, nutraceuticals are taken as DS, and the frequency of its use is marching ahead because of the consumers' curiosity about alternative food and medicines. Moreover, consumers are frustrated with super-specialty expensive, disease treatment approach and are seeking solace by experimenting openly with herbs, vitamins, and other supplements, natural health foods, and food products, marketed for unique health benefits. Most nutraceuticals use well-known vital ingredients for the human body, but many details such as dose, drug-nutraceutical interaction, and the effect of nutraceuticals under certain health conditions remain unpredictable. Many of these are available at Pharmacies, supermarkets, as well as via telemarketing [5, 12–14]. Few imperative nutraceutical products marketed across the global market are given in Table 1.1.

1.2.1 THE SHIFT FROM CURE TO PREVENTION

In 400 BC, Hippocrates said, *"Let food be your medicine and medicine be your food."* Today, as a result of the changing disease pattern, consumer's ambition of remaining fit, and drying up of new product pipelines, proper nutrition is more critical for strengthening our body internally. The nutrients from food are essential for natural processes that continually takes place inside the body. In today's fast-paced and highly demanding lifestyle, people focus more on convenience and are more used to packaged and canned foods. When hunger strikes, it is easier to open a tin or package of ready-made food than a well-prepared fresh food. These convenient ready-made foods can have untoward effects on our health. Hence, nutritionist's advice of nutritious food is not only for satisfying hunger but also for prevention of diseases and maintenance healthier life [15, 16]. Roles of nutrition and diet are shown in Figure 1.1.

TABLE 1.1   List of Some Nutraceuticals in World Market

Product	Source	Purpose
Fuze	Fruits	Antioxidant
Phenorex	Bitter Orange	Hypolipidemic
Fish Oil Plus	Salmon	Brain food
CogniSure	Polypeptide	For Alzheimer's
Calcium plus milk	Milk	For bone health
Bite-amins	Herbal	Anti-mosquito pill
Vita kids bread	MEG-3	Multivitamin
Splenda essentials	Bread (wheat)	Sweetener
Rice protein concentrate	Brown rice	Protein
Rescue water	Fruit	Nutrients
Coral calcium	Calcium and trace minerals	Calcium supplements
GRD	Protein, vitamins, minerals, and carbohydrates	Nutritional supplements
Proteinex	Predigested protein, vitamins, minerals, and carbohydrates	Protein supplement
Calcitriol D-3 Calcirol D-3	Calcium, vitamins	Calcium supplements
Threptin diskettes	Protein and vitamin B	Protein supplement
Chyawanprash	Amla, Ashwagandha, Pippali	Immune booster
Amiriprash (Gold)	Chyawannprash Avaleha, Swarnabhasma, and Ras Sindur	Immuno-modulator
Omega women	Antioxidants, vitamins, phytochemicals	Immune supplement
Celestial healthcare	Dry fruit extract	Immune booster
Weight smart	Vitamins and trace elements	Nutritional supplements
Appetite intercept	Caffeine, tyrosine, and phenylalanine	Appetite suppressants
Chaser	Activated calcium carbonate and vegetable carbon	Hangover supplements
Soya milk	Soy proteins	Nutritional supplement
Proplus	Soy proteins	Nutritional supplement
Snapple-a-day	Vitamins and minerals	Meal replacement beverage
Wellife	Granulated-L-glutamine	Amino acids supplements
PNer plus	Vitamins and other natural supplements.	Neuropathic pain supplements

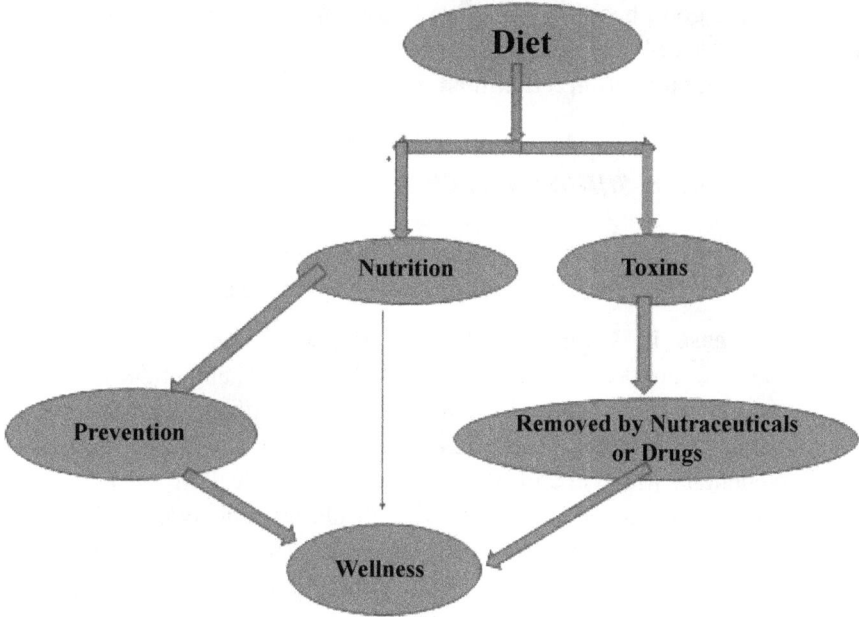

FIGURE 1.1 Role of nutrition and diet.

1.2.2 PREVENTION AND CURE: THE BUZZ WORDS

The primary goal of life should be health and well-being, and the secondary goal should be to cure disease(s) if a patient is hospitalized. The focus of preventive medicine is to avoid hospitalization (Figure 1.2).

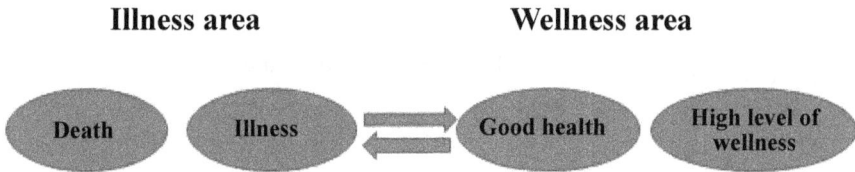

FIGURE 1.2 Health-illness continuum model.

1.2.3 RESPONSIBLE HEALTHCARE: THE SHIFT TOWARD PREVENTION

With changing disease patterns and rising healthcare costs, responsible healthcare, accountable healthcare or, rather, preventive healthcare is the buzzword for good health. People are becoming more aware of prevention and management of diseases. Moreover, rising healthcare costs increase the need to look at prevention rather than cure.

1.2.4   PARADIGM SHIFT: FROM CURE TO PREVENTION [17–19]

Changing trends and lifestyle goals have propelled a shift from cure to health and prevention. Some of the factors responsible for the shift are as follows:

1. **Increase in Chronic Lifestyle Diseases:** The chronic lifestyle diseases are prevalent in developed, developing, and underdeveloped countries. With rapid economic growth, the lifestyle of an average person has gone through massive changes. Increasing urbanization, sedentary lifestyle and wrong food habits are leading to an increase in the prevalence of NCDs. Several chronic lifestyle diseases like T2D, hypertension, hyperlipidemia, overweight/obesity are triggering CVD. The cost of treating infectious disease is a one-time expenditure, but the cost of treating NCDs is life-long and needs regular monitoring. Most of these diseases are prevented or managed to some extent. As these diseases are chronic, people have become aware and are focusing on the prevention of these diseases.

2. **Increasing Awareness Among Consumers:** Millennial consumers are leading the charge and taking the initiative on behalf of their well-being and are prepared to pay premium prices to achieve health and wellness. When it comes to health, people are adopting a proactive approach. The corporate sector is also concentrating on the positive effects of healthy living and managing the health of hyper-stressed employees, along with the general population. The costs of insurance and employee medical claims are at an all-time high and continue to rise. People today are adopting workplace health programs, regular meditation camps, and regardless of age, are adopting a wellness-oriented lifestyle, by concentrating on nutrition, fitness, and controlling work-related stress.

3. **Increasing Healthcare Costs:** The 71st National Sample Survey (NSS), during January–June 2014, conducted a survey which specifically revealed that 58% are private hospitals in contrast to only 42% public hospitals when studied the total hospitalization cases in rural India. The corresponding shares in urban areas were and 68% in private. The NSS findings over the last two decades depict a decline in

the percentage of public hospitals in treating patients. This has created asymmetric healthcare providers and patients giving monopolistic power to few conglomerated private providers resulting in distorted prices in medical treatment and diagnostics. High health care costs, combined with minimal insurance penetration, have resulted in more significant out-of-pocket expenditure for people across India. These increasing costs force people to take precautions and proactive care to prevent diseases and remain healthy. Health professionals focusing on management rather than treatment: Consumer's preference is towards the prevention and maintenance of health and control of diseases; healthcare is transforming from reactive to proactive and predictive care.

4. **Pharmaceutical Firms Venturing into the Health and Food Supplement Sector:** The big Pharma companies are facing a difficult time with patent cliff, generic threat, and low R&D productivity. These multi-national Pharma companies, facing a difficult time, have been systematically expanding into the nutraceutical market owing to its exponential growth in the last few years. Apart from Pharma companies, big FMCG (fast moving consumer goods) companies are also entering the functional foods and functional beverages segment. Thus, boosting the already growing market and further propelling the shift from cure to prevention.

1.2.5   A PARADIGM SHIFT IN FOODS

Food is not only considered as a basic necessity of life and a means of satisfying hunger but also viewed as a way of preventing, managing, and treating (to some extent) ailments. Consumers wanting to manage their healthcare create a demand for food products with associated health benefits.

The shift in food is because:

- Consumers are transformed from passive healthcare recipients to active healthcare consumers.
- People are happily embarrassing Hippocrates' thought of 'let food be thy medicine.' People have increased interest in wellness, self-care, and self-autonomy.
- People have realized the more sensible strategy for living is not antibiotics, but to strengthen our body internally. Treatment with pharmaceuticals is prone to side effects because drugs are xenobiotics,

whereas nutraceuticals are supplementation that can be absorbed and utilized for strengthening and improving vitality.

- Tradition view, food as a means of merely providing healthy growth and development, but today the food has been tailored to replace nutrients lost during cooking, and preventing nutrient deficiencies.
- Advances in nutrition sciences have made the lines between food and medicine fragile, as several types of research are available to prove that the food bio-actives can reduce the risk of chronic diseases, improve quality of life, and promote proper growth and development.

1.2.6   A PARADIGM SHIFT IN SELF-CARE

New self-care shift recognizes the health benefits of food that can coexist with medicines for disease risk/management/treatment. Due to advances in nutrition science, consumers have learned the impact of food on health. Moreover, consumers have started recognizing the shortcomings of cure centric healthcare system, which is expensive, time-consuming, and impersonal.

1.2.7   A PARADIGM SHIFT FROM FOODS TO MEDICAL FOODS AND DIETARY SUPPLEMENTS (DS)

There has been a significant change in the healthcare scenario: The concept "Food" being consumed to stay alive and satisfy hunger has changed to foods having natural functional benefits to human beings to the use of food in the treatment of diseases via healing foods. Figure 1.3 shows the present scenario.

1.3   CATEGORIES OF NUTRACEUTICALS [20, 21]

The hybrid of nutrition and pharmaceutical, Nutraceuticals, are food or part of diet playing a noteworthy function in altering and sustaining normal physiological function that continues to keep the human beings healthy. There are several ways for categorizations exist:

1. Nutraceuticals are often categorized as DS, medicinal food, and pharmaceuticals. According to Dietary Supplement, Health, and Education Act (DSHEA), the DS are the products that are anticipated

to supplement the diet and contain one or more of the following ingredients: herb, vitamin, botanical, mineral, and amino acid. DS are concentrated in capsule, liquid, powder, or pill form. Though the FDA regulates them as foods, their regulation differs from drugs and other foods.

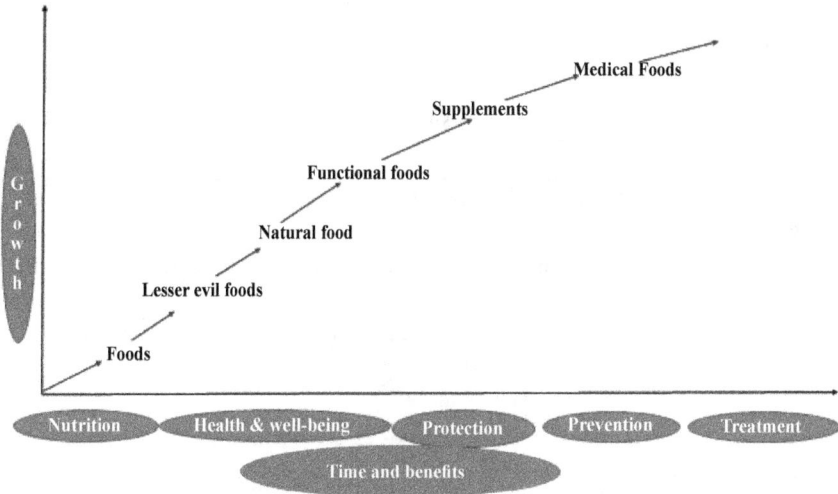

FIGURE 1.3 The changing role of food.

Functional foods are the class of food products that are taken as a diet in order to have valuable consequences that go ahead of basic nutritional function. Medical foods are formulated to devour or manage internally, under the supervision of the physician. The dietary use in the management of medical conditions or disorders with distinctive nutritional requirements is essential.

Pharmaceuticals are valuable components prepared from modified agricultural crops or animals. The term is a combination of "farm" and "pharmaceuticals." Proponents of this concept used modified crops (and even animals) as pharmaceutical factories, with the intention of using the cost-effective technique in healthcare.

2. Considering the promise, the nutraceuticals are categorized as established nutraceuticals and potential nutraceuticals. A potent nutraceutical is one that holds a promise of medical benefit or health benefit. Such a potential nutraceutical becomes an established one after clinical studies, which demonstrate the benefit.

3. Nutraceuticals are non-specific biological therapies used to stop malignant processes, promote wellness, and manage symptoms. They are categorized based on their chemical constituents as Nutrients, Herbal or botanical, and DS. Nutrients are the constituents of feed at a level that will promote wellness, prevent destructive processes, and control symptoms. The chief classes of feed nutrients are vitamins, minerals, fatty acids, and amino acids. Vitamins, minerals, and their associated benefits are listed in Tables 1.2 and 1.3.

TABLE 1.2   Various Vitamins and Their Health Benefits

Vitamins	Health Benefits
Vitamin A_1 Vitamin A_2	Antioxidants, maintenance of healthy skin, vision
Vitamin D	Essential for formation of bones and teeth, helps the body absorb and use calcium.
Vitamin E	Antioxidant, helps form blood cells, muscles, lung, and nerve tissue, boosts the immune system.
Vitamin K	Essential for blood clotting.
Vitamin B_1	Helps to convert food into energy, essential in neurologic functions.
Vitamin B_2	It helps in energy production and other chemical processes in the body, helps maintain healthy eyes, skin, and nerve function.
Vitamin B_3	Helps to convert food into energy. It also maintains proper brain function.
Folic acid	Essential in pregnancy for preventing birth defects, helps in RBC formation, protects against heart diseases.
Nicotinic acid	Required for various nervous system functions
Pyridoxine	Helps to produce essential proteins and convert protein into energy.
Biotin	Required for various metabolic functions.

Herbals are as old as human civilization, and they provide a complete storehouse of remedies to cure acute and chronic diseases. India has the oldest tradition of nature's remedies called Ayurveda. Herbal or botanical products are concentrates and extracts. Herbals as nutraceuticals along with their associated benefits are listed in Table 1.4.

Dietaries supplements are products administered through the mouth that contain dietary ingredients intended to enrich further the food that we eat. Some examples are black cohosh for menopausal

TABLE 1.3 Various Minerals and Their Health Benefits

Mineral	Health Benefits
Calcium	Boosts bone health, lowering high blood pressure, colon cancer, weight management, menopause, premenstrual syndrome (PMS) and cramps.
Magnesium	Boost immune system, treatment of hypertension, cardiovascular disease, osteoporosis, diabetes.
Selenium	Antioxidant, cancer, infectious, and inflammatory disease, immunity
Zinc	Essential for cell reproduction, normal growth and development in children, wound healing, production of sperm and testosterone.
Chromium	Blood glucose control
Iron	The formation of hemoglobin, needed for energy metabolism, prevents anemia, helps to carry and transfer oxygen to tissues.
Copper	Improves brain function, soothes arthritis, helps in skincare, elimination of throat infections, prevents heart diseases and boosts immunity.
Phosphorous	Boost brain function, integral in reducing muscle weakness, improve bone health, dental care, preventing aging.
Iodine	Treats goiter, fibrocystic breast disease, improves hair and skin health
Manganese	Management of body metabolism, prevention of osteoporosis, reduction of fatigue
Molybdenum	Detoxification, metabolism, reproduction
Potassium	Reduces tension in the blood vessels, regulates BP, ensures proper distribution of oxygen to vital organs, protection against cardiovascular diseases, treat low blood sugar.
Silicon	Important for bones health, skin, nail, hair, dental health, relief from sleep disorders, atherosclerosis.
Sodium	Maintains water balance, prevent sunstroke, improve brain function, relieve muscle cramps, prevent premature aging.
Iodide	Important for thyroid function, deficiency can cause goiter, vital for producing T_4.
Boron	Improve bone health, brain function, aging process, and sexual health. Prevent cancer, Alzheimer's disease, and reducing muscle pain.

TABLE 1.4 Common Herbals as Nutraceuticals

Herbals	Health Benefits
Garlic (Dried bulbs of *Allium sativum*, Liliaceae)	Anti-inflammatory, antibacterial, anti-gout, nervine tonic
Maidenhair tree (leaves of *Ginkgo biloba*, Ginkgoaceae)	PAF antagonist, memory enhancer, antioxidant.
Ginger (rhizomes of *Zingiber officinale*, Zingiberaceae)	Stimulant, chronic bronchitis, hyperglycemia, and throat pain.
Echinacea (dried herb of *Echinacea purpurea*, Asteraceae)	Anti-inflammatory, immunomodulatory, antiviral.
Ginseng (dried root of *Panax ginseng*, Araliaceae)	Stimulating immune and nervous system, adaptogenic properties.
Liquorice (dried roots of *Glycyrrhiza glabra*, Leguminosae)	Anti-inflammatory, anti-allergenic, and expectorant.
St. John's wort (dried aerial part of *Hypericum perforatum*, Hypericaceae)	Antidepressant, against HIV and hepatitis-C virus.
Turmeric (rhizome of *Curcuma longa*, Zingiberacae)	Anti-inflammatory, antiarthritic, anticancer, and antiseptic.
Onion (dried bulb of *Alivum cepa* Linn., Liliaceae)	Hypoglycemic activity, antibiotic, and anti-atherosclerosis.
Aloes (dried juice of leaves of *Aloe barbadensis*, Liliaceae)	Dilates capillaries, anti-inflammatory, and emollient, wound healing properties.
Senna (dried leaves of *Cassia angustifolia*, Leguminosae)	Purgative
Asafetida (oleo gum resin of *Ferula assafoetida* L., Umbelliferae)	Stimulant, carminative, expectorant.
Bael (unripe fruits of *Aegle marmelos* Corr., Rutaceae)	Digestive, appetizer, treatment of diarrhea and dysentery.
Brahmi (herbs of *Centella asiatica*, Umbelliferae)	Nervine tonic, spasmolytic, anti-anxiety
Valeriana (dried root of *Valeriana officinalis* Linn., Valerianaceae)	Tranquilizer, migraine, and menstrual pain, intestinal cramps, bronchial spasm.

symptoms, *Ginkgo biloba* for memory loss, glucosamine/chondroitin for arthritis. DS are important in sports nutrition, weight-loss supplements, and meal replacements. Supplement ingredients may contain minerals, herbs, vitamins, other botanicals, enzymes, gland extracts or other dietary substances. They are available in different dosage forms, including tablets, capsules, liquids, powders, extracts, and concentrates.

4. A variety of nutraceuticals are available in the market, which falls in the category of traditional foods and non-traditional foods. Traditional nutraceuticals are natural, whole foods with additional information about their health benefits. There is no change in actual foods apart from the customer's perception of them. Many vegetables, fruits, grains, fish, tea, dairy, and meat products contain several natural constituents (Lycopene, omega-3-fatty acids, etc.) that are beneficial to health beyond basic nutrition. Non-traditional nutraceuticals are the outcome from genetically engineered agri-products to improve the nutritional quality of nutrients enriched food such as calcium-fortified orange juice; cereals with added vitamins, flour with added minerals, and folic acids.

5. The food sources used as nutraceuticals are all-natural and are categorized as dietary fiber (DF), probiotics, prebiotics, polyunsaturated fatty acids (PUFAs), antioxidants, vitamins, polyphenols, and spices (Table 1.5). DF, also known as roughage, consists of lignin and non-digestible carbohydrates that are intrinsic and intact in plants. Functional fiber (FF) consists of isolated, non-digestible carbohydrates that have beneficial effects in humans. Total fiber is the sum of dietary and FF. The adequate intake for fiber defined by the Dietary Reference Intake (DRI) is 38 gm/day for adult men and 25 gm/day for adult women. We usually correlate bacteria with the disease. But our body hosts bacteria, good and bad. Probiotics are live, helpful bacteria and yeasts that are good for health, especially digestive health. Lactobacillus, the most common probiotic, found in yogurt and other fermented foods. Different strains can help with diarrhea and helps in digestion of lactose (Lac), the reducing sugar from milk. *Bifidobacterium*, found in some dairy products, ease the symptoms of irritable bowel syndrome, IBS, and helps in the breakdown of food. Probiotics help to move food through the gut. And, are useful in irritable bowel syndrome, IBS; inflammatory bowel disease, IBD; infectious diarrhea; antibiotic-induced diarrhea. Probiotics are also useful in skin conditions like

eczema; useful in the maintenance of urinary and vaginal health, prevent allergic colds, and maintains oral health.

Prebiotics encourage the activity or growth of microorganisms and add to the well-being of the host. Prebiotics are non-digestible, fiber compounds that pass undigested through the upper part of the GIT and promote the growth or activity of beneficial bacteria that colonize the large bowel by acting as a substrate for them. Prebiotics are neither food nor drugs they are intermediates. All prebiotics are fibers but not all fibers are prebiotics. For food ingredient to be prebiotic, it should be resistance to gastric acidity, cause hydrolysis by various mammalian enzymes, and promotes absorption in the upper GIT; it should get fermented by the intestinal microflora; it should stimulate the growth and/or activity of intestinal bacteria probably linked with the health and well-being. PUFAs are divided into two groups: omega-3 and omega-6 PUFA. These are the essential fatty acids and are intrinsic for physiological integrity, and their source is diet. Damage by free radicals plays a central role in the aging and disease progression process. Antioxidants are the scavengers of free radicals and are the primary line of resistance against them and are vital for maintaining appropriate healthcare and well-being. Oxygen is a highly reactive atom that is competent of fetching element of potentially detrimental molecules universally called "free radicals." These free radicals are proficient of damaging the healthy cells of our body, causing them to lose their function and structure. Antioxidants are capable of stabilizing or deactivating free radicals before they attack cells. Antioxidants are absolutely necessary for maintaining cellular health and well-being. Dietary antioxidants are vitamin C, vitamin E, beta-carotene, and other carotenoids and oxy-carotenoids, lycopene, lutein, and polyphenols.

Polyphenols are natural phytochemical components in plant-based foods, such as cereals, cocoa, coffee, fruits, legumes, tea, vegetables, whole grains, and wine. More than 8,000 polyphenolic compounds, including flavonoids, polymeric lignans, stilbenes, etc., have been recognized in entire plant foods. These compounds are known as the secondary metabolites of the plants, which act as protection alongside ultra-violet radiation, oxidants, and pathogens. Spices are the practically necessary constituent. These are the aromatic vegetable constituents, whole, broken, or ground form, whose function is seasoning rather than nutrition. These impart flavor, aroma, and pungency to foods. But apart from seasoning, spices are nutraceuticals, pharmaceuticals, indigenous medicines, aromatherapy, preservatives, beverages, natural colors, perfumes, dental preparations, cosmetics, and pesticides and thus are economically very important.

TABLE 1.5 Physiological Properties of Dietary Fibers and Their Proposed Health Benefits

Physiological Property	Proposed Effect	Health Benefits
Soluble dietary fiber	Prevent or delays nutrients uptake in the small intestine.	Lower blood cholesterol level.
	Prevents the reabsorption of bile acid.	Prevents the incidences of breast cancer.
	Prevent the digestive enzymes from reaching lipid substrates, inhibits enzyme activity.	Lowers glucose, insulin, and lipid level after a meal.
	Delays gastric emptying and prolonging intestinal phase.	Contribute to safety.
Interaction/ binding	Binding to bile acids	Lower blood cholesterol level.
	Interaction with digestive enzymes	Lowers insulin, glucose, and lipid level after the meal.
Fermentation	Growth of health-promoting bacteria	Protect against inflammation and colorectal cancer.
	Production of short-chain fatty acids	Lowers blood cholesterol level and protect against cancer.
Insoluble dietary fiber	Increase stool weight	Reduce the incidence of colorectal cancer and intestinal diseases.
	Accelerate transit time	Reduce time for nutrients to absorb, lowers glucose, insulin, and lipid level.

1.4 BENEFITS OF NUTRACEUTICALS

With the ever-changing lifestyle, the defense systems are frequently overloaded effects in stress. Moreover, the body's defense mechanism decreases with age. This might result in the progress of age-related diseases. Hence, research has refocused on positive aspects of our diet, with the intention that the consumption within the acceptable Dietary Intakes will keep diseases at bay and allow human beings to maintain a healthy lifestyle.

Bioactive constituents of food or phytochemical-enriched extracts are available commercially in the form of pharmaceutical products (pills, capsules, solutions, gels, powders, granules, etc.). These ranges of products are sold with the intent of treatment/prevention of disease and for the health and well-being of an individual. These products possess multiple therapeutic effects with lacking unwanted side effects. Few quoted examples include:

- The antioxidants, DFs, omega-3-fatty acids, vitamins, and minerals are beneficial in the prevention and treatment of CVD.

- Polyphenols (green tea, grapes) are beneficial in arterial diseases.
- Flavonoids (grapes, apples, cherries, and red wine) fortify the tiny capillaries that carry oxygen and necessary nutrients to all cells.
- Rice bran lowers the serum cholesterol levels in the blood, lowers the level of LDL, and increases the level of HDL in cardiovascular health.
- Rice bran contains both Lutein and Zeaxanthin, which recover the eyesight and lessens the chance of cataracts. Rice bran contains the essential FA, omega-3/6/9 and folic acid, which promotes eye health.
- The lipoic acid, an antioxidant is beneficial for the pharmacotherapy of diabetic neuropathy. DFs from psyllium are valuable in controlling glucose in diabetic patients, and docosahexaenoic acid (DHA) is beneficial in modulating insulin resistance.
- Herbal stimulants from fenugreek, green tea and coffee are beneficial in weight loss program.
- Flavonoids obstruct the enzymes that produce estrogens and decrease the potential risk of estrogen-induced cancers. Soy foods, curcumin possess cancer chemopreventive properties. Lycopene protects against cancer.
- Beetroots, cucumber, spinach, and turmeric are beneficial for anti-tumor activity.
- Curcumin possesses anti-carcinogenic, anti-oxidative, anti-inflammatory properties.
- Linoleic acid (found in green leafy vegetables, nuts, vegetable oils, etc.), is beneficial in treating inflammation and autoimmune diseases.
- Lutein (found in carrots, corn, sweet potatoes, and tomatoes) is useful for the treatment of visual disorders.
- Glucosamine and chondroitin sulfate are used for the treatment of osteoarthritis.
- Curcumin, lutein, and lycopene are beneficial in neutralizing the negative effects of oxidative stress.
- Corn's contribution to heart health lies in its fiber, and significant amount of folate.
- Corn maintains homocysteine, an intermediate in methylation cycle. Homocysteine is unswervingly accountable for the injury of the blood vessel.
- Corn also contains, cryptoxanthin, a natural carotenoid pigment. Cryptoxanthin can decrease the hazard of lung cancer.

1.5 REGULATORY GUIDELINES IN DIFFERENT COUNTRIES

1.5.1 REGULATORY GUIDELINES

After Stephen De Felice MD coined the word, Nutraceuticals in 1989, the world has witnessed the explosive growth of a billion-dollar nutraceutical industry. The regulatory definition of this term has not been finalized, therefore, products available in the market and drugstore or online, without any prescription, are considered food, herbal products, or food supplements. Nutraceutical represents a unique combination of the Pharma and Food industries. Drugs are potent pharmacologically active substances agonizing, antagonizing/modifying physiological/metabolic function, whereas nutraceuticals are food components that not only maintains, supports, normalizes any physiologic/metabolic function, but also potentiates, antagonize/modify physiologic or metabolic functions. Many nutraceuticals are substitutive to medicine and exert a pull on more consumer interest. The goals of nutraceutical regulation are extended to the labeling and safety, with less stress (as compared to pharmaceuticals) on the product attributes and projected applications. This is achieved through good manufacturing practice (GMP) regulations. Table 1.6 highlights the various regulatory guidelines in different nations.

1.5.2 REGULATORY GUIDELINES IN USA [22, 23]

USFDA defines nutraceuticals as DS and the regulations came in 1994. FDA regulates DS and dietary ingredients under diverse series of regulations when compared with those covering "conventional" foods and drug products. Under the Dietary Supplement Health and Education Act (DSHEA), the producers and distributors of DS and dietary constituents are outlawed from marketing products that are misbranded or adulterated.

According to DSHEA, from 1994, it is the manufacturer's accountability to make certain that a nutraceutical is harmless prior to it is marketed. USFDA is in charge of taking action in opposition to any misbranded or adulterated dietary supplement subsequent to its appearance in the market. The industry is liable for assessing the labeling and ensuring the security of their products ahead of marketing to guarantee that they convene all the necessities of DSHEA and FDA regulations. In the USA, health claims of nutraceuticals are authorized under the nutrition labeling and education act (NLEA) of 1990. Health claims depicted a relationship between the food,

TABLE 1.6 Regulatory Guidelines for Some Countries

Country	Regulatory Act	Issues
India	Food Safety and Standard Act (2006)	Manufacture, sale, and import of nutraceuticals
	The Food Safety and Standard Authority of India (FSSAI) (2008)	Food safety and standards
	Food Safety and Standards Rules and Regulations (2009)	Food safety and standards
	The Food Safety and Standard Authority of India (FSSAI) (2010)	Food safety and standards
China	State Food and Drug Administration of China (SFDA) (2003)	Oversees and coordinate the health, food, and drug agencies
	State Food and Drug Administration (SFDA) (2005)	Registration for functional foods
	State Council Legislative Office (SCLO) (2009)	Regulate food products
USA	NLEA (1990)	Nutrition labeling of foods
	DSHEA (1994)	Role of foods
	FDAMA (1997)	Safety of foods, biological products
	FSMA (2011)	Safety of food products
Brazil	National Sanitary Surveillance Agency, ANVISA (2002)	Safety of natural and synthetic products
Canada	Canadian Foods and Drugs Act and Regulation (1953)	Food definition
	Food Directorate of the Health Protection Branch of Health Canada (1996)	Medicinal nutraceuticals
	Canadian Food and Drugs Act (2001)	Describe foods with health benefits
	Natural Health Product Directorate (NHPD) (2003)	Nutraceutical definition
Australia	FSANZ (2003)	Food standards
	Australian Capital Territory-Food Regulation Act (2002)	Modification in food
Europe	Functional Food Science in Europe (FUFOSE) (1996)	Establish a science-based approach for concepts in functional food science

TABLE 1.6 *(Continued)*

Country	Regulatory Act	Issues
	Regulation (EC) no. 258/97 (1997)	Applies to GMP, foods, and food ingredients
	Regulation (EC) No. 1831/2003	For the authorizations of probiotics used as additives
	Regulation (EC) No. 353/2008	Establishes implementing rules for health claims in Regulation EC No. 1924/2006
	Regulation EU No. 383/2010	Authorize food which reduces disease risk and children's health
Japan	FOSHU (1991)	Health claims of specific products
	FHC (2001)	Expanded to tablets and capsules
	FNFC (2005)	Nutraceutical function claims

food component, or dietary supplement elements and decreasing the threat of a disease or health-related condition.

Health claims can be grouped into SSA and FDAMA. SSA (significant scientific agreement): These claims are for conventional foods and DS. SSA establishes nutrient/disease relationship. FDAMA (FDA modernization act): These claims are for conventional food and not for DS:

1. **Qualified Health Claims:** These claims are for conventional foods as well as DS. Any interested party can petition the FDA to issue regulation regarding a health claim of nutraceuticals. FDA evaluates the claim as per the SSA Standards.

2. **Nutrient Content Claims:** Such claims are about the content of certain nutrients or substances in food and are used to depict the percentage of nutrients in a product in relation to the daily intake value.

   Structure/Function claims: the claim was authorized under the DSHEA of 1994. Such claims relate to a positive contribution to health/improvement of function/modifying/preserving the health of an individual.

1.5.3 REGULATORY GUIDELINES IN EUROPEAN COUNTRIES [24–30]

In European countries, the primary step in food regulation was recognized in 1997 with the Green Paper on Food Law, and it was pursued by the White Paper on Food Safety in 2000, which summarized the need for novel and enhanced legislation in the area. These papers led to the General Food Law Regulation [Regulation (EC) No. 178/2002 of the European Parliament and of the Council 2002], which recognized the standard and forecast the formation of a self-governing association called the European Food Safety Authority (EFSA) with the explicit duty of generous systematic guidance based upon technical evaluation of the useful health effects and connected hazard associated to food intake. The mission of EFSA is to "offer the basis for the assurance of a high level of defense of human health and customer attention in relative to food, considering diversity in the delivery of food, including traditional products, while making certain the effectual functioning of the interior market. It establishes ordinary values and duty, the means to offer a strong science base, competent organizational preparations and procedures to underpin decision-making in matters of food and feed safety."

The European Council Regulation (EC) No. 178/2002 defines "food or foodstuff as any material or product, whether processed, partially processed or unprocessed, intended to be, or rationally be expected to be taken by humans." According to this definition, medicinal products cannot be considered food. Food derivatives with a definite favorable consequence on health, such as functional foods and nutraceuticals, can be believed comparable to therapeutic products if their micronutrient content is considered.

Medicinal products are defined by Directive 2001/83/EC of the European Parliament, which was amended by Directive 2004/27/EC of the Council. Medicinal products are defined as "any component or mixture of substances signifying as having properties for treating or averting disease in human beings, or any substance or a mixture of substances that may be employed in or administered to human beings either with a viewpoint to reinstating, accepting or modifying physiological roles by put forth immunological, pharmacological, or metabolic action, or to produce a medical diagnosis."

Food legislation is chiefly under the umbrella of the European Food and Safety Authority (EFSA). This legislation puts a highlight on "food supplements," which are defined as the intense foundation of nutrients (e.g., proteins, vitamins, and minerals) and other materials with a useful nutritional consequence. In order to claim their specific beneficial effects for pathologic conditions, an EFSA positive opinion is required in Europe. This implies a clear-cut relationship substantiated by clinical studies on healthy people. After a positive EFSA opinion, every member state can decide to set specific authorization for the registration of the product before its producing and selling.

The main EU legislation related to food supplements is Directive 2002/46/EC. Innovative products from Europe are alleged to have conceded stringent European development and Quality requirements. As a result, the European Nutraceutical market is considered as a leader and is producing good quality products.

1.5.4 REGULATORY GUIDELINES IN JAPAN [31, 32]

The Japanese community defined functional food early in the 1980s as having three functions, nutrition, sensory (satisfaction), and last is tertiary (physiological). Japan is the first country, which regulated food supplements, the Japanese ministry of health, labor, and welfare (MHLW) set up foods for specified health use (FOSHU), a product-specific approval system in 1991 as a regulatory system to approve the report made on food labels regarding the consequence of food on the human body.

The Council of Pharmaceutical Affairs and Food Hygiene under MHLW, scientifically evaluate food products to be relevant for approval by FOSHU in terms of their efficiency and safety. The regulatory range of FOSHU was widened in 2001 to acknowledge the forms of formulations such as tablets and capsules, in addition to other conventional forms. The MHLW introduced a new regulatory system, 'Foods with Health Claims' in April 2001, which consists of existing FOSHU and newly established foods with nutrient function claims (FNFC). FNFC refers to foods labeled with the functions of their nutritional ingredients. Under the FNFC, 12 vitamins (vitamin A, vitamin B_1, vitamin B_2, vitamin B_6, vitamin B_{12}, vitamin C, vitamin E, vitamin D, biotin, folic acid, pantothenic acid, and niacin) and two minerals (Ca and Fe) are standardized and permitted for use in FNFC products with established upper and lower levels of the daily consumption of these nutrients, to ensure sufficient nutrient intake and safety. And, when the market driven by health-conscious consumers grows, there require stringent regulations to handle the increased demand. In September 2009, authorities created the Consumer Affairs Agency (CAA), which took over the MHLW's responsibility for implementation of laws relating to nutrition labeling and health claims approval. CAA is responsible for the registration approval process of FOSHU products, FOSHU is divided into four subcategories: FOSHU; Qualified FOSHU; Standardized FOSHU; FOSHU with disease risk reduction claim.

FOSHU approval system is voluntary in Japan. Companies are given flexibility to market "health food" without obtaining FOSHU approval on the condition that these products do not bear any health claims or claim physiological effects on the human body. But in order to protect the public from false and misleading claims, CAA encourages industry participation in FOSHU approval system. In Japan, food products are not permitted to bear claims unless they became the part of the regulatory system as FNFC or FOSHU. The approval process for FOSHU takes six months from the day the application reaches to CAA.

1.5.5   REGULATORY GUIDELINES IN INDIA [33]

Nutraceuticals are neither food nor pharmaceuticals, so cannot be regulated as drug nor as food, owing to lack of proper regulatory framework, nutraceuticals in India are not conceptualized in terms of regulations, segments, marketing, manufacturing, imports, and exports. As nutritive pharmaceutical industry is a dynamic, evolving industry, to tap the market potential Indian regulatory system passed Food Safety and Standards Act-2006 (FSSA) which created a special third category- "Foods for Special Dietary Uses/Functional Foods/ Nutraceuticals/Health Supplements" in addition to the first two- "Drugs" and "Conventional Foods." FSSA-2006 put nutraceuticals as a special category of products that fall under the universal umbrella of foods but having specific regulatory requirements. After commencement of FSS Act-2006, several central acts like Prevention of Food Adulteration Act-1954, Fruit Products Order-1955, Meat Food Products Order-1973, Vegetable Oil Products (Control) Order-1947, Edible Oil Packaging (Regulation) Order-1988, Solvent Extracted Oil, De-oiled Meal, and Edible Flour (Control) Order-1967, Milk and Milk Products Order-1992, etc., have been repealed.

1.6 DEMAND FOR NUTRACEUTICALS GLOBALLY

The nutraceutical industry lays fewer than three main segments. It includes functional foods, DS, and herbal/natural products. The global nutraceutical market is showing explosive growth and is expected to touch 285 billion USD, the functional beverages market is projected to touch 105 billion USD, and the functional food business is expected to reach 92.3 billion USD by 2021.

By 2021, the world will have 1 billion populations of 60 plus, and the projected nutraceuticals are going to be more personalize and customize, especially in the developed markets of the world. In the initial years, the nutraceutical industry grew at 7% per annum, for the next few years up to 2010, the growth doubled at 14% per annum. Currently, around 12–15 billion USD is being added every year. Nutraceutical demand will grow with increasing life expectancy, increased risk of diseases like high BP, diabetes, obesity, and cholesterol and high cost associated with healthcare. The USA has the largest and fully matures nutraceutical market projected annually showing 10% growth. The US nutraceutical market comprises of DS (35%) and functional food beverages (65%). US consumers are more health-conscious than other countries and demand personalized and customized nutraceuticals. Current trends in the US are for all-natural, non-modified functional ingredients.

USA has DSHEA, since from 1994, which gives the roadmap for the registration of nutraceuticals/DS in the country for marketing purposes. In India, Food Safety Standards Act-2006, and Food Safety Standard Rules and Regulations-2011 are implemented to avoid the grouping of nutraceutical product either into food or drug. The nutraceuticals used/sold in India are called by the name "Functional Foods for Special Dietary Uses." When a new product wants to enter the nutraceutical market of a country, it must comply with the regulatory framework of that country. In coming years, the successful nutraceutical players are going to be those companies in which functional products are satisfying customers on two counts, conventional, and health value. Future nutraceuticals will have a direct relationship between nutrition and disease.

1.7   CHALLENGES AND OPPORTUNITIES

The area of functional foods and nutraceuticals is new, and numerous breaches subsist in the knowledge foundation. It is extensively established that the health-promoting effects of foods are not from a single component but from a little or numerous components. It creates a pattern change from pharmaceuticals, which is based on the potency or efficiency of a single component. Many bioactive phytochemicals are traditionally ignored, thus lacking in solid scientific footprints. Manufacturers cannot put proper health benefits on their product labels, as such claims need scientific data substantiation, which till date is lacking for many phytochemicals. Government regulatory authorities face challenges in this new group of health products, which lies between foods and drugs. However, all the stakeholders share the common goal of improving the personal and public health through diet modification, to reap the consequent economic and social benefits. The area of functional foods and nutraceuticals is confusing and is lumped together with the area of genetic engineering and biotechnology. Techniques in genetic engineering may be applied to enhance the phytochemical content of food and non-food plants. Although a series of biochemical reactions used by plant materials to synthesize phytochemicals is often not clearly understood, still there is ample potential to harness the plant's sophisticated biochemical machinery to synthesize valuable components and ultimately enhance human health.

Nowadays, many people understand the significant correlation between diet, consumption of quality food and good health, and these people are the best targets of the nutraceutical industry. Furthermore, customers are looking for the best brands to assure product superiority, product quality, and product assurance even if the price is high.

1.8   CONCLUSION

Rapid economic growth due to rampant industrialization have impacted the atmosphere adversely. Vast resources of water, soil, and food are contaminated, leading to potentially harmful effects on the health of the human being. The raised costs of health care resulted in people searching for preventive alternative therapy. Nutraceuticals possess health benefits and disease prevention capability, if taken according to their recommended dietary Intakes; nutraceuticals may help to keep diseases aside and may allow human beings to maintain a healthy lifestyle, quality of life, and longevity.

KEYWORDS

- **Dietary Supplement Health and Education Act**
- **European Food and Safety Authority**
- **foundation for innovation in medicine**
- **functional food**
- **guidelines**
- **regulatory**
- **scenario**

REFERENCES

1. Pushpangadan, P., George, V., Sreedevi, P., Biney, A., & Anzar, S., (2014). Functional foods and nutraceuticals with special focus on mother and child care. *Annl. Phytomed., 3*, 4–24.
2. Kalra, E., (2003). Nutraceutical-definition and introduction. *AAPS Pharm. Sci., 5*, 2, 3.
3. Keservani, R., Kesharwani, R., Vyas, N., Jain, S., Raghuvanshi, R., & Sharma, A., (2010). Nutraceutical and functional food as future food: A review. *Der. Pharmacia. Lett, 2*, 106–116.
4. Palthur, M., Palthur, S., & Chitta, S., (2010). Nutraceuticals: A conceptual definition. *Int. J. Phar. Pharm. Sci., 2*(3), 19–27.
5. Brower, V., (1998). Nutraceuticals: Poised for a healthy slice of the healthcare market. *Nat. Biotechnol., 16*, 728–731.
6. Spreadbury, I., (2012). Comparison with ancestral diets suggests dense acellular carbohydrates promote an inflammatory microbiota and may be the primary dietary cause of leptin resistance and obesity. *Diabetes Metab. Syndr. Obes., 5*, 175–189.
7. Fujita, T., (2000). *Soya Proteins, Water-Soluble Fibers and Gelatins, Basic Amino Acids and /or Basic Peptides as Compositions for Prevention of Obesity* (Vol. 7, p. 5). Jpn Kokai Tokkyo Koho JP 2000001440 A2.
8. Hu, F., (2003). Plant-based foods and prevention of cardiovascular disease: An overview. *Am. J. Clin. Nutr., 78*(suppl), S544–551.

9. Sharma, M., (2013). Functional foods: Marketing 'health' to modern India. *Int. J. Inn. Res. Dev., 2*, 720–739.

10. Ayyagari, R., Grover, V., & Purvis, R., (2011). Technostress: Technological antecedents and implications. *MIS Quarterly, 35*, 831–858.

11. Popkin, B., (2004). The nutrition transition: An overview of world patterns of change. *Nutr. Rev., 62*, S140–S143.

12. Pandey, M., Verma, R., & Saraf, S., (2010). Nutraceuticals: New era of medicine and health. *Asian J. Pharm. Clin. Res., 3*, 11–15.

13. Adelaja, A., & Schilling, B., (1999). Nutraceutical: Blurring the line between food and drugs in the twenty-first century. *Mag. Food Farm. Resour., (14)*, 35–40.

14. Dillard, C., & German, J., (2000). Phytochemicals: Nutraceuticals and human health. *J. Sci. Food Agric., 80*, 1744–1756.

15. Rusu, A., Kuokkanen, K., & Heier, A., (2011). Current trends in the pharmaceutical industry: A case study approach. *Eur. J. Pharm. Sci., 44*, 437–440.

16. Street, A., (2015). Food as pharma: Marketing nutraceuticals to India's rural poor. *Crit. Publ. Health, 25*, 361–372.

17. Clydesdale, F., (1998). Science, education and technology: New frontiers for health. *Crit. Rev. Food Sci. Nutr., 38*, 397–419.

18. Pappachan, M., (2011). Increasing prevalence of lifestyle diseases: High time for action. *Ind. J. Med. Res., 134*(2), 143–145.

19. Singh, A., (2010). Modern medicine: Towards prevention, cure, well-being and longevity. *MSM, 8*(1), 17–29.

20. Hathcock, J., (2001). Dietary supplements: How they are used and regulated. *J. Nutrition, 131*, 1114–1117.

21. Sumeet, G., Devesh, C., Kritika, M., Preeti, S., & Anroop, N., (2010). An overview of nutraceuticals: Current scenario. *Jour. Basic Clin. Pharm., 1*(2), 55–62.

22. Nutrition Labeling and Education Act. Pub. L No. 101-535, 104 Stat 2353.

23. Hasler, C., (2000). The changing face of functional foods. *J. Am. Coll. Nutr, 19*, 499S–506S.

24. Gulati, O., & Ottaway, P., (2006). Legislation relating to nutraceuticals in the European Union with a particular focus on botanical-sourced products. *Toxicol., 221*, 75–87.

25. Regulation (EC) 258/97 of the European Parliament and of the council of 27 January 1997, concerning novel foods and novel food ingredients. *EU Official Journal, 403*, 1–9.

26. Buttiglione, R., & Cox, P., (2003). Regulation (EC) No 1831/2003 of the European Parliament and of the Council on additives for use in animal nutrition. *EU Official Journal, 268*, 29–42.

27. Cox, P., & Roche, D., (2004). Directive 2004/24/EC of the European Parliament and of the council of 31 March, 2004, amending, as regards traditional herbal medicinal products. *EU Official Journal.*

28. Nutrition and health claims, (2006). *Regulation (EC) No 1924/2006 of the European Parliament and of the Council of 20 December 2006 on Nutrition and Health Claims Made on Foods, 15*(18), 244–259.

29. Vassiliou, A., (2008). Commission of regulation (EC) No. 353/2008 of 18 April 2008 establishing implementing rules for applications for authorization of health claims as provided for in article 15 of Regulation (EC) No 1924/2006 of the European Parliament and of the council. *EU Official Journal, 109*, 11–16.

30. Barroso, J., (2010). Commission Regulation (EU) No 383/2010 of 5 May 2010 refusing to authorize a health claim made on foods, other than those referring to the reduction of disease risk and to children's development and health. *EU Official Journal, 113*, 4, 5.
31. Shimizu, T., (2003). Health claims on functional foods: The Japanese regulations and an international comparison. *Nutr. Res. Rev., 16*, 241–252.
32. Ohama, H., Ikeda, F., & Moriyama, H., (2006). Health foods and foods with health claims in Japan. *Toxicol., 221*, 95–111.
33. Palthur, P., Palthur, S. S. S., & Chitta, S. K., (2009). The food safety and standards act, 2006: A paradigm shift in Indian regulatory scenario. *Pharm. Rev., 7*.

CHAPTER 2

Recent Techniques in Isolation of Nutraceuticals from Plants

SUMIT ARORA, SHOBHA UBGADE, and ALOK UBGADE

Department of Pharmacognosy, Gurunanak College of Pharmacy, Nari, Nagpur, Maharashtra, India

ABSTRACT

Nature has its own ways of creating, destroying, and transcending to heal. With the advent of progression encompassing all the spheres; human civilization has evolved, suffered, and sustained. Sufferings have always led to a surge in a directive transformation. Human health is not an exception to the acceptance of healing conferred by nature in the form of available flora and fauna. Food and nutrition both go hand in hand to attain and maintain optimal health. To balance and fill the voids created by any unwanted health suffering or disease; food has now become the medicine as well in the form of nutraceuticals. Nutraceuticals are being explored now extensively for their inherent medicinal importance. However, their consumption as medicinal entity relies on their isolation as an active moiety; which further requires sophisticated technological methods. This chapter principally highlights different techniques working for extraction and isolation of nutraceuticals for their optimum use.

2.1 INTRODUCTION

As of late, the thought of producing advantage of food as wellbeing advancing perspective past its healthy benefit is picking up acknowledgment. Nutraceuticals are the rising class of normal items that makes the relationship among food and wellbeing. "Nutraceutical" was gotten from "nourishment" and "drug." The term Nutraceuticals is portrayed as a "food or its part that gives medical advantages in specifications of avoidance of disease or advancement of wellbeing including its ordinary healthy benefit." The quantity of nutraceutical substances is almost in the hundreds, and probably the most recognizable substances include not many isoflavones, tocotrienols, allyl sulfur mixes, fiber, and carotenoids [1].

As per Western Nutritional Experts, the nourishments that offer best worth to substantial wellbeing incorporate tomato, fish, olive oil, entire wheat bread, and so on the different significant illnesses that are treated with Nutraceutical incorporate heart disease [2], cancer [3], diabetes [4], and so on Presently a day, legitimate planning of food that keeps up the wellbeing has picking up acknowledgment and acknowledgment around the world. Because of this industry managing assembling of food are looking for purchaser requests to change items. Lately, numerous characteristic items from India were use worldwide as nutraceuticals, and its market is extending in the US and Europe [5]. It incorporates enemies of oxidants, pre-biotics, and supportive of biotics, omega-3 unsaturated fats, dietary filaments, etc. [6]. The expanding enthusiasm for the use of food as nutraceuticals prompts the extraction of different normal items from plants. Keeping this in perception, different extraction techniques were used.

Regular ways like Soxhlet extraction, that are utilized for a long time, need tremendous amounts of solvents and are very time consuming [7]. Subsequently, finding new extraction strategies having less extraction time and need of least amounts of dissolvable is of principal significance. The tale extraction technique incorporates microwave and ultrasound helped extraction, quickened dissolvable extraction and supercritical liquid extraction. These methods can have the benefit of more limited extraction time as a result of their likelihood to work at raised temperatures [8]. These tale extraction strategies give advantages to extraction, partition, and seclusion of nutraceuticals from plants.

2.2   MICROWAVE-ASSISTED EXTRACTION (MAE)

Microwaves are electromagnetic waves comprising of an electrical field and a magnetic field. Both of these fields work opposite to one another, and the bearing of engendering fluctuates sinusoidally. Microwave energy is a non-ionizing radiation having a recurrence range somewhere in the range of 300 MHz and 300,000 MHz that causes atomic movement by double systems of relocation of particles and pivot of dipoles. The magnetic field permits the immediate activity of waves onto the material, which halfway assimilates the electromagnetic energy and change them into heat [9, 10]. In correlation with regular warming, the MAE gives focal points where warming shows up directly in the focal point of the body that is being warmed and the warmth infiltrates from internal center to outside while in customary cycle, the warmth enters gradually from external edges to within an object [11].

2.2.1 PRINCIPLES OF MICROWAVE-ASSISTED EXTRACTION (MAE)

In MAE, the energy of microwaves is utilized to warm the separating solvents present with strong examples. These outcomes in the parcel of the objective mix of enthusiasm from the example into the dissolvable. Microwave energy warms up the atoms by ionic conduction and dipole revolution. Ionic conduction and dipole revolution as a rule happens at the same time both in the dissolvable just as in the example, which viably changes over microwave energy to thermal energy. The ionic conduction produces heat because of the opposition of the medium to particle stream. Dipolar polarization (additionally eluded as direction polarization) is the hugest warming component in microwave extraction. At 2.45 GHz, realignment of the dipoles of the dissolvable particles happens inside a quickly changing electronic field, regularly 4,900 million times each second. The dissolvable particles attempt to realign themselves inside the electric field. This prompts vibration, and different impacts giving from this unsettling of atoms, which thus create energy discharge, delivering heat through frictional power and, hence, expanding the temperature. Microwave field requires the presence of a dielectric compound for age of warmth in the example.

The result of microwave energy is administered by the idea of dissolvable and the grid. Appropriate dissolvable choice is the way in to a fruitful extraction. While choosing removing solvents, the significant concern will be given to the microwave-engrossing capability of the dissolvable, which depend on the dipole snapshot of the dissolvable, its interaction with the network just as dissolvable dissolvability of the target atom. Bigger dipole snapshot of a dissolvable permits quicker warming under microwave light. The mixes with high dielectric consistent are fundamentally polar solvents. For instance, hexane is having a dipole snapshot of 0.1 Debye will not warm; on the opposite the CO_2 will warm inside seconds as its dipole second is 2.69 Debye [11–13].

2.2.2   EXTRACTION PRINCIPLE

Since the plant materials are dried before extraction yet at the same time, plant cell contain little dampness that fills in as an objective for microwave warming. Because of microwave impact the dampness gets warmed up and dissipates, that outcomes in incredible tension on the cell divider from inside which at last breaks the cell divider and in this way segment of dynamic constituents of target particles from test to the dissolvable is improved along these lines upgrading the all-out yield [14]. This cycle will be more successful if the plant material is priorly absorbed solvents having higher warming proficiency under microwave. During this cycle, this ascent in temperature can hydrolyze the ether linkages present in cellulosic cell divider which thusly lessens the mechanical quality of cell divider that will upgrade the infiltration intensity of dissolvable into the network [15].

2.2.3   INSTRUMENTATION

Two sorts of MAE frameworks that are commercially utilized incorporates shut extraction vessels which works under controlled tension and temperature, and centered microwaves that work at climatic weight [16]. The shut framework is ideal for extraction under solid conditions, for example, high extraction temperature. The weight in the vessel essentially relies upon the breaking point and volume of the solvents. The engaged framework can be worked at a most extreme temperature controlled by the breaking point of the solvents at environmental weight. Ericsson and Colmsjo revealed a powerful MAE framework, to yield an equal measure of concentrate in a less time as contrasted and Soxhlet extraction method [17].

2.2.4   APPLICATIONS OF MAE

Different specialists have detailed those nutraceuticals can be acquired from plants in a quicker way utilizing MAE when contrasted with ordinary techniques. It was accounted for already that the dynamic nutraceutical puerarin from the spice Radix puerariae could be gotten inside 1 min [18]. A few analysts detailed the extraction season of ginseng saponins was impressively diminished to few moments utilizing MAE; prior extraction time was 12 h [19]. Essentially the alkaloid Cocaine can be acquired inside 30 seconds [20]. Williams et al. detailed that MAE was proficient in recouping 95% of capsaicinoid partition from capsicum organic product in 15 min when contrasted with 2 h and 24 h for the reflux and shaken carafe technique, respectively [21]. The dynamic constituent tanshinones from *Salvia miltiorrhiza* Bunge was extricated inside 2 min utilizing MAE when contrasted with Soxhlet, Ultrasonic, and heat reflux extraction techniques which required 90 min, 75 min, and 45 min, separately [22].

2.3 SONICATION ASSISTED EXTRACTION/ULTRASOUND-ASSISTED EXTRACTION (UAE)

Sonication helped extraction normally alluded to as ultrasound helped extraction (UAE) procedure is developing as the most mainstream extraction strategy broadly. With the taking off energy costs and the drive to downsize ozone harming substance emanations, finding new advances has become basic which will give accumulated quality just as usefulness with extra weight on economy and ecological concerns.

Existing extraction innovations miss the mark regarding speculation and energy: regularly requesting up to half of interests in another plant and over 70% of all out-cycle energy utilized in food ventures [23].

Inside the past couple of years, these downsides have prompted the thought of ultrasound-helped extraction as an improved and effective strategy.

More limited handling period, decreased volume of natural dissolvable, spared energy, and expenses are the most wanted preferences offered by UAE. Likewise, various creative half and half procedures like ultrasound based Soxhlet extraction and Clevenger refining, and blend of ultrasound with various strategies, for example, supercritical liquid, expulsion, and microwave extraction.

Green extraction of common items may be an original plan to satisfy the difficulties of the 21st century. Ultrasound-based extraction procedures assists the cycle and complete extraction happens in a limited capacity to focus time. High reproducibility rates and higher immaculateness of the end result can be promptly accomplished. It is a straightforward cycle that does not request post-treatment of wastewater and requires just a small amount of the energy contribution when contrasted with a customary extraction method [24].

2.3.1 PRINCIPLE

Sound waves having frequencies higher than 20 kHz, causes mechanical vibrations in a strong, fluid, and gas. Sound waves produce extension and pressure inside the medium. Extension will in general bring atoms separated while pressure holds them together. The extension makes rises in a fluid and the air pockets so framed develop lastly breakdown. At the fluid strong interface, pit breakdown is lopsided and delivers rapid planes of fluid. These fluid planes produce extraordinary effect on the outside of solid [25].

Both, proper cell interruption and successful mass exchange are the two main considerations bringing about upgrade of extraction measure in the event of UAE [26]. In differentiation to standard extractions, plant separates diffuse across cell dividers, causing cell break more rapidly [27–30].

2.3.2 MECHANISM

Ultrasound extraction acts through entirely unexpected free or consolidated systems between discontinuity, disintegration, capillarity, detexturation, and sonoporation.

Discontinuity is a cycle which happens because of crashes between the particles and the shockwaves delivered from blasting cavitation rises inside the fluid medium. Fracture of friable solids because of ultrasonic cavitation has been accounted for by a few exploration scientists [31–33].

Disintegration is utilized for a few purposes and is a typical impact of ultrasound [34]. Implosion of cavitation rises on the outside of the leaves begins eroding of the structures of the plant in the extraction medium, a feasible route for the growth of concentrate yield. A report utilizing an ultrasonic test portrayed upgraded the extraction yield with UAE as opposed to ordinary maceration by 5% [35].

Sonocapillary impact alludes to the expansion in degree and pace of entrance of fluid into narrow structures like trenches and pores by use of sonication [36, 37]. In an examination, the yield of absolute polyphenolic content in apple pomace performed by ultrasound was discovered to be improved regarding extraction kinetics [38].

Sonoporation is applied when a porousness of cell film is wanted. For this, high ultrasound frequencies are applied (past 500 kHz) [39, 40]. Be that as it may, a couple of studies additionally center around utilizing low recurrence sound waves for permeabilization of cell wall [41]. Sonoporation can be applied to cell film pores, which may bring about the arrival of cell substance in the extractive medium [42].

Illumination of strong fluid combination by ultrasound waves, a little limited shear powers are delivered in the area of strong issue and fluid. Disturbance and Shear powers happen because of pressure cycles and augmentation of fluid's cavitation bubbles [43]. Post ultrasound extraction had been watched miscellaneously [27].

2.3.3 FACTORS AFFECTING UAE

It is important to place into thought different components that influence the general cycle of the UAE. Plant-related attributes, for example, molecule size, dampness substance, and dissolvable are basic. In addition, other administering factors incorporate recurrence of sound waves, weight, temperature, and sonication time [8, 44].

The general circulation of ultrasonic waves inside an extractor is a key factor in planning an ultrasonic extractor. Increment in the strong substance diminishes the ultrasound force [45].

Dissolvable decision in UAE is chosen by the dissolvability of the objective metabolites in a specific dissolvable and furthermore by certain physical boundaries, for example, fume weight, consistency, and surface strain of the dissolvable. Temperature emphatically impacts the dissolvable properties. An ascent in temperature diminishes both thickness and surface strain, and hoists the fume pressure. An ascent in fume pressure makes more dissolvable fumes go into the air pocket cavity and cavitation bubbles, and upsets the solid and effective breakdown of the air pockets. The blasting of cavitation raises in a powerless way reduces the generally speaking sonication effects [46]. As contrasted and the diverse novel extraction methods like microwave-helped extraction, the ultrasound hardware is a lot less expensive, and its activity is less complex. It very well may be utilized with any dissolvable for removing wide scope of characteristic compounds [47, 48].

2.3.4 INSTRUMENTATION

Two mainstream plans of ultrasound-helped extractors are ultrasonic showers and test. Both these frameworks are upheld on a transducer which goes about as a wellspring of ultrasound power. Ultrasonic showers are modest, effectively accessible, and various examples can be at the same time treated. However, when contrasted with the test frameworks, they show low reproducibility and size. High force ultrasonic tests are commonly favored for doing extraction. There are a few plans of tests accessible with various lengths, distances across, and tip calculations. A large portion of the test producers are made of a titanium combination, on account of its great warm obstruction and against destructive properties. Some more current materials have additionally been examined for ultrasound test tips, for example, Pyrex, and quartz, which are latent in nature and could explain the issue of metal particles release [49].

2.3.5   HYBRID APPARATUS

2.3.5.1   SONO-SOXHLET: ULTRASOUND-ASSISTED SOXHLET EXTRACTION

Sono-Soxhlet: Ultrasound can be applied either outside or inside the extraction chamber to enhance the solid-liquid extraction. Sono-Soxhlet apparatus combines both the merits of ultrasound (enhanced mass transfer and reduction of extraction time) and Soxhlet (extraction repeated by a fresh solvent) [24].

2.3.5.2   SONO-CLEVENGER: ULTRASOUND-ASSISTED CLEVENGER DISTILLATION

The combination of ultrasound with Clevenger distillation has resulted in the development of Sono-Clevenger [50] specifically aimed at getting essential oils from plant materials.

2.3.6   APPLICATIONS OF UAE

Ultrasound-helped extraction has been utilized to remove different nutraceuticals like pomegranate strip [51], Ziziphus lotus organic product [52], tomato pomace [53], grape seeds [54], Pepper [55], rosemary [56], caraway [57], saffron [58], almond oil [48], papaya seed [59], and soybean [28]. Ultrasonication was discovered to be an indispensable pre-treatment for getting exceptional returns of oils from apricot, almond, and rice bran [60]. The pace of extraction of carvone and limonene by UAE utilizing hexane as dissolvable was 1.3—multiple times quicker when contrasted with standard extraction relying upon temperature [27]. Scientists revealed multiple times snappier extraction of ginseng saponins [61]. Ultrasound-helped extraction was found as a proficient technique for extricating bioactive mixes from *Solvia officinalis* [62] and *Hibiscus tiliaceus* L. blossoms [63].

2.4 SUPERCRITICAL FLUID EXTRACTION (SFE)

Extraction procedures offering high proficiency and better selectivity are exceptionally attractive, which is normally undermined if there should be an occurrence of customary extraction methods [64].

The supercritical liquid has attributes of the two gases and fluids. Supercritical state is accomplished once the temperature and furthermore the weight of a substance is raised over its basic worth [8]. Carbon dioxide (CO_2) is the most ordinarily utilized liquid for SFE on account of its low physical constants (Temperature 31.1°C; Pressure 72.8 atm), non-poisonousness, non-combustibility, and accessibility in high virtue with ease.

Supercritical CO_2 is a decent dissolvable for extricating non-polar mixes yet so as to remove polar mixes, polar SF materials are required. Two such effectively utilized polar materials for SFE are Freon-22 (chlorodifluoromethane) [66] and nitrous oxide (N_2O) [67]. Notwithstanding, their application is confined because of their negative properties concerning wellbeing and ecological contemplations.

To acquire an ideal extremity of CO_2-based liquids, modifiers are normally included. Methanol is the most ordinarily utilized modifier and is up to 20% miscible with CO_2.

Some of the major advantages of SFE mentioned are as follows [68]:

- SFs have relatively lower consistency and better diffusivity. In this manner, they can infiltrate more viably into permeable strong materials than fluid solvents and, thus, upgrades the general cycle of mass exchange bringing about quicker extractions.
- The solvation/infiltrating intensity of the liquid can be adjusted by evolving pressure (P) as well as temperature (T); for high selectivity.
- This measure normally is performed at low temperatures, so it might be an ideal procedure to contemplate thermolabile mixes.
- Solutes broke up in supercritical CO_2 can be effortlessly isolated by depressurization.
- Use of naturally antagonistic natural solvents is least.
- Direct coupling with a chromatographic strategy, permits evaluation of profoundly unstable mixes following extraction.

2.4.1 INSTRUMENTATION

SFE is easy to perform and does not need advanced instrumentation [69]. A siphon is needed to gracefully a known weight of extraction liquid to the extraction vessel held over the basic temperature of the liquid. The liquid moves from test and leaves the vessel either by restrictor or controller to disconnected SFE on-line SFE where it is depressurized and vanished leaving the extract [68].

2.4.2 APPLICATIONS OF SFE

Apart from this, it has been used to extract plant materials, particularly lipids, essential oils, and flavors. Some examples are discussed here where various effects using SFE were recorded [64].

The mean extent yields of cedarwood oil utilizing supercritical liquid extraction and steam refining were discovered to be 4.4 and 1.3% [70]. The yield of oil from juniper wood by supercritical CO_2 extraction at 50°C and 10 MPa was 14.7% (w/w), though hydro-refining gave a lesser yield of 11% (w/w) [71]. Moderate supercritical CO_2 conditions (9 MPa and 40°C) may give effective extraction of fennel oil, empowering about 94% of the oil to be separated inside 150 min [72]. Contrasted and hydro-refining, SFE (20 MPa and 50°C) prompted higher centralizations of light oxygenated mixes inside the oil separated from Egyptian marjoram leaves, that gave the oil a prevalent fragrance and cell reinforcement property [73, 74]. Supercritical CO_2 with 15% ethanol as modifier gave more significant returns of Naringin (a glycosylated flavonoid) from *Citrus paradise* [75]. Supercritical CO_2 extraction completed with methanol as modifier in the scope of 3–7% helped in recuperating 3-demethylcolchicine (>97%) and colchicines (>98%) and colchicoside from seeds of *Colchicum autumnale* [76].

2.5   ACCELERATED SOLVENT EXTRACTION (ASE)

ASE is a sort of pressurized dissolvable extraction strategy that is pretty like SFE. The extraction is completed at marginally over the typical breaking point of removing dissolvable; simultaneously, pressure is applied to keep up the dissolvable in fluid state at high temperature. Expanded temperature and raised weight has key function on energy. The fluid condition of the dissolvable causes wellbeing and rushed phytoconstituents extraction from plant material. Likewise, this condition (Increased temperature and raised weight) upgrades the dissemination of dissolvable into the strong grid and the phytoconstituents will move at the quicker rates over the limit layer of strong lattice into the dissolvable [16, 20]. Moreover, raised temperature diminishes the thickness of removing dissolvable in this manner, improving its infiltration power and furthermore upsets the connection among strong and lattice. The dissolvable utilized in ASE is generally natural dissolvable. Yet, a significant number of the natural solvents are having low breaking point, so increment in temperature is not sufficient to improve the extraction proficiency. Accordingly, adequate weight is applied on to the dissolvable during extraction. Boiling water or subcritical water can likewise be used in an ASE gathering called as pressurized heated water extraction or subcritical water extraction, respectively [77]. ASE is considered as a promising elective extraction technique to SFE for the detachment of hydrophilic mixes [78]. Contrasted and conventional Soxhlet extraction, there is a wonderful abatement in the volume of dissolvable and the extraction time for ASE [79].

2.5.1   INSTRUMENTATION

The crude material is facilitated in an extraction cell comprised of hardened steel. An appropriate dissolvable or the combination of solvents siphons through dissolvable supply. By and large, the temperature and weight were kept at 200°C and 10 to 20 megapascals, separately. The ideal outcomes are acquired with this condition kept up for few moments, as it guarantees the most extreme extraction of phytochemicals from therapeutic plant material. The concentrate is at long last gathered into the gathering vial subsequent to cleansing dormant nitrogen gas.

2.5.2   APPLICATIONS OF ACCELERATED SOLVENT EXTRACTION (ASE)

It is regularly utilized technique for the extraction of thermostable natural poisons from ecological frameworks. Restricted uses of ASE have been accessible in the segregation of nutraceuticals. Policosanols have been accounted for as dietary enhancements for cardiovascular wellbeing. The investigation exhibited by Dunford and others that dissolvable sort and temperature affect remove yields and Policosanols content contrasted and different strategies [80, 81]. Already, Plaza et al. detailed that solitary the concentrates got at 200°C had free extremist rummaging potential as contrasted and the concentrate got at room temperature and at 100°C temperature through subcritical water extraction conditions [65].

2.6 CONCLUSION

The need to remove nutraceuticals from plant materials prompts proceeded with discoveries of financially and naturally conceivable extraction advancements. Ordinary strong fluid extraction methods need a larger than average measure of solvents and are tedious. The monstrous measure of dissolvable utilized expands the working expense as well as aims extra natural issues. A few novel extraction strategies are created as a substitute to customary extraction techniques, giving focal points concerning extraction time, yield, dissolvable utilization, and reproducibility.

This part centers around numerous advances utilized for the seclusion and creation of bioactive mixes from normal sources. These days, people are having more mindfulness about the segments present in the nourishments they burn through, leaning toward those acquired from common sources because of undesirable pessimistic impacts of the mixes got by substance union. In any case, more examination is required soon to show the viability of different extraction strategies that needs improvement in the foundation of novel extraction frameworks. Consolidating extraction strategies, for example, High-weight, and microwave energy with traditional Soxhlet extraction prompting a new design of high-weight and microwave-helped Soxhlet extractors. The general extraction selectivity was improved when silica gels couples with supercritical liquid extractions. These aggregate extraction strategies keep up the advantages of conventional Soxhlet extraction, while going around the negative marks of the novel extraction procedures like supercritical liquid, microwave helped ultrasound, and quickened dissolvable extractions [8].

KEYWORDS

- **accelerated solvent extraction**
- **carbon dioxide**
- **microwave-assisted extraction**
- **nitrous oxide**
- **supercritical fluid extraction**
- **ultrasound-assisted extraction**

REFERENCES

1. WILDMAN, R. E. C., (2007). *Handbook of Nutraceuticals and Functional Foods* (2nd edn).
2. Khosravi-Boroujeni, H., Mohammadifard, N., Sarrafzadegan, N., et al., (2012). Potato consumption and cardiovascular disease risk factors among Iranian population. *Int. J. Food Sci. Nutr., 63*(8), 913–920. doi: 10.3109/09637486.2012.690024.
3. Shirzad, H., Burton, R. C., Smart, Y. C., Rafieian-kopaei, M., & Shirzad, M., (2011). Natural cytotoxicity of NC-2+ cells against the growth and metastasis of WEHI-164 fibrosarcoma. *Scand J. Immunol., 73*(2), 85–90. doi: 10.1111/j.1365-3083.2010.02481.x.
4. Introduction to program evaluation for public health programs: A self-study guide. 2011. *Centers Dis. Control. Prev.*
5. Hardy, G., (2000). Nutraceuticals and functional foods: Introduction and meaning. *Nutrition, 16*(7), 688, 689. doi: https://doi.org/10.1016/S0899-9007(00)00332-4.
6. Gokhale, S. B., Kokate, C. K., & Purohit, A. P. (2006). *Textbook of Pharmacognosy* (35th edn.).
7. Luque-De-Castro, M. D., & Garcia-Ayuso, L. E., (1998). Soxhlet extraction of solid materials: An outdated technique with a promising innovative future. *Anal. Chim. Acta, 369*(1, 2), 1–10. https://eurekamag.com/research/009/437/009437607.php (accessed on 30 July 2021).
8. Wang, L., & Weller, C. L., (2006). Recent advances in extraction of nutraceuticals from plants. *Trends Food Sci. Technol., 17*(6), 300–312. doi: https://doi.org/10.1016/j.tifs.2005.12.004.
9. Gedye, R., (1997). Microwave-enhanced chemistry. In: Kingston, H. M., & Stephen, J. H., (eds.), *Fundamentals, Sample Preparation and Applications*. American chemical society: Washington, D.C. xxviii + 772 pp. $109.95. ISBN 0. *J. Am. Chem. Soc., 121*(19), 4729. doi: 10.1021/ja9856046.
10. Zlotorzynski, A., (1995). The application of microwave radiation to analytical and environmental Chemistry. *Crit. Rev. Anal. Chem., 25*(1), 43–76. doi: 10.1080/10408349 508050557.
11. Duarte, F. A., Oliveira, P. V., & Nogueira, A. R. A., (2014). *Microwave-Assisted Extraction* (3rd edn.). Elsevier Inc. doi: 10.1016/B978-0-444-59420-4.00008-8.
12. Camel, V., (2000). Microwave-assisted solvent extraction of environmental samples. *TrAC Trends Anal. Chem., 19*(4), 229–248. doi: https://doi.org/10.1016/S0165-9936 (99)00185-5.
13. Jocelyn, P. J. R., Bélanger, J. M. R., & Stafford, S. S., (1994). Microwave-assisted process (MAP™): A new tool for the analytical laboratory. *TrAC Trends Anal. Chem., 13*(4), 176–184. doi: https://doi.org/10.1016/0165-9936(94)87033-0.
14. Kaufmann, B., Christen, P., & Veuthey, J. L., (2001). Parameters affecting microwave-assisted extraction of withanolides. *Phytochem. Anal., 12*(5), 327–331. doi: 10.1002/pca.599.
15. Mandal, S. C., Mandal, V., & Das, A. K., (2015). *Classification of Extraction Methods*. doi: 10.1016/b978-0-12-802325-9.00006-9.
16. Kaufmann, B., & Christen, P., (2002). Recent extraction techniques for natural products: Microwave-assisted extraction and pressurized solvent extraction. *Phytochem. Anal., 13*(2), 105–113. doi: 10.1002/pca.631.
17. Ericsson, M., & Colmsjö, A., (2000). Dynamic microwave-assisted extraction. *J. Chromatogr. A, 877*(1, 2), 141—151. doi: 10.1016/s0021-9673(00)00246-6.

18. Guo, Z., Jin, Q., Fan, G., Duan, Y., Qin, C., & Wen, M., (2001). Microwave-assisted extraction of effective constituents from a Chinese herbal medicine Radix puerariae. *Anal. Chim. Acta, 436*(1), 41–47. doi: https://doi.org/10.1016/S0003-2670(01)00900-X.

19. Kwon, J. H., Belanger, J., Pare, J. R. J., & Yaylayan, V., (2003). Application of the microwave-assisted process (MAPTM) to the fast excretion of ginseng saponins. *Food Res Int., 36*, 491–498. doi: 10.1016/S0963-9969(02)00197-7.

20. Brachet, A., Christen, P., & Veuthey, J. L., (2002). Focused microwave-assisted extraction of cocaine and benzoylecgonine from coca leaves. *Phytochem Anal., 13*(3), 162–169. doi: 10.1002/pca.637.

21. Williams, O. J., Raghavan, G. S. V., Orsat, V., & Dai, J., (2004). Microwave-assisted extraction of capsaicinoids from capsicum fruit. *J. Food Biochem., 28*(2), 113–122. doi: 10.1111/j.1745-4514.2004.tb00059.x.

22. Pan, X., Niu, G., & Liu, H., (2002). Comparison of microwave-assisted extraction and conventional extraction techniques for the extraction of tanshinones from *Salvia miltiorrhiza* Bunge. *Biochem. Eng. J., 12*(1), 71–77. doi: https://doi.org/10.1016/S1369-703X (02)00039-6.

23. Chemat, F., & Strube, J., (2015). *Green Extraction of Natural Products Related Titles Handbook of Plant Food and Industrial Bioproducts and Natural Food Flavors and Colorants Marketing of Natural Cosmetic Natural Products in Chemical*, 363.

24. Chemat, F., Rombaut, N., Sicaire, A. G., Meullemiestre, A., Fabiano-Tixier, A. S., & Abert-Vian, M., (2017). Ultrasound assisted extraction of food and natural products. Mechanisms, techniques, combinations, protocols and applications. A review. *Ultrason. Sonochem., 34*, 540–560. doi: 10.1016/j.ultsonch.2016.06.035.

25. Luque-García, J. L., & Luque De, C. M. D., (2003). Ultrasound: A powerful tool for leaching. *TrAC Trends Anal. Chem., 22*(1), 41–47. doi: https://doi.org/10.1016/S0165-9936 (03)00102-X.

26. Mason, T. J., Paniwnyk, L., & Lorimer, J. P., (1996). The uses of ultrasound in food technology. *Ultrason. Sonochem., 3*(3), S253–S260. doi: https://doi.org/10.1016/S1350-4177 (96)00034-X.

27. Chemat, S., Lagha, A., AitAmar, H., Bartels, P. V., & Chemat, F., (2004). Comparison of conventional and ultrasound-assisted extraction of carvone and limonene from caraway seeds. *Flavor Fragr. J., 19*(3), 188–195. doi: 10.1002/ffj.1339.

28. Li, H., Pordesimo, L., & Weiss, J., (2004). High intensity ultrasound-assisted extraction of oil from soybeans. *Food Res Int., 37*(7), 731–738. doi: 10.1016/j.foodres.2004.02.016.

29. Toma, M., Vinatoru, M., Paniwnyk, L., & Mason, T. J., (2001). Investigation of the effects of ultrasound on vegetal tissues during solvent extraction. *Ultrason. Sonochem., 8*(2), 137–142. doi: https://doi.org/10.1016/S1350-4177(00)00033-X.

30. Mason, T. J., (1999). *Advances in Sonochemistry*. Elsevier Science.

31. Suslick, K. S., & Price, G. J., (1999). Applications of ultrasound to materials chemistry. *Annu. Rev. Mater. Sci., 29*(1), 295–326. doi: 10.1146/annurev.matsci.29.1.295.

32. Kusters, K. A., Pratsinis, S. E., Thoma, S. G., & Smith, D. M., (1993). Ultrasonic fragmentation of agglomerate powders. *Chem. Eng. Sci., 48*(24), 4119–4127. doi: https://doi.org/10.1016/0009-2509(93)80258-R.

33. Kusters, K. A., Pratsinis, S. E., Thoma, S. G., & Smith, D. M., (1994). Energy—size-reduction laws for ultrasonic fragmentation. *Powder Technol., 80*(3), 253–263. doi: https://doi.org/10.1016/0032-5910(94)02852-4.

34. Suslick, K. S., Fang, M. M., Hyeon, T., & Mdleleni, M. M., (1999). In: Crum, L. A., Mason, T. J., Reisse, J. L., & Suslick, K. S., (eds.), *Applications of Sonochemistry to Materials Synthesis BT-Sonochemistry and Sonoluminescence* (pp. 291–320). Dordrecht: Springer Netherlands. doi: 10.1007/978-94-015-9215-4_24.

35. Petigny, L., Périno-Issartier, S., Wajsman, J., & Chemat, F., (2013). Batch and continuous ultrasound-assisted extraction of boldo leaves (Peumus boldus Mol.). *Int. J. Mol. Sci., 14*(3), 5750–5764. doi: 10.3390/ijms14035750.

36. Mason, T. J., (2015). Some neglected or rejected paths in sonochemistry - a very personal view. *Ultrason. Sonochem., 25*, 89–93. doi: https://doi.org/10.1016/j.ultsonch.2014.11.014.

37. Sankin, G. N., & Malykh, N. V., (2005). Force acting on a cylinder under ultrasonically induced cavitation. *Tech. Phys., 50*(7), 918–923. doi: 10.1134/1.1994974.

38. Pingret, D., Fabiano-Tixier, A. S., Bourvellec, C. L., Renard, C. M. G. C., & Chemat, F., (2012). Lab and pilot-scale ultrasound-assisted water extraction of polyphenols from apple pomace. *J Food Eng., 111*(1), 73–81. doi: https://doi.org/10.1016/j.jfoodeng.2012.01.026.

39. Karshafian, R., Bevan, P. D., Williams, R., Samac, S., & Burns, P. N., (2009). Sonoporation by ultrasound-activated microbubble contrast agents: Effect of acoustic exposure parameters on cell membrane permeability and cell viability. *Ultrasound Med Biol., 35*(5), 847–860. doi: https://doi.org/10.1016/j.ultrasmedbio.2008.10.013.

40. Ohta, S., Suzuki, K., Miyagawa, S., et al., (2009). In: Nakamura, H., (ed.), *Sonoporation in Developmental Biology BT-Electroporation and Sonoporation in Developmental Biology* (pp. 317–326). Tokyo: Springer Japan. doi: 10.1007/978-4-431-09427-2_27.

41. Miller, D. L., Pislaru, S. V., & Greenleaf, J. F., (2002). Sonoporation: Mechanical DNA delivery by ultrasonic cavitation. *Somat. Cell Mol. Genet., 27*(1–6), 115–134. doi: 10.1023/A:1022983907223.

42. Meullemiestre, A., Breil, C., Abert-Vian, M., & Chemat, F., (2016). Microwave, ultrasound, thermal treatments, and bead milling as intensification techniques for extraction of lipids from oleaginous yarrowia lipolytica yeast for a biojetfuel application. *Bioresour Technol., 211*, 190–199. doi: https://doi.org/10.1016/j.biortech.2016.03.040.

43. Vilkhu, K., Manasseh, R., Mawson, R., & Ashokkumar, M., (2011). In: Feng, H., Barbosa-Canovas, G., & Weiss, J., (eds.), *Ultrasonic Recovery and Modification of Food Ingredients BT - Ultrasound Technologies for Food and Bioprocessing* (pp. 345–368). New York, NY: Springer New York. doi: 10.1007/978-1-4419-7472-3_13.

44. Romdhane, M., & Gourdon, C., (2002). Investigation in solid-liquid extraction: Influence of ultrasound. *Chem. Eng. J., 87*(1), 11–19. doi: https://doi.org/10.1016/S1385-8947(01)00206-6.

45. Romdhane, M., Gourdon, C., & Casamatta, G., (1995). Local investigation of some ultrasonic devices by means of a thermal sensor. *Ultrasonics, 33*(3), 221–227. doi: https://doi.org/10.1016/0041-624X(94)00023-I.

46. Santos, H. M., Lodeiro, C., & Capelo-Martínez, J. L., (2009). The power of ultrasound. *Ultrasound Chem. Anal. Appl.*, 1–16. doi: 10.1002/9783527623501.ch1.

47. Zhang, H. F., Yang, X. H., Zhao, L. D., & Wang, Y., (2009). Ultrasonic-assisted extraction of epimedin C from fresh leaves of *Epimedium* and extraction mechanism. *Innov. Food Sci. Emerg. Technol., 10*(1), 54–60. doi: https://doi.org/10.1016/j.ifset.2008.09.007.

48. Zhang, Q. A., Zhang, Z. Q., Yue, X. F., Fan, X. H., Li, T., & Chen, S. F., (2009). Response surface optimization of ultrasound-assisted oil extraction from autoclaved

almond powder. *Food Chem., 116*(2), 513–518. doi: https://doi.org/10.1016/j.foodchem. 2009.02.071.

49. Cravotto, G., Boffa, L., Mantegna, S., Perego, P., Avogadro, M., & Cintas, P., (2008). Improved extraction of vegetable oils under high-intensity ultrasound and/or microwaves. *Ultrason. Sonochem., 15*(5), 898–902. doi: https://doi.org/10.1016/j.ultsonch. 2007.10.009.

50. Pingret, D., Fabiano-Tixier, A. S., & Chemat, F., (2014). An improved ultrasound Clevenger for extraction of essential oils. *Food Anal. Methods, 7*(1), 9–12. doi: 10.1007/ s12161-013–9581-0.

51. Pan, Z., Qu, W., Ma, H., Atungulu, G. G., & McHugh, T. H., (2012). Continuous and pulsed ultrasound-assisted extractions of antioxidants from pomegranate peel. *Ultrason. Sonochem., 19*(2), 365–372. doi: https://doi.org/10.1016/j.ultsonch.2011.05.015.

52. Hammi, K. M., Jdey, A., Abdelly, C., Majdoub, H., & Ksouri, R., (2015). Optimization of ultrasound-assisted extraction of antioxidant compounds from Tunisian *Zizyphus* lotus fruits using response surface methodology. *Food Chem., 184*, 80–89. doi: https:// doi.org/10.1016/j.foodchem.2015.03.047.

53. Luengo, E., Condón-Abanto, S., Condón, S., Álvarez, I., & Raso, J., (2014). Improving the extraction of carotenoids from tomato waste by application of ultrasound under pressure. *Sep. Purif. Technol., 136*, 130–136. doi: https://doi.org/10.1016/j.seppur.2014.09.008.

54. Ghafoor, K., Choi, Y. H., Jeon, J. Y., & Jo, I. H., (2009). Optimization of ultrasound-assisted extraction of phenolic compounds, antioxidants, and anthocyanins from grape (Vitis vinifera) seeds. *J. Agric. Food Chem., 57*(11), 4988–4994. doi: 10.1021/jf9001439.

55. Barbero, G. F., Liazid, A., Palma, M., & Barroso, C. G., (2008). Ultrasound-assisted extraction of capsaicinoids from peppers. *Talanta, 75*(5), 1332–1337. doi: https://doi. org/10.1016/j.talanta.2008.01.046.

56. Jacotet-Navarro, M., Rombaut, N., Fabiano-Tixier, A. S., Danguien, M., Bily, A., & Chemat, F., (2015). Ultrasound versus microwave as green processes for extraction of rosmarinic, carnosic and ursolic acids from rosemary. *Ultrason. Sonochem., 27*, 102–109. doi: https://doi.org/10.1016/j.ultsonch.2015.05.006.

57. Assami, K., Pingret, D., Chemat, S., Meklati, B. Y., & Chemat, F., (2012). Ultrasound induced intensification and selective extraction of essential oil from *Carum carvi* L. seeds. *Chem Eng, Process. Process Intensif., 62*, 99–105. doi: https://doi.org/10.1016/j. cep.2012.09.003.

58. Sereshti, H., Heidari, R., & Samadi, S., (2014). Determination of volatile components of saffron by optimised ultrasound-assisted extraction in tandem with dispersive liquid-liquid microextraction followed by gas chromatography-mass spectrometry. *Food Chem., 143*, 499–505. doi: https://doi.org/10.1016/j.foodchem.2013.08.024.

59. Samaram, S., Mirhosseini, H., Tan, C. P., & Ghazali, H. M., (2014). Ultrasound-assisted extraction and solvent extraction of papaya seed oil: Crystallization and thermal behavior, saturation degree, color and oxidative stability. *Ind. Crops Prod., 52*, 702–708. doi: https://doi.org/10.1016/j.indcrop.2013.11.047.

60. Sharma, A., & Gupta, M. N., (2004). Oil extraction from almond, apricot and rice bran by three-phase partitioning after ultrasonication. *Eur. J. Lipid Sci. Technol., 106*(3), 183–186. doi: 10.1002/ejlt.200300897.

61. Wu, J., Lin, L., & Chau, F., (2001). Ultrasound-assisted extraction of ginseng saponins from ginseng roots and cultured ginseng cells. *Ultrason. Sonochem., 8*(4), 347–352. doi: https://doi.org/10.1016/S1350-4177(01)00066-9.

62. Sališová, M., Toma, Š., & Mason, T. J., (1997). Comparison of conventional and ultrasonically assisted extractions of pharmaceutically active compounds from Salvia officinalis. *Ultrason. Sonochem., 4*(2), 131–134. doi: https://doi.org/10.1016/S1350-4177(97) 00032-1.

63. Melecchi, M. I. S., Martinez, M. M., Abad, F. C., Zini, P. P., Do Nascimento, F. I., & Caramão, E. B., (2002). Chemical composition of *Hibiscus tiliaceus* L. flowers: A study of extraction methods. *J. Sep. Sci., 25*(1, 2), 86–90. doi: 10.1002/1615-9314 (20020101)25:1/2<86::AID-JSSC86>3.0.CO;2-7.

64. Modey, W. K., Mulholland, D. A., & Raynor, M. W., (1996). Analytical supercritical fluid extraction of natural products. *Phytochem. Anal., 7*(1), 1–15. doi: 10.1002/(SICI) 1099-1565(199601)7:1<1::AID-PCA275>3.0.CO;2-U.

65. Plaza, M., Amigo-Benavent, M., Del, C. M. D., Ibáñez, E., & Herrero, M., (2010). Neoformation of antioxidants in glycation model systems treated under subcritical water extraction conditions. *Food Res. Int., 43*(4), 1123–1129. doi: 10.1016/j.foodres. 2010.02.005.

66. Klink, G., Buchs, A., & Gülacar, F. O., (1994). Supercritical fluid extraction of fatty acids and sterols from plant tissues and sediments. *Org. Geochem., 21*(5), 437–441. doi: https://doi.org/10.1016/0146-6380(94)90095-7.

67. Vandana, V., Teja, A. S., & Zalkow, L. H., (1996). Supercritical extraction and HPLC analysis of Taxol from *Taxus brevifolia* using nitrous oxide and nitrous oxide + ethanol mixtures. *Fluid Phase Equilib., 116*(1), 162–169. doi: https://doi.org/10.1016/0378-3812 (96)02991-3.

68. Lang, Q., & Wai, C. M., (2001). Supercritical fluid extraction in herbal and natural product studies: A practical review. *Talanta, 53*(4), 771–782. doi: 10.1016/S0039-9140(00) 00557-9.

69. Vannoort, R. W., Chervet, J. P., Lingeman, H., De Jong, G. J., & Brinkman, U. A. T., (1990). Coupling of supercritical fluid extraction with chromatographic techniques. *J Chromatogr A., 505*(1), 45–77. doi: https://doi.org/10.1016/S0021-9673(01)93068-7.

70. Eller, F. J., & King, J. W., (2000). *Supercritical Carbon Dioxide Extraction of Cedarwood Oil: A Study of Extraction Parameters and Oil Characteristics-F., 231*, 226–231.

71. Marongiu, B., Porcedda, S., Caredda, A., De Gioannis, B., Vargiu, L., & Colla, P. L., (2003). Extraction of *Juniperus oxycedrus* ssp. oxycedrus essential oil by supercritical carbon dioxide: Influence of some process parameters and biological activity. *Flavor Fragr. J., 18*(5), 390–397. doi: 10.1002/ffj.1224.

72. Coelho, J. A. P., Pereira, A. P., Mendes, R. L., & Palavra, A. M. F., (2003). Supercritical carbon dioxide extraction of *Foeniculum vulgare* volatile oil. *Flavor Fragr J., 18*(4), 316–319. doi: 10.1002/ffj.1223.

73. El-Ghorab, A. H., Mansour, A. F., & El-Massry, K. F., (2004). Effect of extraction methods on the chemical composition and antioxidant activity of Egyptian marjoram (Majorana hortensis Moench). *Flavor Fragr. J., 19*(1), 54–61. doi: 10.1002/ffj.1276.

74. Sass-Kiss, A., (1998). A4-Simandi, B. A4-Gao, Y. A4-Boross, F. A4-Vamos-Falusi, Z. AA-S-K. Study on the pilot-scale extraction of onion oleoresin using supercritical CO_2. *J. Sci. Food Agric., 76*(3), 320-326. doi: 10.1002/(SICI)1097-0010(199803)76:3<320:: AID-JSFA916>3.0.CO;2-J.

75. Giannuzzo, A. N., Boggetti, H. J., Nazareno, M. A., & Mishima, H. T., (2003). Supercritical fluid extraction of naringin from the peel of *Citrus* paradisi. *Phytochem. Anal., 14*(4), 221–223. doi: 10.1002/pca.706.

76. Ellington, E., Bastida, J., Viladomat, F., & Codina, C., (2003). Supercritical carbon dioxide extraction of colchicine and related alkaloids from seeds of *Colchicum autumnale* L. *Phytochem. Anal., 14*(3), 164–169. doi: 10.1002/pca.702.

77. Eskilsson, C., Hartonen, K., Mathiasson, L., & Riekkola, M. L., (2004). Pressurized hot water extraction of insecticides from process dust - comparison with supercritical fluid extraction. *J. Sep. Sci., 27*, 59–64. doi: 10.1002/jssc.200301566.

78. Brachet, A., Rudaz, S., Mateus, L., Christen, P., & Veuthey, J. L., (2001). Optimization of accelerated solvent extraction of cocaine and benzoylecgonine from coca leaves. *J. Sep. Sci., 24*, 865–873. doi: 10.1002/1615-9314(20011101)24:10/11<865::AID-JSSC865>3.0.CO;2-U.

79. Richter, B. E., Jones, B. A., Ezzell, J. L., Porter, N. L., Avdalovic, N., & Pohl, C., (1996). Accelerated solvent extraction: A technique for sample preparation. *Anal. Chem., 68*(6), 1033–1039. doi: 10.1021/ac9508199.

80. Dunford, N. T., Irmak, S., & Jonnala, R., (2010). Pressurized solvent extraction of policosanol from wheat straw, germ and bran. *Food Chem., 119*(3), 1246–1249. doi: 10.1016/j.foodchem.2009.07.039.

81. Gil-Chávez, G. J., Villa, J. A., Ayala-Zavala, J. F., et al., (2013). Technologies for extraction and production of bioactive compounds to be used as nutraceuticals and food ingredients: An overview. *Compr. Rev. Food Sci. Food Saf., 12*(1), 5–23. doi: 10.1111/1541-4337.12005.

PART II

Advances in Nanoparticles-Based Nutraceutical Delivery

CHAPTER 3

Solid Lipid Nanoparticles (SLNs): An Emerging Platform for Nutraceutical Delivery

VISHAL C. GURUMUKHI,[1] SANJAYKUMAR B. BARI,[2] and KAUSHALENDRA CHATURVEDI[3]

[1]Department of Pharmaceutics and Quality Assurance, R. C. Patel Institute of Pharmaceutical Education and Research, Shirpur, Dhule, Maharashtra–425405, India, E-mail: vishalgurumukhi1584@gmail.com

[2]H.R Patel Institute of Pharmaceutical Education and Research, Shirpur, Dhule, Maharashtra, India

[3]Lachman Institute for Pharmaceutical Analysis Laboratory at Long Island University, New York, USA

ABSTRACT

Current development in the science of nutraceuticals aims to improve the benefits of functional foods, including minerals, vitamins, and other dietary supplements (DS). Nano-nutraceuticals actively participate in the safe and effective delivery of dietary bioactive. Recent trends in the delivery of nutraceuticals, including medical nutrition, phytonutrients, and nutrition via solid lipid nanoparticles (SLNs), have emerged since the last few decades with the objective of controlled and targeted delivery. SLNs witnesses promising alternatives for various colloidal drug and nutraceuticals delivery systems viz., nanoemulsion, liposomes, and polymeric nanoparticles. The biodegradable and biocompatible nature of SLNs proves itself favorable among other polymeric nanoparticles. Furthermore, SLNs ensure better therapeutics by modifying nutrients release kinetics, bio-distribution, and greater uptake in tissues. Despite the potential ability of SLNs for nutrient delivery, their manufacturing still poses a challenge. USFDA (United States

Food and Drug Administration) in its current guidelines, made it mandatory to implement quality by design (QbD) approach for the manufacturing of pharmaceuticals. The proposed chapter presents insight on SLNs, including basic components, manufacturing techniques, characterization parameters, critical quality attributes (CQAs), and applications towards nutraceutical delivery.

3.1   INTRODUCTION

Nutrients are required continuously to our body for the maintenance, growth, reproduction, and health to prevent and enlarge quality of life. Nutraceuticals are a part of dietary supplements (DS) that involves food and food parts providing medical and health benefits such as prevention and treatment of ailments [1]. Stephen L. DeFelice, was a chairman and founder of Foundation of Innovative Medicine (New York), merging *nutrition* and *pharmaceutical;* and was coined the term Nutraceuticals [1, 2]. According to Health Canada, a nutraceutical is a manufactured good that is quarantined or refined from foods. Since the last few years, quality of life is growing by using nutrients in various forms. The major issue of nutraceuticals is its poor bioavailability which is unable to provide necessary benefit to the body.

To increase the benefit of nutraceuticals in the body via absorption, controlled release of nutrients, health supplements, and bioavailability, the nanotechnology can be used [1].

The advancement in nanotechnology, including nano-nutraceuticals and nano-medicine is arising to change strategies in diagnosis, treatment, and prevention of critical diseases such as cancer by employing recent innovations in this field. These technological innovations, recently named as nanomedicines by the National Institutes of Health (NIH) [3]. Among them, in the early 1990s, the formulation of SLNs has introduced and emerged as the best alternative for conventional drug delivery systems such as emulsion, liposome, and polymeric nanoparticles [4]. SLNs has potential to overcome therapy failures such as poor absorption, rapid metabolism, and elimination of drug. Furthermore, its unique ability to defeat poor drug solubility, unpredictable bioavailability after taken orally and specific targeting [5, 6] make it efficient alternatives for nutraceutical administration.

In this chapter, we explore a detail regarding useful component utilized in the production of SLNs for nutraceutical delivery, preparation method and its characterization. We focused especially on critical quality attributes

(CQAs), which impact for designing of quality products of new efficient and safe nutraceutical formulations via SLNs.

3.1.1 ADVANTAGES AND LIMITATIONS OF SLNS

SLNs possess several advantages over other delivery systems for nutraceuticals, such as good tolerability due to the use of physiological lipids, large scale production, and employed for nutraceutical delivery into the body. The various colloidal carrier systems were in existence, including liposomes, nanoparticles, nano-emulsions, nanosuspensions, micelles, and polymeric microparticles. Particularly, in the case of polymeric nanoparticles; cytotoxicity of tissues if it is drug delivery and lack of suitable commercial technique for production [7] are major limitations.

The potential advantages of SLNs are summarized as [7]:

- Possibility of controlled drug release;
- Nutraceutical carrier;
- High drug/nutrient payload;
- Increased stability;
- Encapsulation of hydrophobic and hydrophilic drug is possible;
- Avoidance of biotoxicity;
- Avoidance of organic solvents;
- Feasibility with large scale preparation and sterilization.

Limitation of SLNs reported recently [8, 9]:

- Low nutrient loading capacity;
- Drug expulsion;
- Drug leakage during storage.

3.2 MISCELLANEOUS TERMS

1. **Nanoparticles (NPs):** A nanoparticles are stable, solid colloidal particles that are generally 10–100 nm in size prepared employing various techniques.
2. **Solid Lipid Nanoparticle (SLNs):** These are considered a novel drug delivery system or nutrient carrier system consists of active drug or nutrient, solid lipid, and surfactant with an average particle diameter fall between 10 and 100 nanometers (nm).

3. **Nanostructured Lipid Carriers (NLCs):** These are composed of both solid and liquid (oils) *lipids* as a core matrix stabilized by surfactant or combination of surfactant.

3.3 SALIENT FEATURES

1. **Regulatory Aspects of Excipients:** The excipients without prior approval from regulatory agencies cannot be utilized in a nutrient delivery system. USFDA has introduced a regulatory guideline for each pharmaceutical excipient to be employed in the preparation of SLNs. Most commonly, excipients with "generally recognized as safe" (GRAS) status are employed for the preparation of NPs. The wide variety of solid lipids, surfactants, and co-surfactants considered as GRAS utilized for designing of SLNs [10–12].

2. **Lab Scale and Large-Scale Production:** SLNs can be prepared by using high-pressure homogenization techniques (hot or cold) either in laboratory-scale or in an industrial scale. Both the methods are quite similar and involve the incorporation of nutrients in melted lipid base. Molten nutrient-lipid matrix is then dispersed in hot surfactant solution with constant stirring to obtain pre-emulsion. Afterward, this is then passed through high-pressure homogenizer 600 bar pressure and at least 4 cycles to obtain SLNs.

    In cold homogenization method, the nutrient containing molten lipid quickly cooled in dry ice or nitrogen gas. The nutrient-lipid matrix is then milled to produce microparticles. These micro-particles are dispersed in a cold solution of emulsifier with constant stirring. The prepared pre-suspension is passed through a high-pressure homogenization (HPH) process at and below room temperature to form the SLNs.

    The pressure applied to the pre-emulsion and homogenization cycle may be varied according to the required particle size. In both the techniques, mechanical activation force is applied to reduce the particle size [13].

3. **High Entrapment Efficiency (EE):** It is an essential feature of SLNs preparation. EE is an ability of SLNs to entrap the maximum amount of nutrient which depends upon the solubility of nutrients in lipid carriers. SLNs produced using cetyl alcohol may give low EE as compared to glyceryl palmitostearate due to imperfections in the crystalline lattice. In general, higher solubility of nutrients in lipid

occurs due to less ordered crystalline lattice structure of lipid [14, 15]. The determination of EE is performed by separating free nutrient from nutrient entrapped in lipid carriers using high-speed ultracentrifugation or Sephadex minicolumn centrifugation technique [16, 17].

4. **Physical and Chemical Stabilization of SLNs:** The SLNs are produced by various methods and needs to be stabilized over the long term. The SLN preparation is stabilized by chemical and physical methods, respectively. Physical stability of SLN can be determined with long storage. For assessment of physical stability, SLNs should be stored at different temperature conditions, i.e., 4–8°C, ambient temperature, and 40°C at 60± 5% relative humidity (RH) for 6 months. The stability is ensured when the particle size of SLNs at all three storage conditions remains unchanged. SLNs are considered to be chemically stable even if the particles have little or no aggregation during long term storage.

Stabilization of SLNs occurs with the incorporation of appropriate surfactant. Most frequently either surfactant alone or in combination with co-surfactant is used for the preparation of SLNs. The combination would produce small size NPs having better storage stability [18].

It was proven to use binary mixtures of surfactants which are much more efficient in stabilization than surfactant alone [15, 19]. Therefore, binary mixtures of surfactants are commonly employed in the production of SLNs [20]. However, several kinds of literature reported the type and amount of surfactant governs the chemical stability of SLNs.

Zeta potential is an important parameter to judge physical stability of SLNs. It provides information of surface charge on SLNs [21].

5. **Drug Release Profile of Active Compounds from SLNs:** The excipients and processing conditions employed in the preparation of SLNs would affect the nutrient release behavior from SLNs. The major problem associated with SLNs is the burst release occurs within 2 h. In addition, nutrient release behaviors are slightly affected by size and shape of SLNs; processing parameters, i.e., temperature, stirring speed, pressure, homogenizing cycle, rotation per min (RPM), etc., and formulation parameters, i.e., type, and amount of surfactant; amount and nature of lipid. However, burst nutrient release from SLNs could be controlled by completely solubilizing the nutrient in the water phase during preparation. Furthermore, SLNs should avoid those surfactants which possess less nutrient solubility or not able to solubilize the nutrient; otherwise it would lead to burst release of nutrient [10, 22].

6. **SLNs Products:** Various SLNs products for nutraceutical delivery including minerals, vitamins, peptides, bioactive phytochemicals, and curcumin (natural polyphenol). Guney et al. [121] successfully prepared ascorbic acid (Vitamin C, AA) known as an antioxidant-loaded SLNs by hot homogenization technique and effective delivery of AA to cancer cells. The particle size was found less than 250 nm and demonstrated for sustained release as well as high EE. By this study, it was inferred that SLNs exhibited more efficient cellular uptake, accumulated in the cytoplasm and induced apoptosis.

    The main features of SLNs for dermal application may be constructive particularly, for cosmetics and pharmaceutics. These are colloidal nano-sized carrier useful for controlled release application for many nutrients, e.g., lipophilic and hydrophilic. SLNs produced by using physiological and biodegradable lipids exhibits low cyto-toxicity and excellent tolerability. The nano-size of SLNs provides close contact to the stratum corneum and thus increases penetration of nutrition into the skin. Furthermore, lipids employed in SLNs have skin hydration effect due to its occlusive properties. The highest occlusion characteristics of SLNs will be ensured by small particle size, low melting, and highly crystalline solid lipids [4].

3.4 BASIC COMPONENTS

3.4.1 *LIPIDS*

The basic components used in SLNs include solid lipid, surfactant, and co-surfactant. The lipid is the main ingredient of SLNs, which governs nutrient material (NM) loading capacity, drug release behavior, and long-term stability. Most commonly employed lipid includes triglycerides (e.g., tristearin), partial glyceride (Imwitor), fatty acids (e.g., stearic acids), steroids (e.g., cholesterols) and waxes (e.g., cetyl palmitate) [7]. These lipids are considered as GRAS, well-tolerated and biocompatible [23].

3.4.1.1 *SELECTION OF LIPIDS*

The selection of suitable lipid is an essential and preliminary step in the preparation of SLNs. Generally, the maximum solubility of drug in given lipid suggests its utilization for preparation of SLNs. Recently, partitioning behavior of drug or nutrient between water and solid lipid (at 10°C above the melting point of the lipid) is performed to selects suitable lipid [24].

The solubilization potential of nutrient in lipid reveals suitable criteria for the selection of appropriate lipid [25]. The quantification of lipid solubility can be speculated by analytical methods. The selection of lipid is significantly essential as it imparts the NM loading, entrapments efficiency, stability, and subsequently controlled release behavior. Moreover, appropriate selection of lipid as a small difference in the composition of lipid and its type can alter the product quality of the lipid nanocarrier [14].

The partitioning behavior of nutrients between lipids (melted lipid) can be speculated by mathematical calculations. Using these calculations, one can speculate the amount of nutrient solubilizes in the lipid phase or water phase [26].

3.4.1.2 POLYMORPHISM

Crystalline solid lipids have its internal arrangement in the appropriate order of units. Due to the kinetics of crystallization and polymorphism of the dispersed lipid, SLNs greatly affect the additional stability aspects. In spite of chemically identical, polymorphs generally have different thermodynamic properties such as melting points, X-ray diffraction (XRD) patterns, and solubility [27].

Kaur et al. reported the main and basic component of SLNs is a solid lipid, which possesses basic properties to establish the loading capacity. The properties of lipid have been described in terms of solubility of the drug in molten lipid; miscibility of drug melt and lipid melt; the physical and chemical structure of solid lipid matrix; and polymorphic state of lipid material, respectively. The higher drug loading lipid capacity could be obtained by solubilizing the drug in molten lipid. Another critical aspect of lipid is polymorphic transformation resulted during the preparation of SLNs. Sometimes, prepared SLNs involves crystallization of lipid through polymorphism where the transformation of α-form of native lipid transform rapidly to β-form with β'-modification [28]. On the other hand, SLNs possess an insufficient drug loading capacity due to drug expulsion after polymorphic transformation during storage [29]. Similar aspect is applicable to the encapsulation of NMs in lipid core as described above.

The DSC and XRD studies highly recommended investigating the crystalline status of the lipid [5]. The DSC reveals melting point and enthalpies (heat change) during the preparation of SLNs. Further, XRD has proved as a tool to investigate the length of long and short spacings of lipid lattice. XRD, wide-angle X-ray scattering, and X-ray photoelectron spectroscopy studies are commonly employed to detect polymorphism in lipids [30–32].

3.4.2 SURFACTANTS

Various compounds exhibiting surfactant properties may be utilized for the production of SLNs with high hydrophilic-lipophilic balance (HLB). These compounds or surfactants are an essential component used in the preparation of SLNs. It is also known as emulsifiers, surface active agents or stabilizers. The surfactants are known to be versatile molecules due to their amphipathic nature. The commonly used surfactants may be classified into anionic, nonionic, and amphoteric according to charge present in the hydrophilic portion of the molecule (after dissociation in aqueous solution). The major determining and significant factor which governs surfactant selection for the preparation of SLNs is safety. Non-ionic surfactants are most frequently used since these are less toxic and chemically inert than ionic surfactants. Surfactants from natural origin are considered to be safe and more commonly employed than synthetic surfactants [11].

The factors that govern surfactant selection for SLNs preparation includes route of administration, HLB value, particle size, lipid modification, and *in vivo* degradation of lipid [33]. A significant role played by surfactant information of nano-sized lipid particles by lowering the interfacial tension [34]. Some examples of surfactants are Caprylocaproyl polyoxyl-8-glycerides [Labrasol®] Polyglyceryl-3 dioleate [Plurol®, Oleique® CC497] Sorbitan esters [Span®] Polyoxyethylene sorbitan fatty acid esters [Tween®] Macrogol fatty acid glycerides [Gelucire® 44/14, Gelucire® 50/13] Polyoxyethylene castor oil derivatives [Cremophor®, Lipocol®] Polyvinyl alcohol tocopherol polyethylene glycol succinate (TPGS) Poloxamer Bile acids (sodium deoxycholate) Phospholipids and PEGylated phospholipids Polyvinylpyrrolidone Cellulose derivatives (hydroxypropylmethylcellulose). Incorporation of co-surfactants or co-stabilizers also enhance stabilization and reduction in size in SLNs production. The example of co-surfactant is diethylene glycol monoethyl ether [Transcutol® HP] Phospholipids Propylene glycol Ethanol Polyethylene glycol Glycofurol Oleoyl/linoleoyl polyoxyl-6-glycerides [Labrafil®] Triacetin [35].

3.4.3 OTHER AGENTS

3.4.3.1 CRYOPROTECTANT

These substances are able to reduce the aggregation between the particles and leads to stabilization of SLNs. This substance is known as cryoprotectant, usually added in the nanoparticle suspension to protect from freezing stress [36] most commonly used cryoprotectants are fructose, glucose, mannitol, trehalose, etc. Sometimes counter ions and surface modifiers listed below [37] are used in SLNs production.

3.4.3.2 COUNTERIONS

1. **Organic Salts:**
   i.   Mono-octyl phosphate;
   ii. Sodium hexadecyl phosphate;
   iii. Mono-decyl phosphate;
   iv. Mono-hexadecyl phosphate.

2. **Ionic Polymers:**
   i.   Dextran sulfate sodium salt.

3.4.3.3 SURFACE MODIFIER

- Dipalmitoyl-phosphatidyl-ethanolamine conjugated with polyethylene glycol 2000 (DPPE-PEG2000);
- Distearoyl-phosphatidyl-ethanolamine-N-poly(ethylene glycol) 2000 (DSPE-PEG2000);
- Stearic acid-PEG 2000 (SA-PEG2000);
- α-methoxy-PEG 2000-carboxylic acid-α-lipoamino acids (mPEG 2000-C-LAA18);
- α-methoxy-PEG 5000-carboxylic acid-α-lipoamino acids (mPEG 5000-C-LAA18);
- Phospholipon 90G [113].

Apart from the above examples, PEG-containing surfactants as surface modifiers, and PEGylated nanoparticles employed as a potential tool to release the drug into the brain. The methoxy-polyethyleneglycol cyanoacrylate-co-hexadecylcyanoacrylate (MePEGCA-HDCA) amphiphilic block-copolymer, newly synthesized, has been employed in the formulation of novel PEGylated polymeric nanoparticles [30]. However, the effect of surface modifiers on SLN surface has been studied earlier. The efficient surface modifier, polyethylene oxide (PEO)-containing nonionic block copolymers can be employed to avoid identification by cells of the mononuclear phagocyte system (MPS). This is used because the cells of the MPS are considered to be a limitation for drug targeting to other sites in the human body when injected intravenously drug carrier [38]. Recently reported N,N,N-Trimethyl chitosan (TMC) has widely been recognized for improvement of absorption, enhanced mucoadhesion, and stabilization characteristics. The outer surface of SLNs, in TMC-coated formulations, adsorbed by polymer film which prevent particle interactions through steric stabilization, results in enhanced stabilization [39].

3.5   METHODS OF MANUFACTURING

3.5.1   HIGH-PRESSURE HOMOGENIZATION

Homogenization is a mechanical process that involves the reduction of particles or droplets into very small (micron) sizes to produce a stable dispersion or emulsion for further analysis. In 1990s, SLNs were discovered by Prof. Rainer H. Müller and Dr. Jörg-Stefan Lucks (Kiel University, North Germany) and Prof. Dr. Maria Gasco (Turin University, Italy). This research group prepared SLNs by using high-pressure homogenization employing microemulsion technique [40].

The high pressure homogenization (HPH) is a unique and cost-effective technique for SLNs production having excellent reproducibility [28], high temporal stability, reduced effect of ionic strength on stability, proper physicochemical modification which results in targeted delivery, high protection of incorporated active molecules, high encapsulation efficiency, reduced bio-toxicity, absence of toxic organic solvent, and suitable for large scale preparation involving minimum cost [41].

The high-pressure homogenization is entirely a mechanical process in which the pre-emulsion is forced at high pressure (100–2,000 Bar) through a narrow gap with the desired cycle.

In this technique, the pressure is applied during the homogenization cycle of a liquid. The mechanical cavitation force at high pressure leads to the reduction of particles or droplets into micro and nano-size range [7]. Usually, the content of lipid in SLNs ranges from 5–10%.

Two approaches are generally employed in high-pressure homogenization methods for the preparation of SLNs, namely hot homogenization and cold homogenization. In the case with hot homogenization SLNs are prepared at elevated temperature conditions and in cold homogenization SLNs are prepared at or below room temperature.

A preliminary step involves in both approaches is identical, i.e., dispersing NM into the molten state of native lipid. The molten state of lipid can be achieved by raising temperature to 5–10°C above a melting temperature of lipid. On the other hand, the solution containing surfactant maintained at the same temperature could be added slowly and drop-wise to enhance uniform mixing coupled with high-speed stirring results in the formation of pre-emulsion. This pre-emulsion is then subjected to high-pressure homogenization with the desired pressure and homogenization cycle to get the desired particle size range:

1. **Hot High-Pressure Homogenization (Hot HPH):** The primary step involves the dispersion or dissolution of nutrient in a molten lipid followed by high pressure (100–700 Bar or more) of the homogenizer may be applied to get the particle of the desired size. The homogenizer works with applied pressure and pushes the liquid through a narrow gap on a very short distance with a very high velocity (over 1,000 km/h) [5]. The resulting mechanical shear stress and cavitational forces divide the particle and thereby reduce them into submicron size [7], keeping in mind rise in temperature during the HPH processing [42]. Prior to the application in a high-pressure homogenizer, a pre-emulsion of active ingredient loaded lipid melt produced in combining with aqueous surfactant phase high-speed homogenizer equipment (Ultra-turrax). This process produced a uniform particle size of dispersion. The pre-emulsion with uniform particle size produced an excellent final product. Thus, pre-emulsion is produced at a high temperature above the lipid's melting point [5]. Afterward, the dispersion is placed for subsequent cooling at room temperature or below room temperature which results in re-crystallization of dispersion and SLNs formation. Figure 3.1 illustrates the preparation of SLNs employing hot high-pressure homogenization (Hot HPH) technique.

2. **Cold Homogenization:** Hot HPH has several advantages for preparation of SLNs, but still suffer from few limitations [43], i.e., NM degradation due to elevated temperature, increase in complexity of crystallization step of dispersion leading to supercooled melt and

drug distribution into aqueous phase of formulation due to homogenization process. In view to overcome these limitations, a cold homogenization method has been developed for thermolabile NM. This method involves the basic step similar to hot homogenization, i.e., involving dispersion or solubilization of an active agent into molten lipid at a temperature 5°C or 10°C above the melting point of lipid. Nonetheless, the remaining processing steps are different [44].

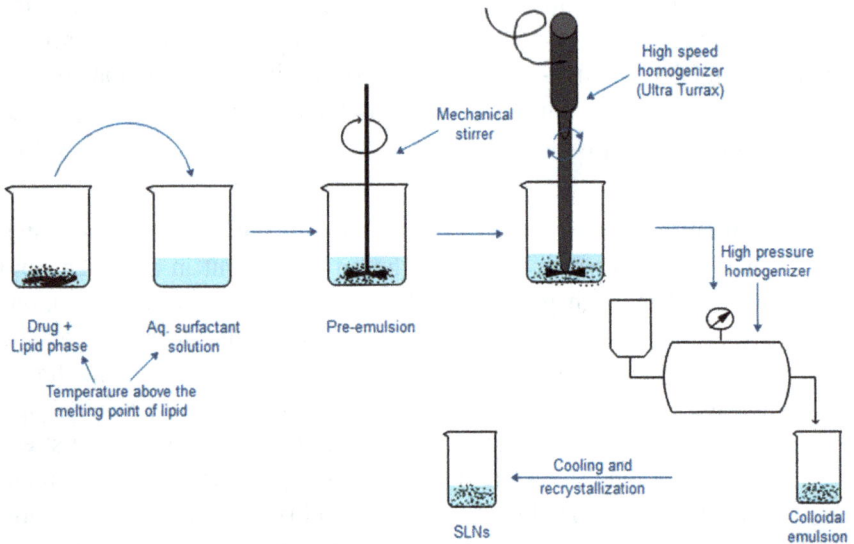

FIGURE 3.1   A schematic representation of hot high pressure homogenization techniques for preparation of SLNs.

The active drug-containing molten lipid quickly cooled in dry ice or liquid nitrogen. The homogeneous distribution of drug in molten lipid matrix and solidification of nanoparticles is the function of high cooling rate. The solid particles consisting of NM and lipid matrix is milled to produce particles. The desired particle size achieved using mortar or ball milling are in the range of 50–100 μm. The obtained solid lipid particles are dispersed in a cold surfactant solution to form a pre-suspension. It is then passed through the high-pressure homogenization process at and below room temperature to obtain the SLNs. In comparison to hot homogenization, bigger particle size and increased in size distribution are obtained in cold homogenization process [5, 44].

Cold homogenization is used to involve the homogenization of solid lipids as opposed to a lipid melt in hot homogenization. High energy input is required to produce the desired size SLNs. Thus, hot homogenization techniques itself is more efficient resulting in smaller and monodisperse particle [45]. Figure 3.2 represents the cold homogenization method for preparation of SLNs.

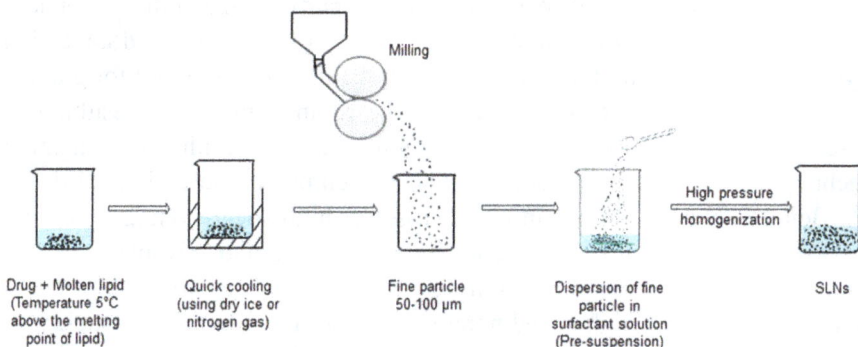

FIGURE 3.2   The schematic representation of cold homogenization techniques for preparation of SLNs.

3.5.2 HIGH SHEAR HOMOGENIZATION AND/OR ULTRASONICATION TECHNIQUE

High shear homogenization followed by ultrasonication is dispersing techniques used in the preparation of SLNs. This technique produced sound waves which can be used to reduce homogeneous particle size in a range from 80–800 nm [46]. Sonication is a process of utilization of sound energy generated by sonicator to agitate particles and reduce particle size for SLNs preparation. In general, sounds waves (ultrasonic frequencies) are used in order to breakdown particles into a smaller size, known as ultra-sonication. Ultrasonic bath or ultrasonic probe equipment are most frequently employed in the laboratory for preparation of SLNs. Ultrasonic bath is employed for large volumes of diluted lipid dispersions whereas, the probe sonicator is more suitable for dispersions that require more energy in a small volume (e.g., high concentration of lipids). Probe sonicator provides high energy to lipid dispersions but sometimes overheating causes lipid degradation of lipid dispersion. This issue can be overcome by advanced control mode which adjusts automatically ultrasonic pulse length to prevent the sample from overheating [42].

In order to obtain SLNs dispersion, lipidic matrix phase dispersed in a warm aqueous phase containing emulsifier by high shear homogenization followed by ultrasonication. The initial step involves melting the lipid at a temperature of 5°C or 10°C above the melting point. At the same time, the aqueous surfactant phase also warmed at the same temperature provided to the lipidic phase. Melted lipidic phase consequently dispersed slowly in the aqueous phase at the same temperature under high-speed stirring with a homogenizer to produce dispersion. Next, the particle size in the dispersion/emulsion is reduced by sonication under controlled temperature and sonication cycle. After processing through sonication, the dispersion placed for gradual cooling at room temperature or below the room temperature resulting in re-crystallization of dispersion and SLNs formation. The ultracentrifugation technique subsequently applied to obtain concentrated lipidic SLNs [45].

Being common equipment on a lab-scale, high shear homogenizer and sonication have an easy production process is a grand advantage of this method. Metal contamination during ultrasonication is noticeable disadvantage. Moreover, high-speed homogenizer produces broader particle size distribution leads to particle growth on storage. A high surfactant concentration could participate to improve stability [47]. However, a high amount of surfactant concentration reported as disadvantageous [48]. The schematic representation of this method is presented in Figure 3.3.

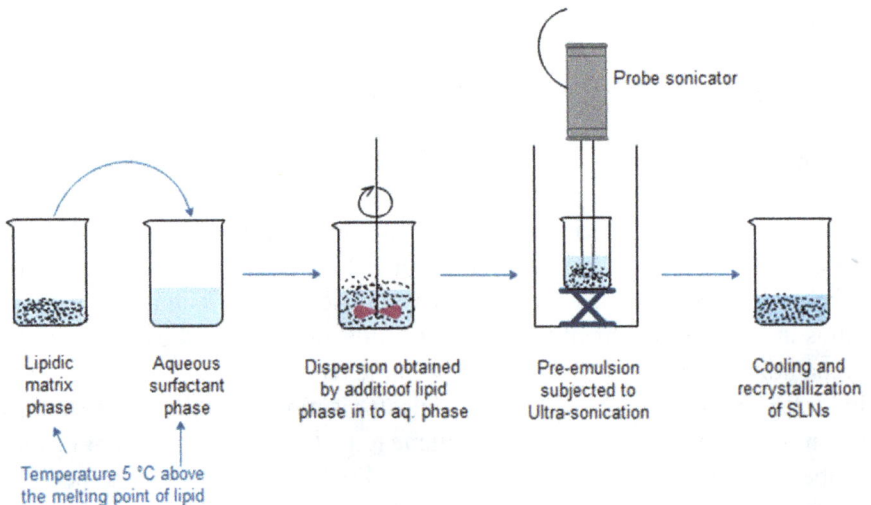

Probe sonicator

Lipidic matrix phase — Aqueous surfactant phase — Dispersion obtained by additioof lipid phase in to aq. phase — Pre-emulsion subjected to Ultra-sonication — Cooling and recrystallization of SLNs

Temperature 5 °C above the melting point of lipid

FIGURE 3.3   The schematic representation of high shear homogenization/ultra-sonication technique for preparation of SLNs.

3.5.3 MICRO-EMULSION

Gasco and co-workers were developed SLN using micro-emulsion technique [46]. Basically, the microemulsion is based on a two-phase system comprised inner and outer phase prepared for SLNs. In this technique, the lipid phase and aqueous phase are prepared separately. The lipid phase is melted, and the drug is incorporated subsequently in a molten lipid. Secondly, the aqueous phase is prepared with a mixture of surfactant and co-surfactant(s). The aqueous phase temperature should be kept as equal to that of melted lipid. A transparent and thermodynamically stable system is produced when the hot aqueous phase mixed in hot lipidic phase in the correct ratio for microemulsion formation. This is the prerequisite for the formation of SLNs. This hot microemulsion is then added so as to disperse completely in a cold aqueous medium (2–5°C) at a 1:25 to 1:50 ratio (microemulsion: water, v/v) under constant stirring. This dispersion leads to instant re-crystallization of oil droplets in a cold aqueous medium [49, 50]. Figures 3.4 illustrates the preparation of SLNs employing the micro-emulsion technique.

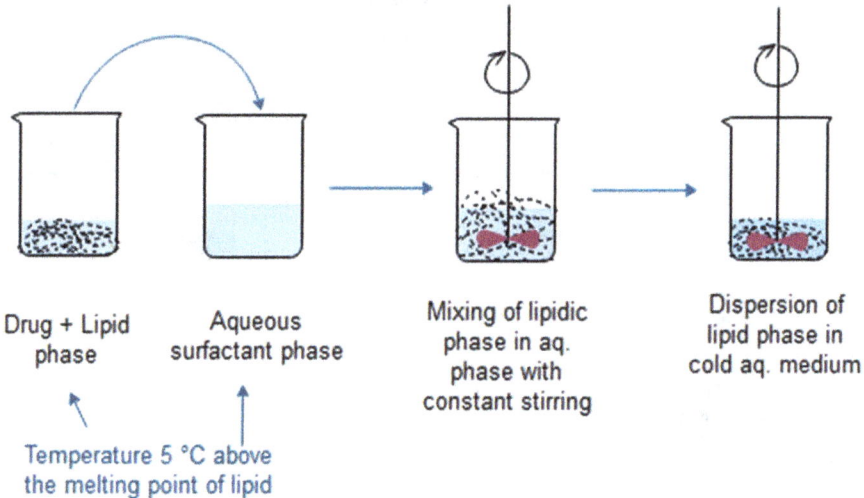

Drug + Lipid phase

Aqueous surfactant phase

Mixing of lipidic phase in aq. phase with constant stirring

Dispersion of lipid phase in cold aq. medium

Temperature 5 °C above the melting point of lipid

FIGURE 3.4 The schematic representation of micro-emulsion technique for preparation of SLNs.

SLNs obtained after re-crystallization employing micro-emulsion technique are spherically uniform in shape with narrow size distribution. The final dispersion of SLNs is diluted in an aqueous medium. The use of high concentration of surfactant or co-surfactant alone or in combination is a major drawback of this technique. However, SLNs concentrations can be achieved through ultrafiltration, lyophilization or other relevant methods [45].

3.5.4 SOLVENT EMULSIFICATION-EVAPORATION TECHNIQUE

The solvent emulsification-evaporation technique involves evaporation of water-immiscible solvent after emulsification. In this technique, organic solvent (water-immiscible solvent, e.g., toluene, chloroform) is prepared by dissolving hydrophobic drug and lipid. The organic phase is then emulsified by adding into an aqueous phase containing surfactant and stabilizer under constant stirring using a magnetic stirrer or high-speed homogenizer. The temperature of both the phases should be kept at 10°C above the melting point of lipid. Stirring is continued up to the nano-suspension formation and organic solvent present in the formulation is removed, at room temperature, by stirring followed by vacuum drying under reduced pressure. The organic solvent is then evaporated solvent diffuses into a continuous phase [51]. The solvent emulsification-evaporation technique is depicted in Figure 3.5.

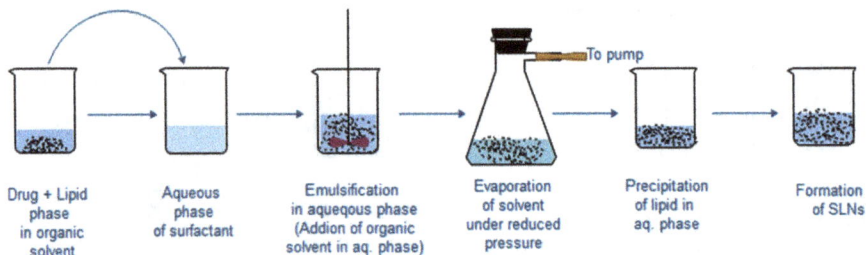

| Drug + Lipid phase in organic solvent | Aqueous phase of surfactant | Emulsification in aqueous phase (Addion of organic solvent in aq. phase) | Evaporation of solvent under reduced pressure | Precipitation of lipid in aq. phase | Formation of SLNs |

FIGURE 3.5   The schematic representation of solvent emulsification-evaporation technique for preparation of SLNs.

This technique is further classified into single and double emulsification-evaporation based on nutrient solubility in water-immiscible solvent. Former is employed only when the active NM is to be encapsulated shows the solubility in water-immiscible solvent (i.e., organic phase) and later is employed intended for insoluble behavior of active NM in a water-immiscible solvent. Such substance is dissolved in the aqueous phase and emulsified in an organic phase containing lipid and other ingredients [52].

3.5.5 *SOLVENT INJECTION TECHNIQUE*

The solvent injection method is very similar to the solvent diffusion method [53]. Figure 3.6 gives a graphic presentation of steps involved in solvent injection technique. The water-miscible organic solvent or its mixture employed in the preparation of SLNs. In this method, lipids are dissolved in water-miscible organic solvent viz. acetone, ethanol, methanol, and isopropanol and injected quickly into aqueous surfactant solution under stirring continuously. After solvent distribution into continuous aqueous surfactant solution, a precipitate of SLNs is produced. The particle size of SLNs depends upon the velocity of the diffusion of the solvent across the lipid-solvent interface into the aqueous phase.

Jain et al. produced SLNs recently employing solvent injection method produce average particle size 140 to 220 nm with enhanced rigidity of SLNs. The obtained size range is a result of diffusion of solvent across-solvent lipid phase in medium followed by solvent evaporation [54]. Furthermore, the particle size obtained by this method is depending on the velocity of the distribution process. Higher velocity produces smaller particle size [55].

Muller-Goymann and Schubert produced the SLNs by a solvent injection process and reported that the rise in diameter of particle is due to a fall of the diffusion rate of the solute molecules in the outer phase in the lipid-solvent phase [56]. The major benefit of this method is easy handling and fast process without any major equipment. However, use of organic solvent is a disadvantage.

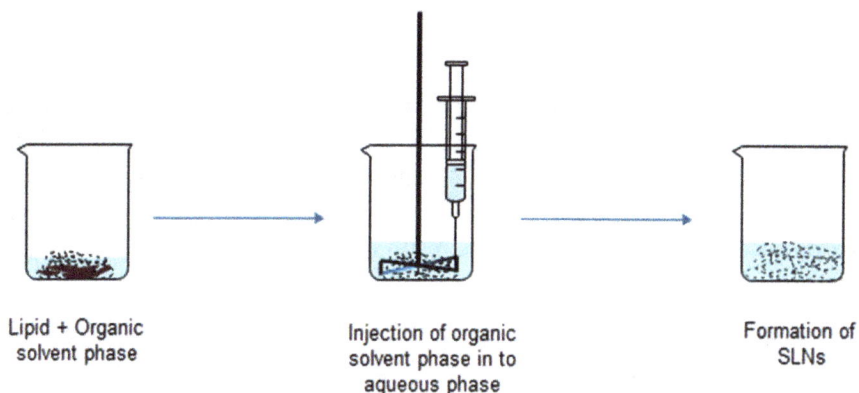

Lipid + Organic
solvent phase

Injection of organic
solvent phase in to
aqueous phase

Formation of
SLNs

FIGURE 3.6 The schematic representation of solvent injection technique for preparation of SLNs.

3.5.6 DOUBLE EMULSION

Cortesi et al. and his research group were the first who described the double emulsion method for liposphere preparation [57]. Here, two emulsification steps are required for the preparation of warm w/o/w double microemulsion. The main fact of this method is to solubilize a hydrophilic drug molecule in the internal aqueous phase of w/o/w double emulsion with the help of surfactants. In the initial step, an aqueous solution of drug (inner phase) is needed to disperse in a mixture of melted lipid, surfactant, and co-surfactant under stirring continuously with high shear homogenization equipment. The temperature should be kept slightly higher than above the melting point of lipid. At this point, transparent system is formed which further dispersed in a mixture of water, surfactant, and co-surfactant, in a second step, results in the formation of clear w/o/w double emulsion system. This system kept under mechanical agitation to form SLNs [58, 59]. A schematic showing the steps in the double emulsion is depicted in Figure 3.7.

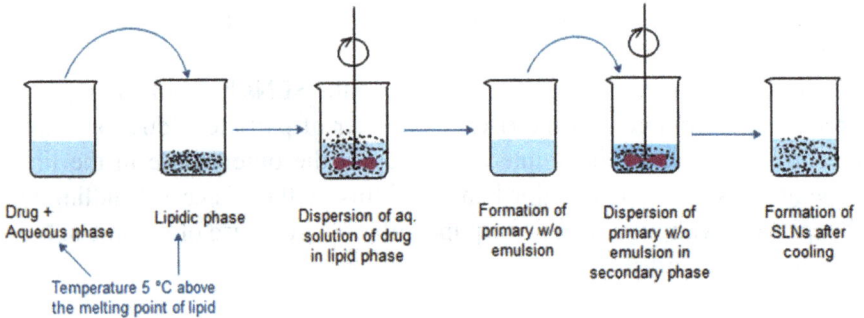

Drug +
Aqueous phase   Lipidic phase   Dispersion of aq.   Formation of   Dispersion of   Formation of
                                          solution of drug   primary w/o   primary w/o   SLNs after
                                          in lipid phase   emulsion   emulsion in   cooling
                                                                                          secondary phase

Temperature 5 °C above
the melting point of lipid

FIGURE 3.7   Schematic representation of double emulsion technique for preparation of SLNs.

The double emulsion technique is mainly used for the preparation of SLNs encapsulated with a hydrophilic drug. However, hydrophilic drug interactions with solvent and excipients affect the preparation by this technique [46]. The product obtained by this method may endure the main toxicological problems could be the result of solvent residue [60].

3.6 CRITICAL QUALITY ATTRIBUTES (CQAS)

The relevant CQAs of the SLNs formulation can be justified by quality risk management system and experimentation. The general CQAs of the

SLNs formulation should be considered during product development. These properties are constitutional to the formulation that affect the manufacturing process. Hereinafter, are described some of the critical common quality attributes that should be considered during the SLNs development.

3.6.1   PARTICLE SIZE

The particle size of SLNs is considered as highly critical since the smaller particle size allows better penetration through GI epithelial lining and paracellular pathways. The size of particles depends upon the amount and chemical nature of surfactant and co-surfactant in SLNs formulation.

3.6.2   POLYDISPERSITY INDEX (PDI)

Polydispersity index (PDI) is the ratio of standard deviation to mean particle size of SLNs. The consistent particle size of SLNs is desired for good content uniformity of NM and its stability. The PDI value (>300) indicates dispersion of particles having a uniform particle size, however, PDI (<300) denote non-uniformity in the formulation, therefore PDI is considered as CQAs in the formulation of SLNs.

3.6.3   ZETA POTENTIAL

Zeta potential is an essential factor for the stability of SLNs. The SLNs formulation having high zeta potential value confers better physical stability by preventing particle aggregation. The negative zeta potential value of SLNs usually occurs due to the charge present on lipid and surfactant molecules. Therefore, the zeta potential is considered as CQAs in the formulation of SLNs.

3.6.4   ENTRAPMENT EFFICIENCY (%)

Entrapment efficiency (EE) of SLNs is a crucial factor in the formulation of SLNs. It is defined as the amount of nutrient entrapped in lipid matrix to the theoretical amount incorporated into SLNs. EE is an essential parameter in the study of nutrient release behavior or diffusion of drug/NM across a biological membrane. EE is depending upon the lipid solubility of nutrients, nature of lipid and; the type and concentration of surfactant utilized in the formulation of SLNs. EE due to formulation aspect is considered as CQAs in the design of SLNs.

3.7   CHARACTERIZATION TECHNIQUES

Solid lipid nanoparticles (SLNs) are the colloidal nutraceuticals delivery system, which is made using intermediate molecular weight triglycerides or waxes [61]. SLNs are designed to provide three must characteristics such as colloidal or smaller particle size, solid dosage form delivery, and lipid matrix. These three characteristics all together provide nutraceutical delivery which has improved nutrient solubility, so the dissolution, biocompatibility, and if designed such then controlled release profile for the nutrients. SLNs key component which decides its improved property is the particles which are in NM ranges. However, the particles in NM ranges can create difficulties in characterizing SLNs. These difficulties relate to the nutrient solubility and its solid-state stability. Smaller particles can increase the solubility of the NM beyond its saturation solubility leading to crystallization or polymorphism. Therefore, it is essential to have a detailed protocol for characterizing the complex SLN formulations. Different techniques are used to characterize and establish the stability of SLNs. These techniques and methods are based on the thermal behaviors, crystallinity, solid-state stability, particle size distribution, surface characteristics and structural properties of nanoparticles [62–64]. This chapter provides the outlined information and critical aspects of analytical techniques commonly used in the characterization of nanoparticle dispersion.

3.7.1   PARTICLE SIZE ANALYSIS

SLNs have particle sizes less than 1 μm, and in the case of targeted drug delivery, particle sizes are kept between 50 and 300 nm. The particle size of SLN is one of the first indicators to provide information about the formulation's stability [10]. Nanoparticles have a high surface area that leads to the generation of high surface free energy [65], which could lead to the potential problem of particle aggregation. Therefore, particle size determination provides the information on the particle aggregation led to formulations physical instability [27]. Formulation factors such as dispersing medium, surfactant, and co-surfactant influences the sizes and crystallization.

Similarly, processing parameters such as production techniques, homogenization time, sonication time, temperature, and lyophilization influence the particle size, crystallization, and polymorphism [5, 66, 67]. Therefore, formulation and processing parameters are carefully analyzed before employing for the large batch production. The presence of higher lipid surfactant ratio decreases the particle size indicating a higher amount of surfactant may help to stabilize the formulation [68].

If nutrient entrapment is higher than 1% can cause an increase in particle size. Therefore, it is preferred nutrient entrapment value less than 1%.

Light scattering methods are often used for particle size distribution analysis. Light scattering methods employees two primary methods which are laser diffraction (LD) and photon correlation spectroscopy.

LD and dynamic light scattering (DLS) are the two widely employed analytical techniques to characterize particle sizes of SLN [69]. Both methods differ in their working principle. LD method uses a laser beam passing through a sample and collects light intensity data at different scattering angles away from the axis of the laser beam (Figure 3.8). Mie light scattering theory and mathematical models were applied to intensity data to find out the particle size. The advantages of this LD method are that it is simple, fast, non-destructive, and covers a broad range of particles such as 100 nm to several millimeters [70]. Average time required is less than 1 min. to analyze the sample. However, the LD method has some disadvantages which could lead to wrong result interpretation or the data collection. Some of these disadvantages are associated with either instruments capability or sample property. Instrument related factors are accuracy, low resolving power, and multiple scattering effects. Sample associated factors such as strong absorbing particles can present problems because they may not produce good scattering, and second is the incapability of the system for treating mixture. A mixture containing components which have different optical properties could lead to wrong interpretation. Based on the sample property and physical nature, the minimum amount required to carry out analysis may vary. Approximately 1–2 gm of samples and >5 gm of sample required to in case of dispersion and dry powder samples, respectively.

In DLS, the Brownian motion or random thermal movement of submicron particles are measured as a function of time [71]. A laser beam is passed through the sample, and light is scattered by particles in suspension. In suspension, submicron particles diffusion causes the fluctuation in scattering intensity at a certain angle (Figure 3.9). Moreover, the scattered light intensity signal is used to attribute the information related to the Brownian movement of the particles, which is subsequently used to measure the particle size. Smaller particles have a faster Brownian motion which causes higher fluctuation in light scattering and opposite in cases of larger particles. This property of particles helps to measure the particle size. DLS method is the fast, non-destructive, and a minimal amount of sample requirement. Compared to LD, this method can be effectively used to analyze mixtures. However, a significant drawback of DLS is that it assumes all particles and spherical, which is practically difficult. Also, the method does not provide size distribution data, but instead, it gives data which is related to mean size and polydispersity of the suspension [72].

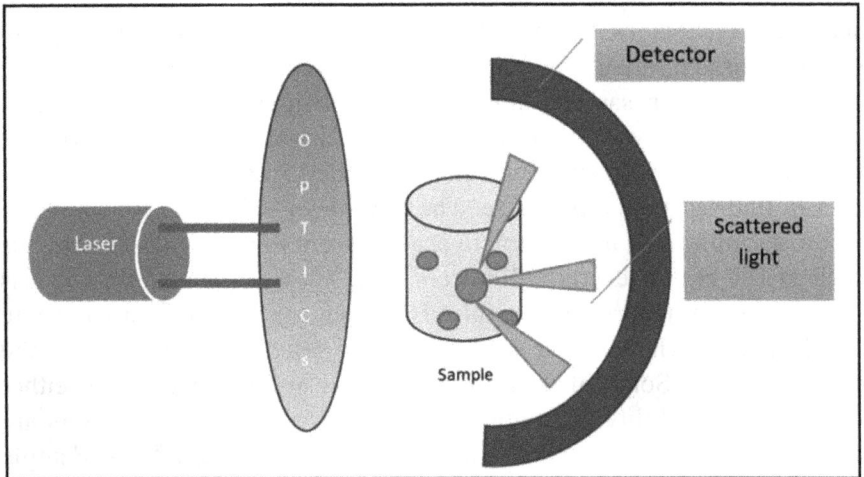

FIGURE 3.8   Schematic representation of laser diffraction for particle size distribution.

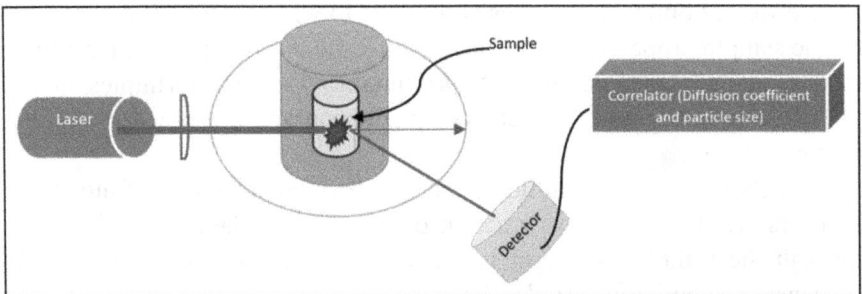

FIGURE 3.9   Schematic representation of DLS for particle size distribution.

3.7.2 *MORPHOLOGY AND STRUCTURAL PROPERTIES OF SLN*

Morphology and structural properties of SLN formulations are critical in establishing product characteristics of the formulation. Morphology is the study of the size, shape, and structure of the components present in the sample. While structural properties of the SLNs are more about the interior structures of formulation, such as properties of the different components which are present in the inner core of the formulation. SLNs are either in a spherical shape or non-spherical particles, and the shape of the particle can significantly influence the NM loading capacity and nutrient releasing mechanism in SLNs [73, 74]. This indicates that the shape of the particle that have an effect on the stability of the formulation because the spherical particles have limited specific area on the other hand, non-spherical particles has a larger surface area. This decides the amount of surfactant is needed to stabilize the formulation. As described in the previous section that LD and DLS may not be sensitive enough to differentiate between the anisometric and spherical particles. This made it very important to corroborate the results of particle size analysis with the electron microscopy. Microstructure analysis of SLNs is critical because of the excipient's material properties. The surfactant is the crucial ingredient in stabilizing the nanoparticles. However, it is possible that the surfactant starts self-assembling in dispersion and forms some new colloidal structures [75]. These colloidal structures are nothing but the micelles, and micelles have a lipophilic domain which can trap the nutrient molecule. This can affect the drug/nutrient release mechanism; therefore, it is essential to understand the microstructure of developed formulations.

The morphology and microstructure properties of SLNs can be analyzed using the electron microscopy. This involves the use of an electron beam instead of a light beam. In electron microscopy, sample, and electrons from the electron beam start interacting with each other via electrostatic forces, i.e., Coulomb forces. This results in the scattering of electrons, and these electrons are collected to project a two-dimensional image of the sample. Scanning electron microscopy (SEM), transmission electron microscopy (TEM) and atomic force microscopy (AFM) are the widely preferred imaging techniques to characterize SLNs [76].

3.7.2.1 *SCANNING ELECTRON MICROSCOPY (SEM)*

SEM is one of the most commonly preferred instrumental techniques for imaging analysis. SEM is most commonly used of morphological studies such as shape analysis and surface characteristics. The electron beam attributed to acquire the SEM image using the sample surface scan. An electron starts deflecting at a large number of elastic scattering when the electrons are passed through the sample [77]. The energy change caused by the electron deflections is detected by the detector, which further translated into the two-dimensional image (Figure 3.10). SEM has been employed to take pictures when SLNs are in dry powder form as well as when SLNs are in contact with the dissolution media [78–80]. However, the major issue with SEM is sample preparation. If the sample has very high surface charges that will affect the image quality also the use of vacuum in sample analysis may affect the nanoparticles leading to ambiguity in the observation.

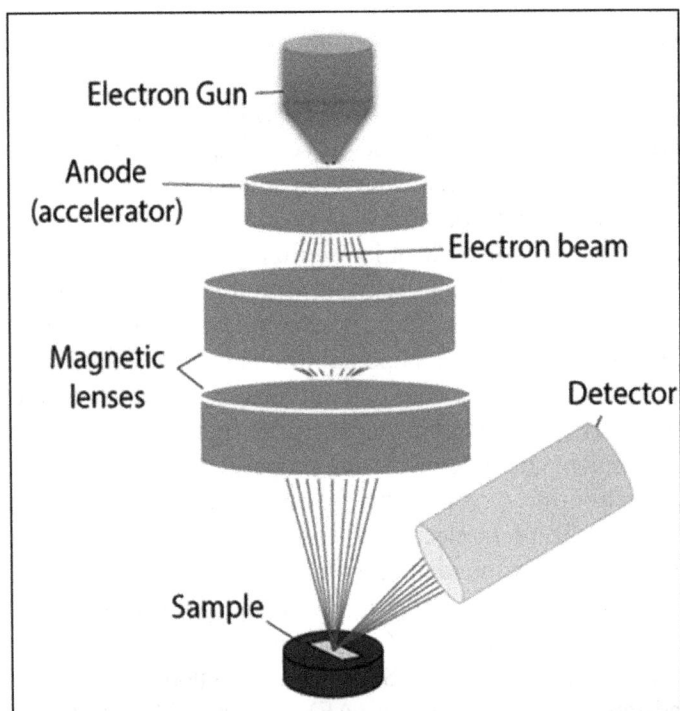

FIGURE 3.10   Schematic representation of SEM.

3.7.2.2   *TRANSMISSION ELECTRON MICROSCOPY (TEM)*

TEM is often used in morphological and microstructure studies of nanoparticles. The TEM contains an illumination system, which drives the electron from a gun to the samples. Then the sample is screened by several lenses [81]. The transmission electron microscope contains objective, condenser, intermediate, and projector lenses (Figure 3.11). Different techniques have been used to prepare samples for the TEM analysis, such as negative staining, freeze-fracture and vitrification [82]. Negative staining technique involves the use of heavy metal salts. A small drop of the heavy metal salt is added onto the sample and sprayed onto the TEM sample assembly subsequently dried, and imaging is performed. Staining technique is fast, simple, and requires very less effort in making a sample. However, staining followed by drying may generate artifacts which are difficult to separate from the real colloidal part. The second method for sample preparation is the freeze-fracture method. In this method, sample dispersion is placed between two metal slides and then vitrified by rapid freezing in liquid nitrogen or liquid propane. Afterward, a frozen sample is fractured by using a vacuum or constant cooling. Fracture planes may further etch by sublimation of the frozen water under vacuum. Freeze-fracture TEM is very useful in analyzing the size, shape, and microstructure of the SLNs. In the past, this technique is successfully used to characterize different types of drug delivery which are lipid-based. TEM was used to visualize the changes in particle morphology due to phase separation. Also, the researcher has been employing TEM to detect the polymorphic transition. Even though the freeze-fracture method has been successfully used, but it is important to keep in mind that particles are fractured randomly which are further analyzed. Therefore, a sufficiently large number of particles must be investigated before reaching to any conclusion pertaining to the size, shape, and structure of the SLN. The second factor which could lead to uncertainty in results are the issues related to the solvent re-deposition.

3.7.2.3 ATOMIC FORCE MICROSCOPY (AFM)

AFM is a topography technique and widely accepted in the pharmaceutical world [83, 84]. The reason for the preference of AFM over other scanning technique is that the system can provide microstructural details of the sample with insights on intermolecular forces at the NM scale. AFM can be employed in a wide spectrum of applications such as pharmaceuticals, biologicals, and polymers. AFM system can be modified based on the requirement such as force modulation microscopy for determining mechanical properties of solid substances. AFM provides the application of capturing images at NM level without moving sample, switching tips, and relocating the scanning area.

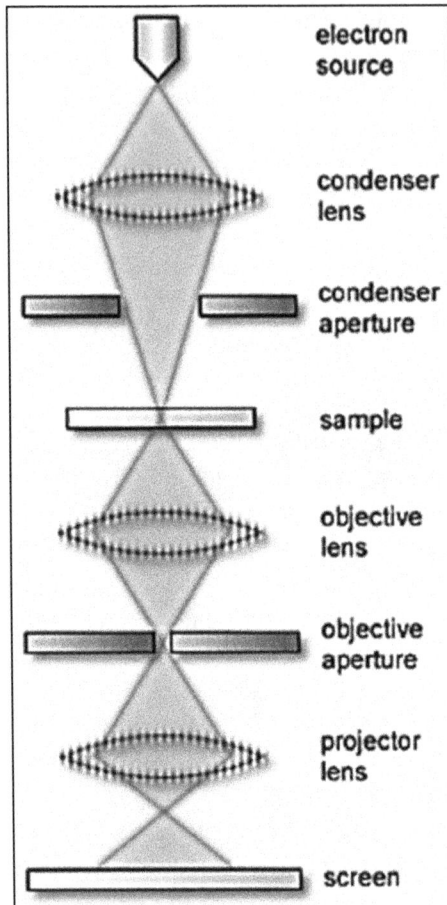

FIGURE 3.11   Schematic representation of TEM.

As depicted in Figure 3.12, three major components in the AFM system are cantilever; tip mounted to a piezoelectric actuator (PZA) and detector [85]. The purpose of using PZA is to provide constant pressure and constant height of tip which is may or may not in contact with the sample. During sample scan tip is moves up and down as it moves forward with scanning. This produces the deflection in the incident beam, which is ultimately detected by the detectors. Typically, AFM measurements can be carried out in three ways based on the requirements, which are 1) Contact mode 2) non-contact mode 3) Tapping mode [86]. AFM tips and cantilevers are fabricated using Si or Si_3NO_4 AFM has been used for investigating the morphology of SLNs. Probe contact mode needs the contact between the tip and the sample that could lead to distortion in samples. Therefore, the non-contact mode is used for imaging of SLN [78]. However, the non-contact mode resolution reduces to as low as 2 nm. There are no special precautions required to prepare the samples for AFM scanning, which makes it advantageous over SEM and TEM.

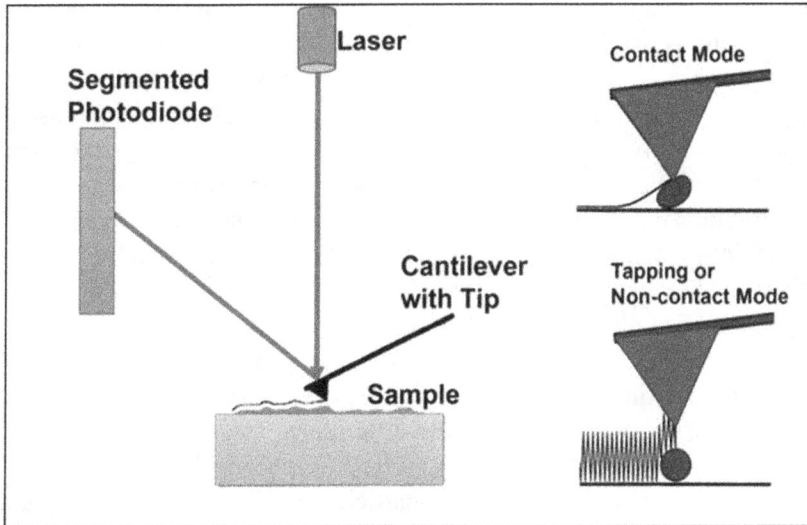

FIGURE 3.12   Schematic representation of AFM.

3.7.3   SOLID STATE CHARACTERISTICS OF SLN

Lipids, drug or NM, and other excipients are processed through multiple processes to prepare SLN. This manufacturing process involves steps like heating and mechanical agitation, which generally produces large amount of stress on to the particles [87–89]. Under these stress conditions, drug/ nutrient have a tendency to change its crystallinity or the polymorphic form [90, 91]. Also, the drug particles are in NM particle size ranges, and the solid property of the formulation will control the stability as well as the release of the drug from the formulation. The crystallinity of the lipid particles is often addressed for the modified release properties. Therefore, it is very important to characterize the SLN for their solid-state properties, specifically properties related to crystallinity and the possible polymorphic transitions. Prepared hot nanoemulsions using a solid lipid in the hydrophobic phase of the dispersions must be cooled down the critical crystallization temperature of the lipid to crystallize and form nanoparticles [92]. However, if the critical crystallization temperature is not reached, then lipids are in a liquid state. This led to the formation of supercooled emulsion than the desired product with lipid nanoparticles. This indicates that the special thermal treatment is necessary to confirm that particles formed are in the solid-state [93]. The critical crystallization temperature is affected by the other components which are present in the dispersion. The presence of drug/NM effects lowers the crystallinity of lipids. Therefore, an excess amount of drug/nutrient will lead to a less crystalline formulation. It is possible to see the changes after the initial solidification of SLN. The solid lipids which are used in this case generally show the polymorphism over time. During the storage, these nanoparticles transform into stable polymorph, which may not always be desirable. This is because polymorphic transitions are generally led to changes in the shapes of the nanoparticles. And as mentioned in previous sections, if the physiological or microstructure of the formulation is altered that can significantly affect the stability and performance of the formulation. A most common example is of drug/NM expulsion from the nanoparticle over the storage time. During the storage, the lipid has a tendency to change its crystalline form into more stable crystalline. This transition leads to a change in the crystal shape so the particle shape which could lead to the expulsion of drug/NM from the nanoparticle. Therefore, it is very important to address the crystallinity and polymorphism in SLNs.

Differential scanning calorimetry (DSC) powder X-ray diffraction (PXRD) mostly preferred analytical techniques to characterize crystallinity and polymorphism of the SLN [94–96]. Thermal analysis of SLN requires careful investigation to assess the solid-state properties of the formulation. Such as DSC is very sensitive and best technique to determine crystallinity [97]. However, the polymorphic transition can be seen if it is carefully investigated. Therefore, in this case, PXRD is the best technique. PXRD can provide the structural information of the solid component so the polymorphic transition of the nanoparticles. It is recommended that formulation should be analyzed in its final dosage form in DSC. XRD provides flexibility towards the sample preparation. However, if the sample requires dilution before analysis that could lead to uncertainty in the observation from the DSC and XRD.

3.7.3.1 X-RAY DIFFRACTION (XRD)

Solid-state in SLN tends to change its crystalline form over time, and that could negatively affect the formulation performance towards stability and therapeutic. PXRD is the best analytical instrumental system to analyze this behavior of SLN. XRD is based on the diffraction phenomenon, which is generated because of the interaction between the X-ray and the crystal lattice [98, 99]. The diffractogram displays the peaks at the specific angular position of the X-ray. This provides the information on the structural arrangement of the molecule in the crystal. XRD is used to distinguish the solid, crystalline nature or amorphous nature, and identification of the polymorphic form of the lipid matrix in the formulation. XRD is also used to study the phase separation in SLN.

3.7.3.2   DIFFERENTIAL SCANNING CALORIMETRY (DSC)

Differential scanning calorimetry (DSC) is a thermodynamic tool for assessing the heat energy absorbed or liberated during the various transitions in the sample, which occurs in upon controlled heating, cooling, or isothermal conditions. In DSC analysis difference in the amount of heat/energy required to raise the temperature of a sample and reference mounted in instrument is measured associated with temperature [100, 101]. The phenomena causing this enthalpic transition include phase transitions or thermal degradation of the sample. Phase transitions of a sample can include polymorphic transitions, crystallization, melting or vaporization/sublimation of sample specimen. The most important part of the DSC instrument is the DSC cell in which sample and reference pans are placed as the experiment is performed. This DSC cell includes multiple factors such as proper calibration and cleaning of the contaminated cell, which can affect the results significantly, and therefore, it is vital for the analyst to make sure the experimental protocol involves the checking of all these components. The essential DSC cell components are the sample pan, reference pan, a source of heat energy and a path having known thermal resistance (Figure 3.13).

DSC is preferably used to determine the crystallinity of solid components in lipid nanoparticles [102, 103]. In DSC if SLN is treated as a sample, then the amount of heat required to raise the temperature of crystalline material compared to the non-crystalline material will be higher. Moreover, this difference in the heat requirement is used to assess the crystallinity of the lipid nanoparticles. DSC can be employed to understand enantiotropic or monotropy of the system. This could provide the information on the polymorphism in lipids.

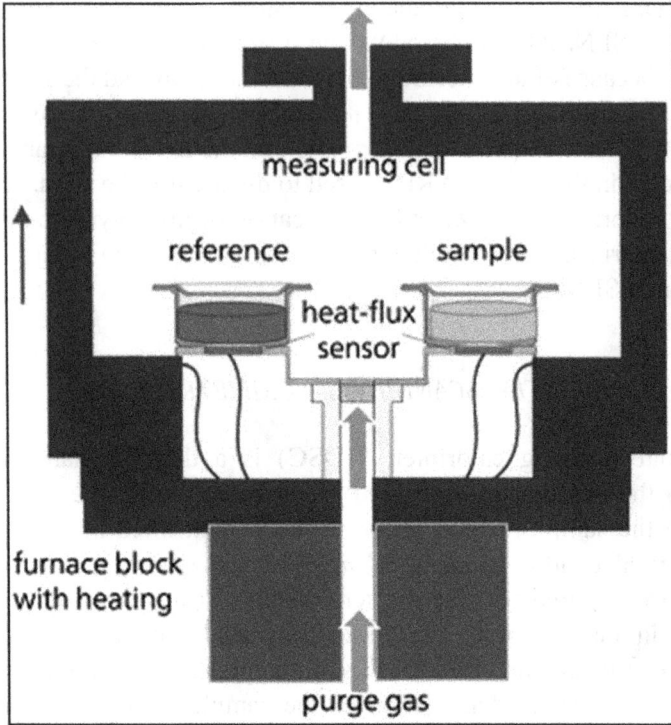

FIGURE 3.13   Schematic representation of DSC.

3.7.4   *STRUCTURAL ANALYSIS OF SLN*

The presence of multiple components such as surfactant, lipid, and excipients in SLN could result in the generation of new colloidal structure, which is not warranted. Moreover, the presence of this colloidal structure can negatively affect product performances. The use of spectroscopic techniques such as nuclear magnetic resonance (NMR) and Fourier transform infrared (FT-IR) spectroscopy can provide the options to evaluate the presence of any other colloidal species in the system. Also, these methods can be employed to find out the nature of the interaction between nutrients and excipients.

3.7.4.1   *NUCLEAR MAGNETIC RESONANCE (NMR)*

The proton NMR spectroscopy is based on the amount of energy need to cause a nuclear spin as a function of the magnetic environment experienced by the nucleus [104]. Typical application of NMR spectroscopy in SLN is the characterization of lipid nanoparticles, presenting the insight on the liquid lipid contained in SLN and the nutrient [105–107]. The associations between drugs and the lipid carrier can be studied with the help of NMR. Preparation of SLN involves the intense mixing between drug and solid lipid, and this could change the lipid crystal. The changes in mobility, mixing behavior and the colloidal structures of lipid can be analyzed using the NMR.

3.7.4.2 FOURIER TRANSFORM INFRARED (FT-IR) SPECTROSCOPY

FT-IR is the modification in traditional IR spectrophotometer. This modification provides many advantages over the conventional IR spectrophotometer such as sensitivity, variable temperature set up, less sample analyzing time and inline measurements [108]. The working principle involves detecting the transmitted radiation. The process involves the sending of IR radiation from a source to an interferometer to modify the radiation afterward it passes through the sample and the transmitted light is detected by the detector (Figure 3.14). Every molecule or functional group absorbs the IR radiation at a fixed wavelength which further leads to vibration of molecules [109]. These wavelengths or the frequency numbers are used as a fingerprint for detecting compatibility between two or more chemical components, the effect of temperature and moisture [110, 111]. In a dispersion conformational information about lipid molecules is analyzed with the help of FT-IR. Thus, the chemical incompatibility, excipient interaction or the changes due to the storage or the manufacturing steps can be easily analyzed using the FT-IR [112].

3.8 CONCLUSION

Thus, the present chapter describes various aspects of SLNs for nutraceutical delivery to improve the health. The SLNs exhibit significant potential and probable for an extensive range of applications in both the food and pharmaceutical industries in large scale production. SLNs offers various nutrients such as carbohydrates, lipids, vitamins, antimicrobial, antioxidants, minerals, flavors, phytosterols (PS), and probiotics to encapsulate to present several benefits. SLNs facilitate to improve the solubility, stability, and bioavailability of active ingredients.

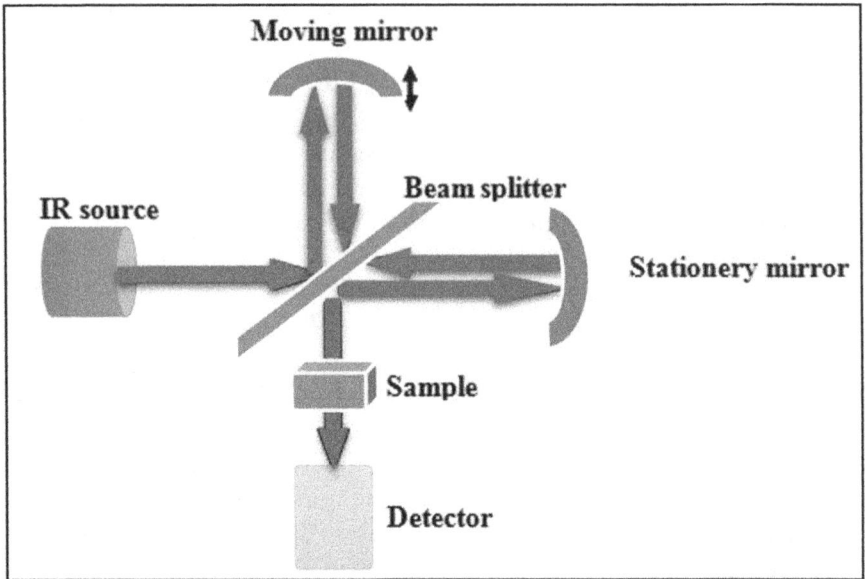

FIGURE 3.14   Schematic representation of FT-IR.

Thus, in this chapter, we presented overall coverage of essential components to prepare SLNs, its characterizations, critical attributes which impart to produce quality products. In addition, stability and controlled release of nutrients should be fulfilled by SLNs along with safety.

KEYWORDS

- **entrapment efficiency**
- **generally recognized as safe**
- **high-pressure homogenization**
- **nanoparticles**
- **nanostructured lipid carriers**
- **national institutes of health**
- **relative humidity**
- **rotation per min**

REFERENCES

1. Zanella, M., et al., (2015). Nutraceuticals and nanotechnology. *Agro Food Industry Hi-Tech, 26*(5, S), 26–31.
2. Garg, T., et al., (2016). Colloidal systems: An excellent carrier for nutrient delivery *Nutrient Delivery*. Elsevier Inc. doi: 10.1016/b978-0-12-804304-2.00018-4.
3. Singh, R., & Lillard, J. W., (2009). Nanoparticle-based targeted drug delivery. *Experimental and Molecular Pathology*, 215–223. Elsevier Inc. doi: 10.1016/j.yexmp.2008.12.004.
4. Pardeike, J., Hommoss, A., & Müller, R. H., (2009). Lipid nanoparticles (SLN, NLC) in cosmetic and pharmaceutical dermal products. *International Journal of Pharmaceutics*, 170–184. doi: 10.1016/j.ijpharm.2008.10.003.
5. Mehnert, W., & Mäder, K., (2012). Solid lipid nanoparticles: Production, characterization and applications. *Advanced Drug Delivery Reviews*, 83–101. Elsevier B.V. doi: 10.1016/j. addr.2012.09.021.
6. Campardelli, R., et al., (2013). Lipid nanoparticles production by supercritical fluid assisted emulsion-diffusion. *Journal of Supercritical Fluids, 82*, 34–40. Elsevier B.V. doi: 10.1016/j.supflu.2013.05.020.
7. Mäder, K., & Mehnert, W., (2001). Solid lipid nanoparticles: Production, characterization and applications. *Advanced Drug Delivery Reviews, 47*(2, 3), 165–196. doi: 10.1016/ S0169-409X(01)00105-3.
8. Kaur, I. P., et al., (2008a). Potential of solid lipid nanoparticles in brain targeting. *Journal of Controlled Release, 127*(2), 97–109. doi: 10.1016/j.jconrel.2007.12.018.
9. Zhang, X., et al., (2010). Formulation optimization of dihydroartemisinin nanostructured lipid carrier using response surface methodology. *Powder Technology, 197*(1, 2), 120–128. Elsevier B.V. doi: 10.1016/j.powtec.2009.09.004.
10. Müller, R. H., Radtke, M., & Wissing, S. A., (2002). Solid lipid nanoparticles (SLN) and nanostructured lipid carriers (NLC) in cosmetic and dermatological preparations. In: *Advanced Drug Delivery Reviews* (pp. 131–155). doi: 10.1016/S0169-409X(02)00118-7.
11. Gursoy, R. N., & Benita, S., (2004). Self-emulsifying drug delivery systems (SEDDS) for improved oral delivery of lipophilic drugs. *Biomedicine and Pharmacotherapy, 58*(3), 173–182. doi: 10.1016/j.biopha.2004.02.001.
12. Aditya, N. P., et al., (2014). Development and evaluation of lipid nanocarriers for quercetin delivery: A comparative study of solid lipid nanoparticles (SLN), nanostructured lipid carriers (NLC), and lipid nanoemulsions (LNE). *LWT - Food Science and Technology, 59*, 115–121. doi: 10.1016/j.lwt.2014.04.058.
13. Gastaldi, L., et al., (2014). Solid lipid nanoparticles as vehicles of drugs to the brain: Current state of the art. *European Journal of Pharmaceutics and Biopharmaceutics*, 433–444. Elsevier B.V. doi: 10.1016/j.ejpb.2014.05.004.
14. Pathak, K., Keshri, L., & Shah, M., (2011). Lipid nanocarriers: Influence of lipids on product development and pharmacokinetics. *Critical Reviews™ in Therapeutic Drug Carrier Systems, 28*(4), 357–393. doi: 10.1615/CritRevTherDrugCarrierSyst.v28.i4.20.
15. Patel, G. V., et al., (2014). Nanosuspension of efavirenz for improved oral bioavailability: Formulation optimization, *in vitro*, *in situ*, and *in vivo* evaluation. In: Patel, G. V., Patel, V. B., Pathak, A., & Rajput, S. J., (2014). *Nanosuspension of Efavirenz for Improved Oral Bioavailability: Form; Drug Development and Industrial Pharmacy* (Vol. 40, No. 1, pp. 80–91). doi: 10.3109/03639045.2012.746362.

16. Kumbhar, D. D., & Pokharkar, V. B., (2013). Engineering of a nanostructured lipid carrier for the poorly water-soluble drug, bicalutamide: Physicochemical investigations. *Colloids and Surfaces A: Physicochemical and Engineering Aspects, 416*, 32–42. Elsevier B.V. doi: 10.1016/j.colsurfa.2012.10.031.

17. Ranpise, N. S., Korabu, S. S., & Ghodake, V. N., (2014). Second generation lipid nanoparticles (NLC) as an oral drug carrier for delivery of lercanidipine hydrochloride. *Colloids and Surfaces B: Biointerfaces, 116*, 81–87. Elsevier B.V. doi: 10.1016/j.colsurfb.2013.12.012.

18. Negi, L. M., Jaggi, M., & Talegaonkar, S., (2014a). Development of protocol for screening the formulation components and the assessment of common quality problems of nanostructured lipid carriers. *International Journal of Pharmaceutics, 461*(1, 2), 403–410. doi: 10.1016/j.ijpharm.2013.12.006.

19. Jose, S., et al., (2014). *In vivo* pharmacokinetics and biodistribution of resveratrol-loaded solid lipid nanoparticles for brain delivery. *International Journal of Pharmaceutics*. doi: 10.1016/j.ijpharm.2014.08.003.

20. Shete, H., & Patravale, V., (2013). Long-chain lipid based tamoxifen NLC. Part I: Preformulation studies, formulation development, and physicochemical characterization. *International Journal of Pharmaceutics, 454*(1), 573–583. Elsevier B.V. doi: 10.1016/j.ijpharm.2013.03.034.

21. Radomska-Soukharev, A., & Müller, R. H., (2006). Chemical stability of lipid excipients in SLN-production of test formulations, characterization and short-term stability. *Pharmazie, 61*(5), 425–430.

22. Gohla, S., Mader, K., & Muller, R. H., (2000). *Solid Lipid Nanoparticles (SLN) for Controlled Drug Delivery: A Review of the State of the Art.*, 50.

23. Shah, M. R., Imran, M., & Ullah, S., (2017). *Lipid-Based Nanocarriers for Drug Delivery and Diagnosis, Lipid-Based Nanocarriers for Drug Delivery and Diagnosis.* doi: https://doi.org/10.1016/B978-0-323-52729-3.00005-6.

24. Negi, L. M., Jaggi, M., & Talegaonkar, S., (2014b). Development of protocol for screening the formulation components and the assessment of common quality problems of nanostructured lipid carriers. *International Journal of Pharmaceutics, 461*(1, 2), 403–410. Elsevier B.V. doi: 10.1016/j.ijpharm.2013.12.006.

25. Joshi, M., & Patravale, V., (2008). Nanostructured lipid carrier (NLC) based gel of celecoxib. *International Journal of Pharmaceutics, 346*(1, 2), 124–132. doi: 10.1016/j.ijpharm.2007.05.060.

26. Chalikwar, S. S., et al., (2012). Formulation and evaluation of nimodipine-loaded solid lipid nanoparticles delivered via lymphatic transport system. *Colloids and Surfaces B: Biointerfaces, 97*, 109–116. Elsevier B.V. doi: 10.1016/j.colsurfb.2012.04.027.

27. Heurtault, B., et al., (2003). Physico-chemical stability of colloidal lipid particles. *Biomaterials*, 4283–4300. doi: 10.1016/S0142-9612(03)00331-4.

28. Kaur, I. P., et al., (2008b). Potential of solid lipid nanoparticles in brain targeting. *Journal of Controlled Release*, 97–109. doi: 10.1016/j.jconrel.2007.12.018.

29. Almeida, A. J., & Souto, E., (2007). Solid lipid nanoparticles as a drug delivery system for peptides and proteins. *Advanced Drug Delivery Reviews*, 478–490. doi: 10.1016/j.addr.2007.04.007.

30. Blasi, P., et al., (2007). Solid lipid nanoparticles for targeted brain drug delivery. *Advanced Drug Delivery Reviews*, 454–477. doi: 10.1016/j.addr.2007.04.011.

31. Feng, L., & Mumper, R. J., (2013). A critical review of lipid-based nanoparticles for taxane delivery. *Cancer Letters*, 157–175. Elsevier Ireland Ltd. doi: 10.1016/j.canlet.2012.07.006.

32. Lin, C. H., et al., (2017). Recent advances in oral delivery of drugs and bioactive natural products using solid lipid nanoparticles as the carriers. *Journal of Food and Drug Analysis, 25*(2), 219–234. Elsevier Ltd. doi: 10.1016/j.jfda.2017.02.001.

33. Shah, R., Eldridge, D., & Palombo, E. H. I., (2015). Composition and Structure. In: *Lipid Nanoparticles: Production, Characterization and Stability.* doi: 10.1007/978-3-319-10711-0.

34. Morsy, S., (2014). Role of surfactants in nanotechnology and their applications. *Int. J. Curr. Microbiol. App. Sci., 3*(5), 237–260. Available at: http://www.ijcmas.com/vol-3–5/Salwa M.I. Morsy.pdf.

35. Desai, P. P., Date, A. A., & Patravale, V. B., (2012). Overcoming poor oral bioavailability using nanoparticle formulations-opportunities and limitations. *Drug Discovery Today: Technologies, 9*(2), e87–e95. Elsevier Ltd. doi: 10.1016/j.ddtec.2011.12.001.

36. Abdelwahed, W., et al., (2006). Freeze-drying of nanoparticles: formulation, process and storage considerations. *Advanced Drug Delivery Reviews, 58*(15), 1688–1713. doi: 10.1016/j.addr.2006.09.017.

37. Shah, R., et al., (2015). *Lipid Nanoparticles: Production, Characterization and Stability* (pp. 11–23). doi: 10.1007/978-3-319-10711-0.

38. Li, X. W., et al., (2008). Effect of poly(ethylene glycol) stearate on the phase behavior of monocaprate/tween80/water system and characterization of poly(ethylene glycol) stearate-modified solid lipid nanoparticles. *Colloids and Surfaces A: Physicochemical and Engineering Aspects, 317*(1–3), 352–359. doi: 10.1016/j.colsurfa.2007.11.011.

39. Kulkarni, A. D., et al., (2017). N,N,N-Trimethyl chitosan: An advanced polymer with myriad of opportunities in nanomedicine. *Carbohydrate Polymers, 157*, 875–902. Elsevier Ltd. doi: 10.1016/j.carbpol.2016.10.041.

40. Müller, R. H., (2007). Lipid nanoparticles: Recent advances. *Advanced Drug Delivery Reviews*, 375–376. doi: 10.1016/j.addr.2007.05.002.

41. Shahgaldian, P., et al., (2003). Para-acyl-calixarene based solid lipid nanoparticles (SLNs): A detailed study of preparation and stability parameters. *International Journal of Pharmaceutics, 253*(1, 2), 23–38. doi: 10.1016/S0378-5173(02)00639-7.

42. Pardeshi, C., et al., (2012). Solid lipid based nanocarriers: An overview/nanonosači na bazi čvrstih lipida: Pregled. *Acta Pharmaceutica, 62*(4). doi: 10.2478/v10007-012-0040-z.

43. Elgart, A., et al., (2012). Lipospheres and pro-nano lipospheres for delivery of poorly water-soluble compounds. In: *Chemistry and Physics of Lipids* (pp. 438–453). Elsevier Ireland Ltd. doi: 10.1016/j.chemphyslip.2012.01.007.

44. Mishra, B., Patel, B. B., & Tiwari, S., (2010). Colloidal nanocarriers: A review on formulation technology, types and applications toward targeted drug delivery. *Nanomedicine: Nanotechnology, Biology, and Medicine*, 9–24. Elsevier Inc. doi: 10.1016/j.nano.2009.04.008.

45. Ganesan, P., & Narayanasamy, D., (2017). Lipid nanoparticles: Different preparation techniques, characterization, hurdles, and strategies for the production of solid lipid nanoparticles and nanostructured lipid carriers for oral drug delivery. *Sustainable Chemistry and Pharmacy, 6*, 37–56. Elsevier. doi: 10.1016/j.scp.2017.07.002.

46. Kumar, S., & Randhawa, J. K., (2013). High melting lipid based approach for drug delivery: Solid lipid nanoparticles. *Materials Science and Engineering C.*, 1842–1852. Elsevier B.V. doi: 10.1016/j.msec.2013.01.037.

47. Wissing, S. A., Kayser, O., & Müller, R. H., (2004). Solid lipid nanoparticles for parenteral drug delivery. *Advanced Drug Delivery Reviews*, 1257–1272. doi: 10.1016/j.addr.2003.12.002.

48. Naseri, N., Valizadeh, H., & Zakeri-Milani, P., (2015). Solid lipid nanoparticles and nanostructured lipid carriers: Structure preparation and application. *Advanced Pharmaceutical Bulletin, 5*(3), 305–313. doi: 10.15171/apb.2015.043.

49. Shah, R. M., et al., (2014). Physicochemical characterization of solid lipid nanoparticles (SLNs) prepared by a novel microemulsion technique. *Journal of Colloid and Interface Science, 428*, 286–294. Elsevier Inc. doi: 10.1016/j.jcis.2014.04.057.

50. Jaiswal, P., Gidwani, B., & Vyas, A., (2016). Nanostructured lipid carriers and their current application in targeted drug delivery. *Artificial Cells, Nanomedicine, and Biotechnology, 44*(1), 27–40. doi: 10.3109/21691401.2014.909822.

51. Hari, B. N. V., et al., (2016). Engineered nanoparticles of efavirenz using methacrylate copolymer (Eudragit-E100) and its biological effects *in-vivo*. *Materials Science and Engineering C, 67*, 522–532. Elsevier B.V. doi: 10.1016/j.msec.2016.05.064.

52. Hadinoto, K., Sundaresan, A., & Cheow, W. S., (2013). Lipid-polymer hybrid nanoparticles as a new generation therapeutic delivery platform: A review. *European Journal of Pharmaceutics and Biopharmaceutics, 85*(3 PART A), 427–443. Elsevier B.V. doi: 10.1016/j.ejpb.2013.07.002.

53. Das, S., & Chaudhury, A., (2011). Recent advances in lipid nanoparticle formulations with solid matrix for oral drug delivery. *AAPS PharmSciTech, 12*(1), 62–76. doi: 10.1208/s12249-010-9563-0.

54. Jain, A. K., et al., (2014). Adapalene loaded solid lipid nanoparticles gel: An effective approach for acne treatment. *Colloids and Surfaces B: Biointerfaces, 121*, 222–229. Elsevier B.V. doi: 10.1016/j.colsurfb.2014.05.041.

55. Kaur, S., et al., (2015). Nanostructured lipid carrier (NLC): The new generation of lipid nanoparticles. *Asian Pac. J. Health Sci., 2*(22), 76–93.

56. Schubert, M. A., & Müller-Goymann, C. C. (2003). Solvent injection as a new approach for manufacturing lipid nanoparticles - evaluation of the method and process parameters. *European Journal of Pharmaceutics and Biopharmaceutics, 55*, 125–131. doi: 10.1016/ S0.

57. Cortesi, R., et al., (2002). Production of lipospheres as carriers for bioactive compounds. *Biomaterials, 23*(11), 2283–2294. doi: 10.1016/S0142-9612(01)00362-3.

58. Severino, P., et al., (2014). Solid lipid nanoparticles for hydrophilic biotech drugs: Optimization and cell viability studies (Caco-2 & HEPG-2 cell lines). *European Journal of Medicinal Chemistry, 81*, 28–34. Elsevier Masson SAS. doi: 10.1016/j.ejmech. 2014.04.084.

59. Shi, L. L., et al., (2015). Optimization of process variables of zanamivir-loaded solid lipid nanoparticles and the prediction of their cellular transport in Caco-2 cell model. *International Journal of Pharmaceutics, 478*(1), 60–69. Elsevier B.V. doi: 10.1016/j. ijpharm.2014.11.017.

60. Li, Q., et al., (2017). A review of the structure, preparation, and application of NLCs, PNPs, and PLNs. *Nanomaterials, 7*(6), 122. doi: 10.3390/nano7060122.

61. Üner, M., & Yener, G., (2007). Importance of solid lipid nanoparticles (SLN) in various administration routes and future perspective. *International Journal of Nanomedicine, 2*(3), 289–300.

62. Hu, F. Q., et al., (2002). Preparation of solid lipid nanoparticles with clobetasol propionate by a novel solvent diffusion method in aqueous system and physicochemical characterization. *International Journal of Pharmaceutics, 239*(1,2), 121–128. doi: 10.1016/ S0378-5173(02)00081-9.

63. Gaumet, M., et al., (2008). Nanoparticles for drug delivery: The need for precision in reporting particle size parameters. *European Journal of Pharmaceutics and Biopharmaceutics, 69*(1), 1–9. doi: 10.1016/j.ejpb.2007.08.001.
64. Jorgensen, L., Martins, S., & Van De, W. M., (2009). Analysis of protein physical stability in lipid based delivery systems—the challenges of lipid drug delivery systems. *Journal of Biomedical Nanotechnology, 5*(4), 401–408.
65. Otsuka, H., Nagasaki, Y., & Kataoka, K., (2012). PEGylated nanoparticles for biological and pharmaceutical applications. *Advanced Drug Delivery Reviews, 64*, 246–255. doi: 10.1016/j.addr.2012.09.022.
66. Zur, M. A., Schwarz, C., & Mehnert, W., (1998). Solid lipid nanoparticles (SLN) for controlled drug delivery-drug release and release mechanism. *European Journal of Pharmaceutics and Biopharmaceutics, 45*(2), 149–155. doi: 10.1016/S0939-6411(97) 00150-1.
67. Bunjes, H., Koch, M. H., & Westesen, K., (2003). Influence of emulsifiers on the crystallization of solid lipid nanoparticles. *Journal of Pharmaceutical Sciences, 92*(7), 1509–1520.
68. Heike, B., Michel, H. J. K., & Kirsten, W., (2002). Effects of surfactants on the crystallization and polymorphism of lipid nanoparticles. *Progr. Colloid Polym. Sci., 121*, 7–10.
69. Kathe, N., Henriksen, B., & Chauhan, H., (2014). Physicochemical characterization techniques for solid lipid nanoparticles: Principles and limitations. *Drug Development and Industrial Pharmacy, 40*(12), 1565–1575. doi: 10.3109/03639045.2014.909840.
70. Brar, S. K., & Verma, M., (2011). Measurement of nanoparticles by light-scattering techniques. *TrAC - Trends in Analytical Chemistry, 30*(1), 4–17. Elsevier Ltd. doi: 10.1016/ j.trac.2010.08.008.
71. Hassan, P. A., Rana, S., & Verma, G., (2015). Making sense of Brownian motion: Colloid characterization by dynamic light scattering. *Langmuir, 31*(1), 3–12. doi: 10.1021/ la501789z.
72. Filipe, V., Hawe, A., & Jiskoot, W., (2010). Critical evaluation of nanoparticle tracking analysis (NTA) by nano sight for the measurement of nanoparticles and protein aggregates. *Pharmaceutical Research, 27*(5), 796–810. doi: 10.1007/s11095-010-0073-2.
73. Bunjes, H., Koch, M. H. J., & Westesen, K., (2000). Effect of particle size on colloidal solid triglycerides. *Langmuir, 16*(12), 5234–5241. doi: 10.1021/la990856l.
74. Saupe, A., Wissing, S. A., Lenk, A., Schmidt, C., & Müller, R. H., (2005). Solid lipid nanoparticles (SLN) and nanostructured lipid carriers (NLC)-structural investigations on two different carrier systems. *Bio-Medical Materials and Engineering, 15*(5), 393–402.
75. Helgason, T., et al., (2009). Effect of surfactant surface coverage on formation of solid lipid nanoparticles (SLN). *Journal of Colloid and Interface Science, 334*(1), 75–81. Elsevier Inc. doi: 10.1016/j.jcis.2009.03.012.
76. Saupe, A., Gordon, K. C., & Rades, T., (2006). Structural investigations on nanoemulsions, solid lipid nanoparticles and nanostructured lipid carriers by cryo-field emission scanning electron microscopy and Raman spectroscopy. *International Journal of Pharmaceutics, 314*(1), 56–62. doi: 10.1016/j.ijpharm.2006.01.022.
77. Goldstein, J., (1920). Scanning electron microscopy and x-ray microanalysis. *Notes and Queries, s12–VII*(121), 110. doi: 10.1093/nq/s12-VII.121.110-j.
78. Dubes, A., et al., (2003). Scanning electron microscopy and atomic force microscopy imaging of solid lipid nanoparticles derived from amphiphilic cyclodextrins. *European*

Journal of Pharmaceutics and Biopharmaceutics, 55(3), 279–282. doi: 10.1016/S0939-6411(03)00020-1.

79. Dolatabadi, J. E. N., Hamishehkar, H., & Valizadeh, H., (2015). Development of dry powder inhaler formulation loaded with alendronate solid lipid nanoparticles: Solid-state characterization and aerosol dispersion performance. *Drug Development and Industrial Pharmacy, 41*(9), 1431–1437. doi: 10.3109/03639045.2014.956111.

80. Singh, S., Dobhal, A. K., Jain, A., Pandit, J. K., & Chakraborty, S., (2010). Formulation and evaluation of solid lipid nanoparticles of a water-soluble drug: Zidovudine. *Chemical and Pharmaceutical Bulletin, 58*(5), 650–655.

81. Cowley, J. M., (1969). Image contrast in a transmission scanning electron microscope. *Applied Physics Letters, 15*(2), 58–59. doi: 10.1063/1.1652901.

82. Bozzola, J. J., & Russell, L. D., (1999). *Electron Microscopy: Principles and Techniques for Biologists.* Jones & Bartlett Learning.

83. Dingler, A., et al., (1999). Solid lipid nanoparticles (SLN(TM)/lipopearls(TM))-a pharmaceutical and cosmetic carrier for the application of vitamin E in dermal products. *Journal of Microencapsulation, 16*(6), 751–767. doi: 10.1080/026520499288690.

84. Begat, P., et al., (2004). The cohesive-adhesive balances in dry powder inhaler formulations I: Direct quantification by atomic force microscopy. *Pharmaceutical Research, 21*(9), 1591–1597. doi: 10.1023/B:PHAM.0000041453.24419.8a.

85. Giessibl, F. J., (2003). Advances in atomic force microscopy. *RevModPhys, 75*, 949. doi: 10.1103/RevModPhys.75.949.

86. Boussu, K., et al., (2005). Roughness and hydrophobicity studies of nanofiltration membranes using different modes of AFM. *Journal of Colloid and Interface Science, 286*(2), 632–638. doi: 10.1016/j.jcis.2005.01.095.

87. Lippacher, A., Müller, R. H., & Mäder, K., (2001). Preparation of semisolid drug carriers for topical application based on solid lipid nanoparticles. *International Journal of Pharmaceutics, 214*(1), 9–12. doi: 10.1016/S0378-5173(00)00623-2.

88. Souto, E. B., et al., (2004). Evaluation of the physical stability of SLN and NLC before and after incorporation into hydrogel formulations. *European Journal of Pharmaceutics and Biopharmaceutics, 58*(1), 83–90. doi: 10.1016/j.ejpb.2004.02.015.

89. Mukherjee, S., Ray, S., & Thakur, R. S., (2009). Solid lipid nanoparticles: A modern formulation approach in drug delivery system. *Indian Journal of Pharmaceutical Sciences, 71*(4), 349.

90. Morris, K. R., et al., (2001). Theoretical approaches to physical transformations of active pharmaceutical ingredients during manufacturing processes. *Advanced Drug Delivery Reviews, 48*(1), 91–114. doi: 10.1016/S0169-409X(01)00100-4.

91. Geoff, G. Z. Z., Devalina, L., Eric, A. S., & Qiu, Y. (2004). Solid-phase transformation considerations during process development and manufacture of solid oral dosage forms: A review. *Advanced Drug Delivery Reviews, 56*, 371–390. doi: 10.1016/j.addr.2003.10.009.

92. Heike, B., Kirsten, W., & Koch, M. H. (1996). Crystallization-tendency-and-polymorphic-transitions-in-triglyceride-nanoparticles. *International Journal of Pharmaceutics, 129*, 159–173.

93. Westesen, K., Bunjes, H., & Koch, M. H. J., (1997). Physicochemical characterization of lipid nanoparticles and evaluation of their drug loading capacity and sustained release potential. *Journal of Controlled Release, 48*(2, 3), 223–236. doi: 10.1016/S0168-3659(97)00046-1.

94. Ruktanonchai, U., et al., (2008). The effect of cetyl palmitate crystallinity on physical properties of gamma-oryzanol encapsulated in solid lipid nanoparticles. *Nanotechnology, 19*(9). doi: 10.1088/0957-4484/19/9/095701.

95. Sanjula, B., et al., (2009). Effect of poloxamer 188 on lymphatic uptake of carvedilol-loaded solid lipid nanoparticles for bioavailability enhancement. *Journal of Drug Targeting, 17*(3), 249–256. doi: 10.1080/10611860902718672.

96. Manoj, K. R., & Achint, J. S. S., (2011). Studies on binary lipid matrix-based solid lipid nanoparticles of repaglinide: *In vitro* and *in vivo* evaluation. *Journal of Pharmaceutical Sciences, 100*(6), 2366–2377. doi: 10.1002/jps.

97. Chaturvedi, K., et al., (2018). Influence of processing methods on physico-mechanical properties of ibuprofen/HPC-SSL formulation. *Pharmaceutical Development and Technology, 23*(10), 1108–1116. Taylor & Francis. doi: 10.1080/10837450.2018.1425430.

98. Goldstein, J. I., Newbury, D. E., Michael, J. R., Ritchie, N. W., Scott, J. H. J., & Joy, D. C., (2017). *Scanning Electron Microscopy and X-Ray Microanalysis.* Springer.

99. Yamamoto, K., Tsutsumi, S., & Ikeda, Y., (2012). Establishment of cocrystal cocktail grinding method for rational screening of pharmaceutical cocrystals. *International Journal of Pharmaceutics, 437*(1, 2), 162–171. Elsevier B.V. doi: 10.1016/j.ijpharm. 2012.07.038.

100. Jin, Y., & Wunderlich, B., (1993). Single-run heat capacity measurement by DSC: Principle, experimental and data analysis. *Thermochimica Acta, 226*(C), 155–161. doi: 10.1016/0040-6031(93)80216-W.

101. Ozawa, T., & Kanari, K., (1995). Linearity and non-linearity in DSC: A critique on modulated DSC. *Thermochimica Acta, 253*(C), 183–188. doi: 10.1016/0040-6031(94)02088-6.

102. Siekmann, B., & Westesen, K., (1994). Thermoanalysis of the recrystallization process of melt-homogenized glyceride nanoparticles. *Colloids and Surfaces B: Biointerfaces, 3*(3), 159–175. doi: 10.1016/0927-7765(94)80063-4.

103. Kovačević, A. B., et al., (2014). Solid lipid nanoparticles (SLN) stabilized with poly-hydroxy surfactants: Preparation, characterization and physical stability investigation. *Colloids and Surfaces A: Physicochemical and Engineering Aspects, 444*, 15–25. doi: 10.1016/j.colsurfa.2013.12.023.

104. Jackman, L. M., & Sternhell, S., (2013). *Application of Nuclear Magnetic Resonance Spectroscopy in Organic Chemistry: International Series in Organic Chemistry.* Elsevier.

105. Jenning, V., Mäder, K., & Gohla, S. H., (2000). Solid lipid nanoparticles (SLN) based on binary mixtures of liquid and solid lipids: A (1)H-NMR study. *International Journal of Pharmaceutics, 205*, 15–21. doi: 10.1016/S0378-5173(00)00462-2.

106. Jenning, V., Thünemann, A. F., & Gohla, S. H., (2000). Characterization of a novel solid lipid nanoparticle carrier system based on binary mixtures of liquid and solid lipids. *International Journal of Pharmaceutics, 199*(2), 167–177.

107. Jores, K., et al., (2004). Investigations on the structure of solid lipid nanoparticles (SLN) and oil-loaded solid lipid nanoparticles by photon correlation spectroscopy, field-flow fractionation and transmission electron microscopy. *Journal of Controlled Release, 95*(2), 217–227. doi: 10.1016/j.jconrel.2003.11.012.

108. Chopin, T., & Whalen, E., (1993). A new and rapid method for carrageenan identification by FT IR diffuse reflectance spectroscopy directly on dried, ground algal material. *Carbohydrate Research, 246*(1), 51–59. doi: 10.1016/0008-6215(93)84023-Y.

109. Stuart, B., (2005). Infrared spectroscopy. *Kirk-Othmer Encyclopedia of Chemical Technology.*

110. Dugar, R. P., Gajera, B. Y., & Dave, R. H., (2016). Fusion method for solubility and dissolution rate enhancement of ibuprofen using block copolymer poloxamer 407. *AAPS PharmSciTech, 17*(6), 1428–1440. doi: 10.1208/s12249-016-0482-6.

111. Gajera, B. Y., Dugar, R. P., & Dave, R. H., (2016). Formulation development and optimization of ibuprofen poloxamer melt granules using hydrophilic excipients. *British Journal of Pharmaceutical Research, 13*(6), 1–19. doi: 10.9734/BJPR/2016/29048.

112. Bunaciu, A. A., Aboul-Enein, H. Y., & Fleschin, S., (2010). Application of Fourier transform infrared spectrophotometry in pharmaceutical drugs analysis. *Applied Spectroscopy Reviews, 45*(3), 206–219.

113. Attama, A. A., et al., (2007). Solid lipid nanodispersions containing mixed lipid core and a polar heterolipid: Characterization. *European Journal of Pharmaceutics and Biopharmaceutics, 67*(1), 48–57. doi: 10.1016/j.ejpb.2006.12.004.

114. Fang, R. H., et al., (2010). Quick synthesis of lipid-polymer hybrid nanoparticles with low polydispersity using a single-step sonication method. *Langmuir, 26*(22), 16958–16962. doi: 10.1021/la103576a.

115. Gidwani, B., et al., (2016). Factorial design and a practical approach for gastro-retentive drug delivery system. *Research Journal of Pharmacy and Technology, 9*(6). doi: 10.5958/0974-360X.2016.00122.0.

116. Patil-Gadhe, A., & Pokharkar, V., (2014). Montelukast-loaded nanostructured lipid carriers: Part I oral bioavailability improvement. *European Journal of Pharmaceutics and Biopharmaceutics, 88*(1), 160–168. Elsevier B.V. doi: 10.1016/j.ejpb.2014.05.019.

117. Watt, I. M. (1997). The Principles and Practice of Electron Microscopy. Cambridge University Press.

118. Reed, S. J. B., (2005). *Electron Microprobe Analysis and Scanning Electron Microscopy in Geology*. Cambridge University Press.

119. Vasconcelos, T., et al., (2016). Amorphous solid dispersions: Rational selection of a manufacturing process. *Advanced Drug Delivery Reviews*, 85–101. doi: 10.1016/j.addr.2016.01.012.

120. Yasir, M., et al., (2010). Biopharmaceutical classification system: An account. *International Journal of PharmTech Research, 2*(3), 1681–1690.

121. Güney, G., Kutlu, H. M., & Genç, L. (2014). Preparation and characterization of ascorbic acid loaded solid lipid nanoparticles and investigation of their apoptotic effects. *Colloids and Surfaces B: Biointerfaces, 121*, 270–280.

CHAPTER 4

Fabrication Methods of Therapeutic Nanoparticles: Potential Opportunities and Challenges in Drug Delivery and Nutraceutical Delivery

SWAPNIL G. PATIL,[1] SURENDRA G. GATTANI,[1] KIRAN PATIL,[2] SHASHIKANT BAGADE,[2] and DEBARSHI KAR MAHAPATRA[3]

[1]School of Pharmacy, S.R.T.M. University, Vishnupuri, Nanded–431606, Maharashtra, India

[2]NMIMS, School of Pharmacy and Technology Management, Shirpur, Maharashtra, India

[3]Department of Pharmaceutical Chemistry, Dadasaheb Balpande College of Pharmacy, Nagpur–440037, Maharashtra, India

ABSTRACT

Recently, nanotechnologies and nanomaterials fascinate remarkable attention in recent researches. New physical properties and novel technologies, both in device manufacture and sample preparation evoke on account of the development of nanoscience. Nanotechnology has created a potential impression in numerous fields like medicine, including immunology, cardiology, endocrinology, ophthalmology, oncology, pulmonology, etc. Moreover, it is extremely utilized in specified areas like brain targeting, tumor targeting, and gene delivery. Nanotechnology has provided various significant systems, devices, and materials for better pharmaceutical applications. Nano-pharmaceuticals reveal the huge prospective in drug delivery as a carrier for three-dimensional and the progressive provision of bioactive and diagnostics. There has been a significant research interest in the drug delivery area using numerous particulate delivery systems as carriers for small and large molecules. Alteration and improvement of pharmacokinetic and pharmacodynamics properties of several types of drug molecules are emerged by particulate systems like nanoparticles. Polymeric nanoparticles have been broadly studied as particulate carriers in the pharmaceutical and medical fields because they show promising effects of drug delivery system resulting from their controlled and sustained release properties, sub-cellular size, biocompatibility with tissue and cells. This review summarizes various conventional and recent techniques of nano-fabrication along with specific opportunities and challenges in the fabrication of nanoparticles: (i) conventional techniques comprising three different methods such as the dispersion of preformed polymers, the polymerization of monomers and Ionic gelation method of hydrophilic polymers. (ii) Advance techniques comprising of spray drying, sol-gel, high pressure homogenization (HPH), desolvation of macromolecules and dialysis.

4.1 INTRODUCTION

Nanotechnology is a branch of science which deals with planning and manufacturing on enormous expansion of Nanostructural materials [1]. During the past few years, nanotechnology, and Nanoscience studies have rapidly developed in a broad range of product domains [3]. The advancement in nanotechnology is being predicted at various levels, such as materials, systems, and devices [2]. The nanomaterial parade distinctive features because of their variations in size-dependent physicochemical properties [1–3]. It has also demonstrated that nanoparticles procure a great prospective as a drug carrier. Nanotechnology should not be observed as one method that exclusively affects specific targeted areas. It does not merely mean the exact tiny structures and products. The features characterized by nanoscale structures are assimilated into large surface as well as bulk material [3, 4]. Nanoencapsulation of medicinal drugs increases drug efficacy, specificity, tolerability, and therapeutic index of corresponding drugs. Pharmaceutical nanoparticles are defined as solid, subnanosized colloidal microscopic structures made up of synthetic and semisynthetic polymer having a size range between 10 and 1,000 nm [4, 5], as shown in Figure 4.1. There are various forms of nanoparticles such as polymeric and metal nanoparticles, liposomes, micelles, dendrimers, quantum dots, microcapsules, lipoproteins cells, cell ghost and many different nanoassemblies [6, 7]. Nanoparticles have unique physicochemical properties which have shown promising drug delivery system to the desired sites in the body [7]. It enhances the drug release, improves the bioavailability and solubility, and also minimizes the toxicity as well as drug degradation [6–8]. Due to expanded contact region for van der Waals attraction, nanoparticles show strong adhesion [9]. It is necessary to comprehend the pharmaceutically relevant properties of nanoparticles so as to achieve the better development of the novel drug delivery systems. The major challenge for the development of nanoparticles as a drug delivery system is the control of particle size, surface properties and time release of active moiety get the site-specific action at the desired proportion and dose. Polymeric nanoparticle offers some distinct advantages over other nanocarriers, like they increase the drugs/protein stability and shows useful controlled release properties [10–12]. Various prominent features and applications of the nanosystem are given in Table 4.1.

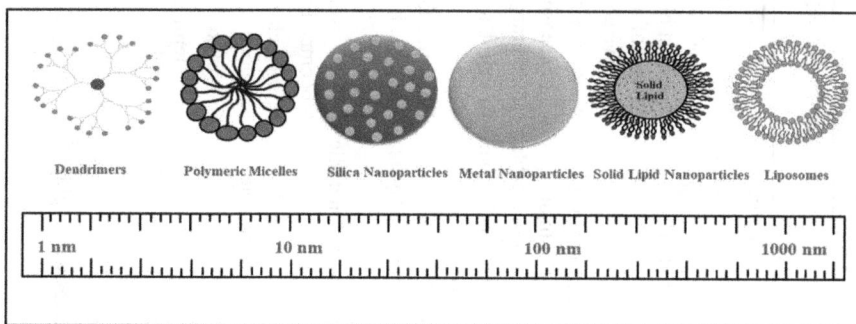

FIGURE 4.1 Nanoscale.

4.1.1 ADVANTAGES OF NANOPARTICLES AS DRUG DELIVERY SYSTEM [3, 10, 13–16]

- Nanoparticles having the properties like particle size and surface characteristics are easily manipulated for active and passive drug targeting the following parenteral administration.
- The surface of nanoparticles can be adapted to alter the bio-distribution of drugs to achieve maximum therapeutic efficacy with minimal adverse effects.
- Release rate and degradation characteristics of the particles can be readily modulated by varying matrix components.
- Nanoparticles show higher loading capacity of drug without any chemical reaction and thus increase the stability of the drug.
- Site-specific targeting can be achieved with ligands on the surface of Particles or with magnetic guidance.

TABLE 4.1 Types, Characterization, and Potential Application of Nanosystem [6, 7, 10]

Types of Nanosystem	Size	Characterization	Potential Application
Polymeric nanoparticles	10–1,000 nm	Solid, biodegradable encapsulated nanoparticle composed of synthetic or natural polymer.	Excellent carrier for controlled and sustained delivery of drugs. Stealth and surface modified can be used for active and passive delivery of bioactives.
Solid lipid nanoparticles	10–1,000 nm	Submicron colloid carriers, composed of physiological lipid.	Excellent biocompatibility, control release and high content of drug, enhanced bioavailability of entrapped bioactive compounds.
Inorganic nanoparticles	<100 nm	Mainly metallic nanoparticle, gold, and silver colloids, very small in size, resulting in high surface area available for functionalization, stable.	Applied in drug and gene delivery, tissue engineering, highly sensitive diagnostic assay, thermal ablation, radiotherapy enhancement.
Carbon nanoparticles	<100 nm	Hollow cage spherical nature pure carbon, known as fullerene.	Antiviral, antibacterial, photodynamic, and anti-tumor effect.
Carbon nanotubes	0.5–3 diameter and 20–1,000 length	Third allotropic crystalline form of carbon sheets either single (SWCNTs) or multiple layers (MWCNTs).	DNA mutation detection, disease protein biomarker detection, high tensile strength useful in tissue engineering, as a carrier for gene and peptic delivery.
Nanoshell	<50 nm	Dielectric code covered by a thin layer of metallic shell.	Broad wavelength-tunable optical properties, biocompatibility, tumor specific imaging.
Nanowires		In nanowire the diameter is of in order of nanometer, but the length can be in micrometer	Special electronic properties. Useful in stem cell engineering, surgery, and diagnosis.
Nanocrystal	2–9.5 nm	Crystalline structure nanoparticle.	Improved formulation for poorly soluble drugs.
Quantum dots (QD)	2–9.5 nm	Smallest in this series that contain a tiny droplet of free electrons, bright fluorescence, narrow emission, broad UV excitation and high photostability	Long term multiple color imaging of liver cell; DNA hybridization, immunoassay; receptor-mediated endocytosis; tumor and lymph node visualization
Dendrimers	<10 nm	Mono disperses globular molecules with highly branched	Used in photodynamic therapy, used for diagnostic application in X-ray or MRI, used for controlled release drug delivery, tissue engineering, transdermal drug delivery.

- Nanoparticles are biodegradable and it does not accumulate in the body and thus are free of risk.
- Effective drug accumulation at the specific targeted sites can be achieved by nanoparticles by penetrating them through capillaries.
- Oral, nasal, parenteral, intraocular routes are administered through nanoparticles.

4.1.2   LIMITATIONS OF NANOPARTICLES [10, 17–19]

- Aggregation of particles is observed because of the smaller size and large surface area of the particle and hence formulation of nanoparticles is difficult in liquid and dry forms.
- Limited drug loading capacity and very reactive in the cellular environment due to small size of the nanoparticles.
- Inflammatory reaction can be contributed by nanoparticles, due to the impairment of macrophages to phagocytes.
- Due to minute particles, problems can arise for an individual by inhaling those minute asbestos particles.
- Nanotechnology is costly, and manufacturing of nanocarriers can cost a lot of money. These are more challenging to manufacture, which makes the product made with nanotechnology most likely costlier.

4.2   PREPARATION OF NANOPARTICLES

Nanoparticles can be prepared by selecting a suitable method which is based on the various characteristics of biodegradable polymers and the active drug which is to be loaded [3, 4, 20]. Biodegradable polymers provide biocompatible or nontoxic by-products which are degradable *in vivo*, either enzymatically or non-enzymatically. Biodegradable polymers are absorbed as well as eliminated through normal physiological pathways [21]. Biodegradable polymers are categorized into three classes such as natural, synthetic, and semisynthetic. Various examples used as natural biodegradable polymers are gelatin, alginate, albumin, collagen, starch, dextran, chitosan (CHT), chitin, while synthetic biodegradable polymers are having examples like polylactic acid, poly(orthoester), polyhydroxybutyrate, plo.hydroxyvalerate, and polyanhydride [3, 5, 21–23]. CHT, alginate, and hyaluronic acids are naturally occurring biodegradable polymers which can be modified to produce semisynthetic biodegradable polymers. Thus, for the biodegradable delivery system, the polymers should essentially meet various parameters such as permeability, size of nanoparticles required, biodegradability, biocompatibility, drug release profile, toxicity, and tensile strength [22, 24].

The various techniques used for preparing nanoparticles are [7, 24, 25]:

   i.   Dispersion of preformed polymers;
   ii.   Polymerization of various monomers;
   iii.   Ionic gelation method of hydrophilic polymers.

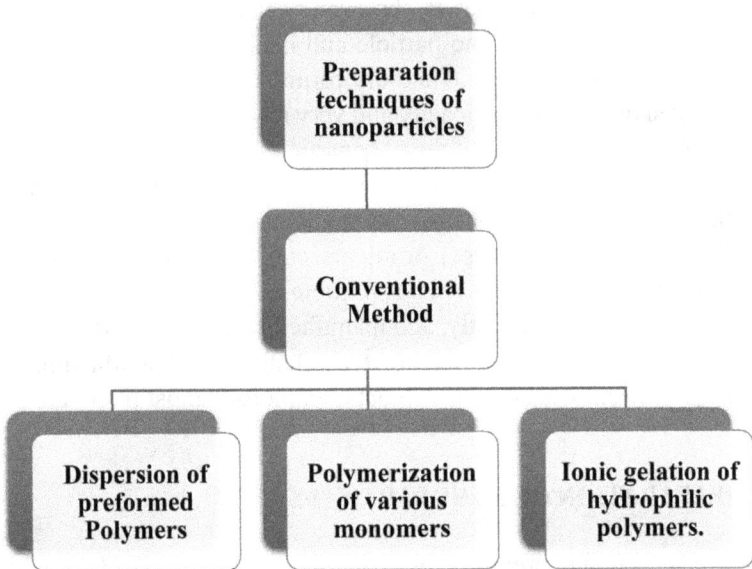

```
                    ┌─────────────────┐
                    │   Preparation   │
                    │  techniques of  │
                    │  nanoparticles  │
                    └─────────────────┘
                             │
                    ┌─────────────────┐
                    │  Conventional   │
                    │     Method      │
                    └─────────────────┘
                             │
        ┌────────────────────┼────────────────────┐
┌───────────────┐   ┌───────────────┐   ┌───────────────┐
│ Dispersion of │   │ Polymerization│   │Ionic gelation │
│   preformed   │   │  of various   │   │ of hydrophilic│
│   Polymers    │   │   monomers    │   │   polymers.   │
└───────────────┘   └───────────────┘   └───────────────┘
```

4.2.1   NANOPARTICLES PREPARED FROM DISPERSION OF PREFORMED POLYMERS

Various preformed polymers are used for the nanoparticle's fabrication, which can be formed either dispersing a polymer-drug phase into an external phase or by phase inversion technique, whereby the external phase is firstly mixed with the internal phase containing the drug and polymer [25]. Polymers with various categories are used for the nanoparticle fabrication which are as follows: poly(lactic acid) (PLA); poly(D, L-glycolide), PLG; poly (D,L-lactide-co-glycolide) (PLGA) and poly(cyanoacrylate) (PCA) [24–27]. This technique is used in many ways such as discussed below.

4.2.1.1 SOLVENT EVAPORATION METHOD

Solvent evaporation technique is the commonly used method for preparing biodegradable and non-degradable microspheres [7, 25, 28]. This method involves various polymers as well as the drug (hydrophilic or hydrophobic), which are dispersed in suitable solvents (methylene chloride, chloroform, ethyl acetate). The formation of o/w emulsion is achieved by further emulsifying the above solution within the external aqueous phase having surfactant like gelatin, polysorbate-80, polyvinyl alcohol, poloxamer-188 to form an oil-in-water (O/W) [25, 29] as shown in Figure 4.2. The stable form of O/W emulsion is evaporated or homogenized by increasing the pressure or the temperature under high shear by using suitable equipment for homogenization (e.g., microfluidizer, ultrasonication) [24, 25, 30, 31]. The size of particles can be adjusted by monitoring various parameters like stirring speed, viscosity of both the phase, i.e., organic and aqueous phase, various categories and quantities of the dispersing agent and temperature [32]. Various types of emulsion are used, oil/water emulsion exist in various choices as water can be used as nonsolvent; which simplifies the process and therefore process is improved economically, as it removes the requirement of recycling, the washing step is simplified and the accumulation of the particles are minimized [32, 33]. Modification can be achieved to alter this method by formulating the emulsion with partly mutual soluble solvents and eliminating the volatile organic solvent containing a precipitation by extraction [33, 34].

Nanoparticles can also be formed by phase inversion. In this method, an aqueous phase is dispersed into the drug containing polymer solution in order to form water in oil emulsion. Phase inversion occurs upon further addition of water. Various emulsifier combinations can be used. One popular method, which has been used to prepare commercial aqueous ethylcellulose dispersion (Surelease) for coating purposes, is based on the *in-situ* formation of an emulsifying agent. Fatty acids, such as oleic or stearic acid, are added to the polymer melt. The aqueous phase containing an alkaline agent is added to the organic polymer phase, resulting in the ionization of the fatty acids at the interface [25, 35].

4.2.1.2 DOUBLE EMULSION SOLVENT EVAPORATION METHOD/ SPONTANEOUS EMULSIFICATION

Recently, emulsion solvent evaporation technique has been further modified and a double emulsion of water/oil/water type has been proposed for the

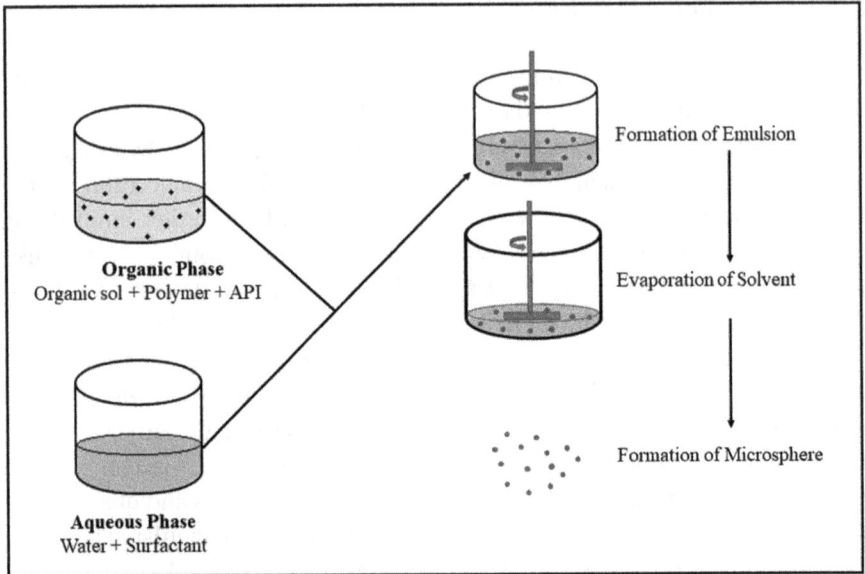

FIGURE 4.2   Solvent evaporation technique.

fabrication of nanoparticles [31, 36]. This technique includes drug in the aqueous phase which is further added to the organic phase containing polymer to form water in oil emulsion under high shear homogenization. Further, under continuous stirring, the above solution is dispersed within the secondary aqueous phase for the formation of the w/o/w emulsion [7, 36], as shown in Figure 4.3. Saturation of two liquids, i.e., polymer-solvent and water are achieved by mixing them together in equal volume. After the phase separation, the bottom layer consisting of solvent saturated water and the top layer containing water-saturated organic solvent is collected [33]. By evaporating the organic solvent nanoparticle are synthesized and then collected by repetitive washing of buffer by ultracentrifugation method and are lyophilized [36]. Quintanar-Guerrero et al. proposed that the Nanoparticles can be prepared from a pure diffusion mechanism [37]. Various types of solvents can be used benzyl alcohol, propylene carbonate [38] ethyl acetate [34, 39], isopropyl acetate, methyl acetate, methyl ethyl ketone [40], benzyl alcohol, butyl lactate [41] and isovaleric acid [42]. Different kinds of surfactant are pluronic F68, PVA (polyvinyl alcohol), and sodium taurodeoxycholate, which is used for the addition in the aqueous phase [38, 39, 42, 43] while soy lecithin surfactant is commonly used for the addition in the organic phase. Various types of surfactants can persuade different sizes of the particle [32, 44]. The total quantity of surfactant used for the nanoparticle preparation has an effect on the properties (drug release profile, zeta potential) [45] of the NPs. Particle agglomeration and high polydispersity can be achieved due to low concentration of surfactants [31, 46]. But using excessive surfactants reduces the drug loading capacity because of the strong interaction between the drugs and surfactants. Hence, surfactant used with suitable concentration leads to successful fabrication of nanoparticles. Alternative methods such as the probe sonicator can be used to achieve higher energy in the formed emulsion to form mono-dispersed emulsion [31, 47]. Various parameters such as mode, time, and power of sonicator are important for the preparation of emulsions [31].

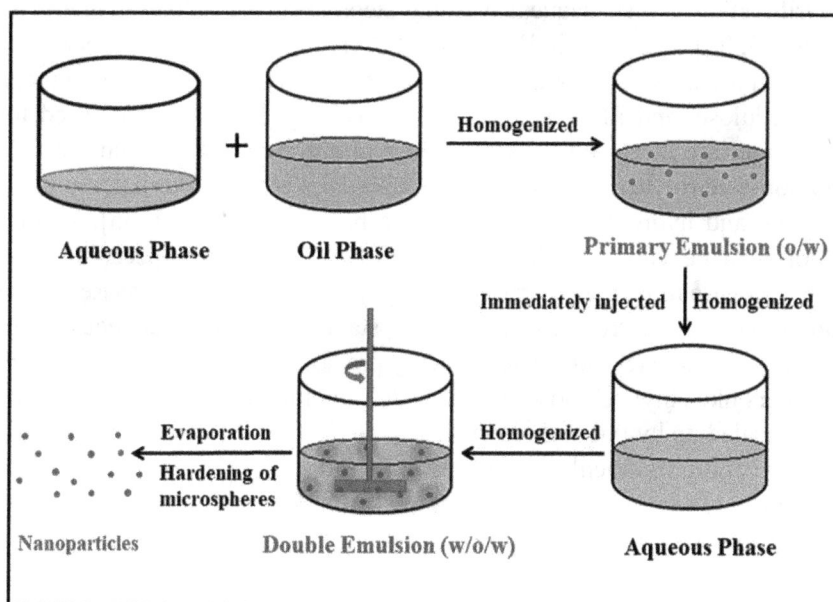

FIGURE 4.3 Double emulsion solvent evaporation technique.

4.2.1.3 *SALTING OUT METHOD*

The modification to the solvent evaporation technique is the "salting-out" procedure [25, 31, 48, 49]. The salting-out process is the most frequently adopted processes used to prepare nanoparticles [25, 49, 50]. The formulated nanoparticles can be achieved by the addition of an aqueous phase containing [36] an electrolyte or non-electrolyte to a dispersion of the organic solvent consisting of polymer as well as drug under continuous stirring to form oil in water emulsion [25]. Poly(vinyl alcohol) has been added to the aqueous phase to act as viscosity-enhancing and emulsifying agent [25]. The saturation of the aqueous phase decreases the acetone miscibility [31, 36] and water by a salting-out process [7, 33, 51] and the oil in water emulsion is achieved. After the formation of an internal organic phase droplet, water is added to allow proper distribution of the organic solvent into the external phase and precipitation of the polymer results in the fabrication of the nanoparticle. The solubility/miscibility of acetone with external phase are thereby gradually increased up to complete miscibility by diluting the initially saturated aqueous phase with water. The salt or non-electrolyte can be removed by centrifugation and subsequent washing steps from the polymeric nanoparticles [25, 31], as shown in Figure 4.4. For the fabrication of nanoparticles, various polymers such as acetate phthalate, methacrylic acid copolymers, ethylcellulose, and PLA are used [7, 25, 31, 52]. Various agents used for salting out are electrolytes like magnesium chloride and calcium chloride and non-electrolytes like sucrose and colloidal stabilizer like polyvinylpyrrolidone and hydroxyethylcellulose have been used [31, 49, 55]. Various factors can be varied in this technique, such as stirring speed, internal/external phase ratio, concentration of polymer used for organic phase, nature and amount of electrolyte and nature of stabilizer used for aqueous phase [7]. High proficiency can be achieved by preparing nanospheres of different polymers like ethyl cellulose and PLA, Poly(methacrylic) acid, and it can be easily scaled up by this technique [7, 25, 53–55].

Prevention from chlorinated solvents and commonly used surfactant with the conventional solvent evaporation techniques are the benefits of the salting-out technique [7, 25].

4.2.1.4 SOLVENT DISPLACEMENT/NANOPRECIPITATION

Solvent evaporation technique has various difficulties in the fabrication of nanoparticles; hence a new procedure for nanoparticles preparation by co-precipitation technique was established [56].

This methodology relies on the interfacial deposition of a polymer following removal of a semi-polar solvent miscible with water from a lipophilic solution [57, 58]. The principle of this method for the preparation of nanoparticles is called as Marangoni effect [31, 59]. The solvent displacement method comprises of a drug and a polymer in an organic phase which is dispersed entirely in the external aqueous phase. The above solution immediately dispersed in an external phase and due to which complete miscibility of each phase and instantaneous precipitation of the polymer is obtained. Thus, neither separation nor extraction of the solvent is essential for the polymer precipitation. After the nanoparticle fabrication, the remaining solvent gets eliminated and the free-flowing nanoparticles will be achieved under reduced pressure. This method is particularly useful for the drugs that are slightly soluble in water. If the drug is highly hydrophilic, it diffuses out into the external aqueous phase as nanocrystals, which further grow during storage. In the case of hydrophilic polymer, polymer in an aqueous phase is emulsified in the oil phase. The precipitation of polymer proceeds in addition of acetone [33, 36] as in Figure 4.5.

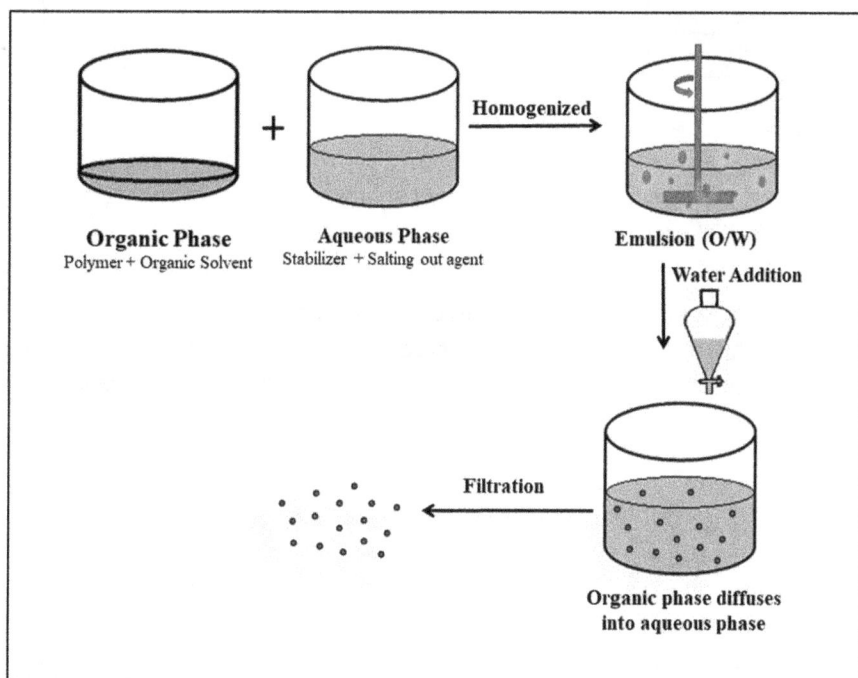

FIGURE 4.4 Salting out technique.

Various types of polymers such as peptides and non-polymer material, including amphiphilic cyclodextrins (CD) and drugs can be used to fabricate nanoparticles by this technique [60–64]. Material to be nanoprecipitated depends on the various solubility properties and hence instead of water it is being substituted by ethanol, methanol, or propanol [65]. In broad, nanoparticles can be fabricated by encapsulating the active ingredient to aqueous polymer solution by adding one phase to another by continuous stirring [33, 66–68].

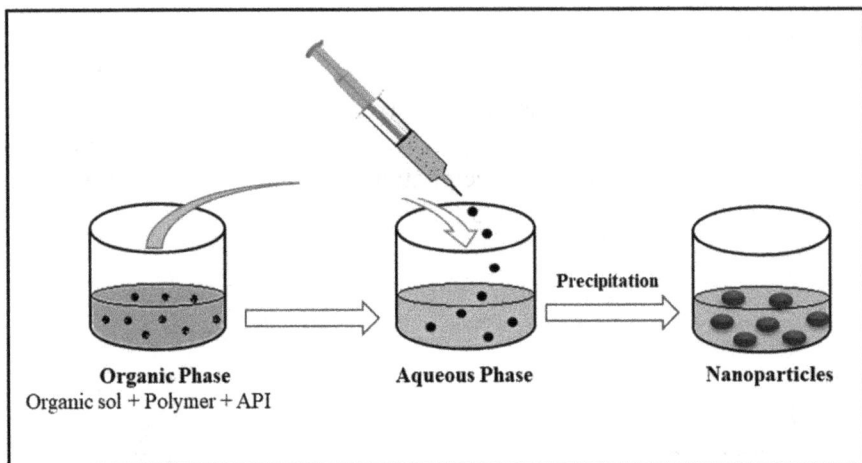

FIGURE 4.5   Solvent displacement technique.

In this method, the drug is dissolved in a small volume of appropriate oil and then diluted in the organic solvent (acetone/ethanol/methanol). When the organic solution is dispersed in the aqueous phase, the polymer precipitates around the nanodroplets, forming a reservoir system [33, 36].

4.2.1.5   SUPERCRITICAL FLUID (SCF) TECHNOLOGY

Techniques using supercritical fluid (SCF) have emerged recently as a promising method for the fabrication of microparticles with ecological and processing benefits [69]. The fabrication and systematic strategy of a particulate system including nanoparticles is being empowered by the application of novel technologies, such as SCF technology. A fluid is supercritical when it is compressed beyond its critical pressure (P_c) and heated beyond its critical temperature (T_c) [70, 71]. SCF technology is a significant method for the fabrication of nanoparticles. In several industrial applications, the conventional recrystallization and milling process are replaced due to quality and the purity of the nanoparticles and ecological advantages [71–73]. Conventional methods for the formulation of nanoparticles have disadvantages such as extreme solvent used, thermal, and chemical degradation, physical changes, and also having difficulty by controlling the parameters like particle size and particle size distribution during manufacturing [74]. However, in addition to density, diffusivity of the SCF's is higher than that of liquid solvents and can be easily varied. Rapid equilibration of the fluid is the advantage achieved by SCF because of high diffusivity and low viscosity [71, 74, 75], as shown in Figure 4.6.

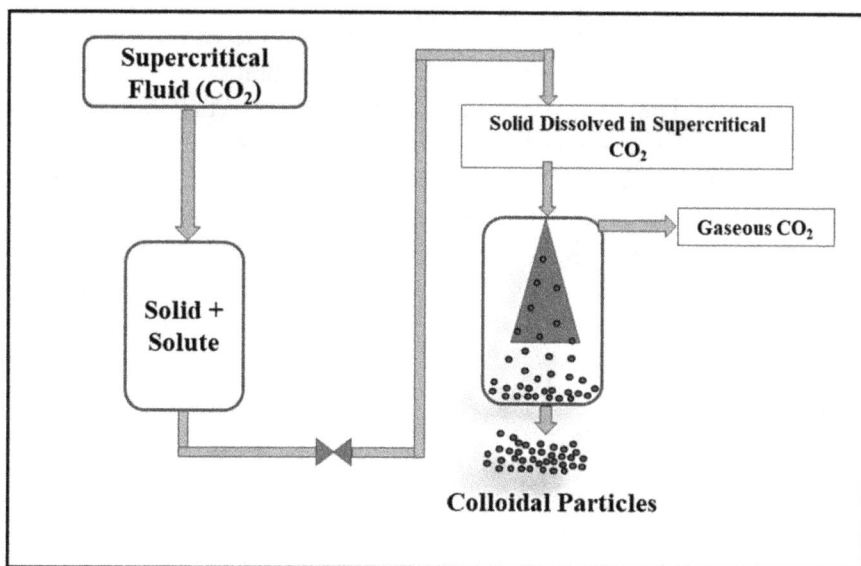

FIGURE 4.6 Supercritical fluid technology.

The design of active ingredient (active molecules and carriers) has been taken into consideration by various processes using SCF technology. Two techniques are categorized such as methods for solubilizing the active drug, the SF is used as solvent and the other method where SF is used like antisolvent, and can be interacted with an organic solution to form a precipitate of active molecule [69, 72, 74].

Supercritical CO_2 has given more attention to formulating the pharmaceutical nanoparticle because it is inflammable, non-hazardous, safe, and cheap, and has a mild critical temperature [71, 72, 75]. In presence of supercritical CO_2 (ScCO_2), the growth of particles takes place at near ambient temperatures in a nonoxidizing temperature and the application of high shear forces is not required. Hence it is essential for the encapsulation of labile particles [69].

1. **Techniques Using the Supercritical Fluid as a Solvent**

    i. **Rapid Expansion of Supercritical Solutions (RESS):** This technique involves the active pharmaceutical ingredient (API)/ drugs which are dissolved in the SCF CO_2 [69] and decrease in the pressure to ambient, the API/drug can be precipitated to produce the nanoparticles [71]. The depressurization can be achieved rapidly in a low-pressure chamber by heating the capillary nozzle [69, 71, 76, 77]. Hence it leads to an increase in the rate of nucleation and high supersaturation can be occurred. On adding the individual molecules on the surface by a condensation mechanism leads to the growth of nuclei. Growth of the particles occurs due to the mechanism of coagulation leading to the collision and sticking of the particles to each other [69, 75]. Expansion is a mechanical perturbation traveling at supersonic velocity, ensuring a supersaturation and uniform conditions [78]. RESS process is very useful as the particles obtained are free of organic solvents and the high-pressure part of the equipment is inexpensive [69]. Also, surfactant or nucleating media are not required for the activation of nucleation [71]. Polymer solubility can be improved by various cosolvents like ethanol, methanol, DCM, butyl acetate, acetone, chlorodifluoromethane, but the removal of the above solvents is difficult from the resulting particles, and it increases the cost and also harms ecological system [69, 79].

2. **Techniques Using the Supercritical Fluid as an Antisolvent:**

    i. **Supercritical Fluid Antisolvent (SAS):** In industry, the liquid antisolvent process is used in large scale. SCF antisolvents suggest the substitutes for these processes by determining the residual organic solvent. This technique is apt for processing insoluble mechanisms in $ScCO_2$ for which RESS is not applicable, or for encapsulating material sensitive to the high shear stress caused by RESS. The prospect with low solubility of supercritical CO_2 were developed by its antisolvent action for the fabrication of nanoparticles. The organic solvent is prepared by adding an API, and then the solution is injected into supercritical carbon dioxide

(ScCo$_2$). When the injection of the drug solution is complete, a washing step is carried out to eliminate the organic solvent so as to avoid it from condensing during the depressurizing step. After the removal of the residual solvent, the pressure is lowered to the atmospheric pressure, and the collection of the particles is carried out by the filtration process. Particle growth after the formation of nuclei in SAS leads to the failure in the fabrication of nanoparticles and has to accept a narrow size distribution. In RESS, reduction of pressure is high, whereas in SAS; diffusivity of Supercritical CO$_2$ is high. For the fabrication of nanoparticles having a size less than 300 nm, the antisolvent action needs to be even faster than SAS [69, 80, 81].

4.2.2 POLYMERIZATION TECHNIQUE OF VARIOUS MONOMERS

This method involves the formation of nanoparticles by dissolving the drug by polymerization of monomers in the aqueous solution [3, 7, 21, 80, 81]. Further, the drug particles are then incorporated in an aqueous solution followed by the suspension, which is filtered to eliminate the impurities like stabilizers and surfactants which are used earlier [21, 37, 82]. This nanosuspension is polymerized by ultracentrifugation and re-suspending agent and the nanoparticles are collected [3, 7, 21, 72]. Polymerization techniques are described by two processes as in subsections.

4.2.2.1 EMULSION POLYMERIZATION

Emulsion polymerization is fastest and frequently used procedure for the preparation of nanoparticles from monomers. In this method, a monomer gets mixed with an immiscible external aqueous phase comprising a surfactant. The monomer molecules diffuse from the emulsion droplets through the aqueous phase to the micelles. The solubilized monomer molecules within the micelle are then polymerized to form the polymer dispersion. Due to anionic polymerization monomer radical collides with another monomer molecules leading to the polymerization. After the polymerization reaction, the emulsifier molecules stabilize the colloidal polymer dispersion against physical instability (coagulation, flocculation, coalescence) [25, 72, 83] as shown in Figure 4.7.

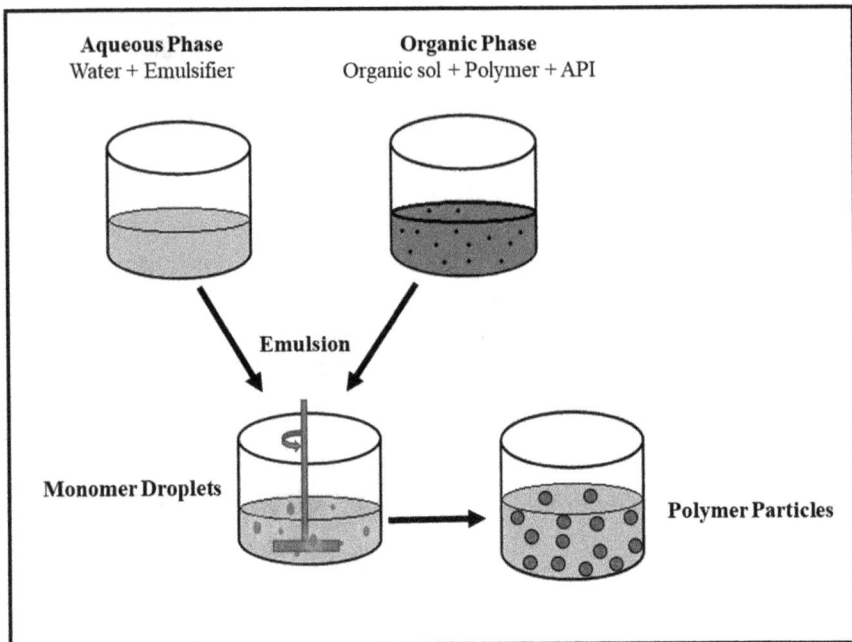

FIGURE 4.7   Emulsion polymerization.

4.2.2.2   INTERFACIAL POLYMERIZATION

It is a unique prominent technique which is being used to prepare polymer nanoparticle [84, 85]. In this method monomer and drug are dispersed in water-miscible solvent (e.g., ethanol) and an oil (e.g., Miglyol, ethyl oleate, phospholipids). The above solvent is then dispersed in an external aqueous phase with stabilizer under agitation, which rapidly diffuses in the aqueous phase, and the monomer polymerizes at the droplet/water interface by the anionic polymerization.

During the process, the solution containing oil leads to polymerization at the interface and not through the droplet. The water-miscible cosolvent forms the nanocapsules. The monomer is transported to the interface by diffusion of cosolvent from oil to external aqueous phase. The ethanol is then removed under vacuum, which can be used further to concentrate the polymer dispersion. After the solvent removal, nanoparticles (nanocapsules) are filtered and collected [83–85], as shown in Figure 4.8.

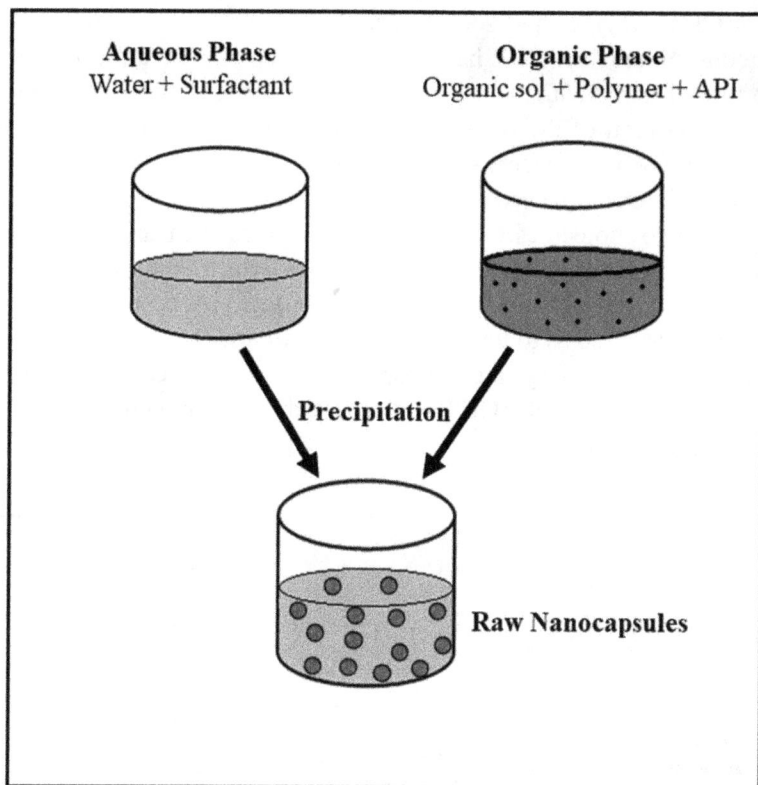

FIGURE 4.8 Interfacial polymerization.

4.2.3   COACERVATION OR IONIC GELATION METHOD OF HYDROPHILIC POLYMERS

Recently biodegradable nanoparticles can be prepared from biodegradable polymer like CHT, gelatin, and sodium alginate having features like biocompatibility and non-hazardous. This technique can be used to formulate hydrophilic polymer-based nanoparticles, where the ionic chelation refers to the material undergoing transition from liquid to gel due to ionic interaction conditions at room temperature. CHT is a gelling polysaccharide agent which is used for the fabrication of nanoparticles by the ionic deletion process. These ionic gels can be formed by the addition of little amount of polyphosphate ions like tri-polyphosphate. This technique includes a two aqueous phase such as CHT polymer and sodium tripolyphosphate under agitation. Due to the constant stirring, CHT having amino group possess a positive charge which further reacts with the tripolyphosphate having negative charge which leads coacervation of the particles having a nanometer (nm) size range as shown in Figure 4.9. Coacervation formation can be attributed when there is electrostatic interaction between two aqueous phases take place. The interaction of the two molecules due to ionic force, results in the conversion of liquid phase to gel phase at room temperature, which is known as an ionic deletion method. Crosslinking agents (e.g., Glutaraldehyde) can be added during the process so as to harden the nanoparticles. Nanoparticles having a physicochemical property like the particle size and surface charge could be controlled by changing the CHT and crosslinking agent concentration, and also the pH value (Table 4.2) [7, 21, 31, 33, 83, 85–87].

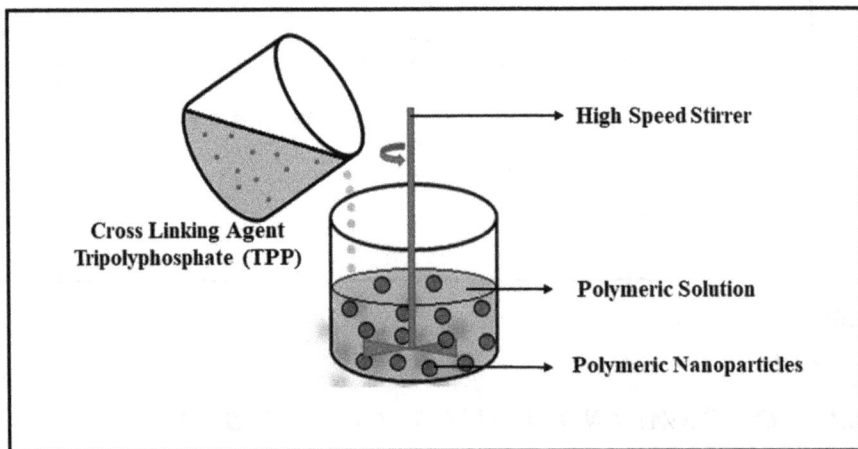

FIGURE 4.9   Ionic gelation method.

4.3   ADVANCE METHODS FOR PREPARATION OF NANOPARTICLES

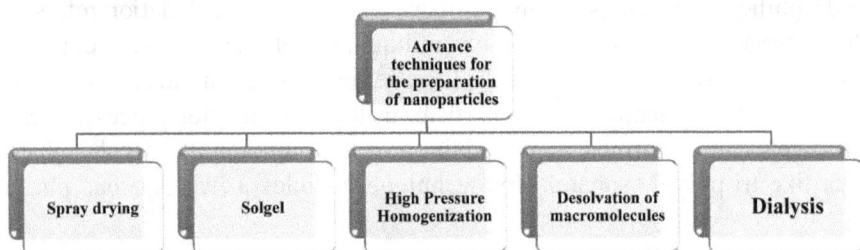

TABLE 4.2 Fabrication of Various Drug and Polymer Nanoparticles by Using Conventional Techniques

Conventional Method	Drug	Material	References
Solvent evaporation	Praziquantel, Metformin, Halperidol, Doxirubicin	PLGA, PLA, ethylcellulose	[88–91]
Double emulsion evaporation	Doxirubicin, Docetaxel	PLGA, PVA	[90, 92]
Salting out	Cabazitaxel	Human serum albumin	[93]
Nanoprecipitation	Cytarabine, Doxirubicin	PLGA, pluronic F68, bovine serum albumin	[94, 95]
Supercritical fluid technology (RESS)	Ibuprofen, Carbamazepine	Stearic acid, carbon oxide	[96, 97]
Supercritical fluid technology (SAS)	5-fluorouracil, 10-Hydroxycamptothecin (HCPT)	L-PLA, carbon oxide	[98, 99]
Emulsion polymerization	Doxorubicin	Poly(butyl cyanoacrylate)	[100]
Interfacial polymerization	Triamcinolone acetonide, Lomustine	Polymethylcyanoacrylate (PMCA), PLGA	[101, 102]
Ionic gelation of hydrophilic polymers	5 fluorouracil, Vincristine	Chitosan, sodium tripolyphosphate, folic acid	[103, 104]

4.3.1   SPRAY DRYING TECHNIQUE

Spray techniques are easy and simple, one-step method which is suitable for preparing nanoparticles. This method is cast-off for encapsulating an active ingredient within the defensive shell [105]. In this method, liquid gets converted into dry particles under continuous process. This is technique has the rapid results and is inexpensive, and controls the physicochemical properties of the nanoparticles by changing the process parameters such as flow rate, nozzle geometry, inlet air temperature, and solution viscosity) [33, 106].

The spray drying technique is established on the principle of nebulization which depends upon the atomization of a solution, including APIs and carrier molecules, by means of compressed air or nitrogen through a desiccating chamber, and warm air is used for the drying. This is achieved by three steps:

- Aerosolformation;
- Interaction of aerosol with hot air and drying of the aerosol; and
- Separation of the dried product and the air charged with the solvent.

This method is applied to prepare nanoparticles by spraying the complex liquid mixture consisting of an API which is dissolved in either organic or in aqueous polymer solution as shown in Figure 4.10. Nanoparticles fabricated by spray drying techniques are determined by the primary preparation, whether it is in the solution, suspension, or emulsion form. Water-soluble and water-insoluble, heat-resistant, or heat-resistant and heat-sensitive drugs are encapsulated by the spray drying technique. Various biodegradable polymers are used for this technique are PLA, Eudragit, gelatin, PLGA, polysaccharides [31, 33, 69, 105].

This technique is an inexpensive, single step, continuous process and easy to scale up as compared to ionic gelation and emulsification methods. It is less dependent on solubility parameters of the drug and the polymer and also can be used without organic solvents [69].

4.3.2   SOL-GEL TECHNIQUE

Sol-gel technique is used for fabricating small particles in material chemistry, used for metal oxide synthesis [107]. Sol-gel thin-film processing shows various benefits like low-temperature which simplifies the fabrication and gives accurate microstructural and chemical control. The sol-gel derived film provides a high degree of biocompatibility and specific surface area and the external surface which simplifies the function by appropriate biomolecules

[108]. Sol-gel technique has the ability to control the size, distribution, and morphology of the particles by controlling various reaction parameters. Graham introduced the solgel term during his work on silica sols in 1864. This technique proposed a low temperature process for manufacturing of purely inorganic or organic materials. This procedure depends on the hydrolysis and condensation reaction of organometallic compounds in acidic solution, which gives the benefits for the production of nanoparticles comprising of excellent mechanism of the reaction kinetics, ease of compositional alterations, customizable microstructure, introduction of various functional groups, etc.

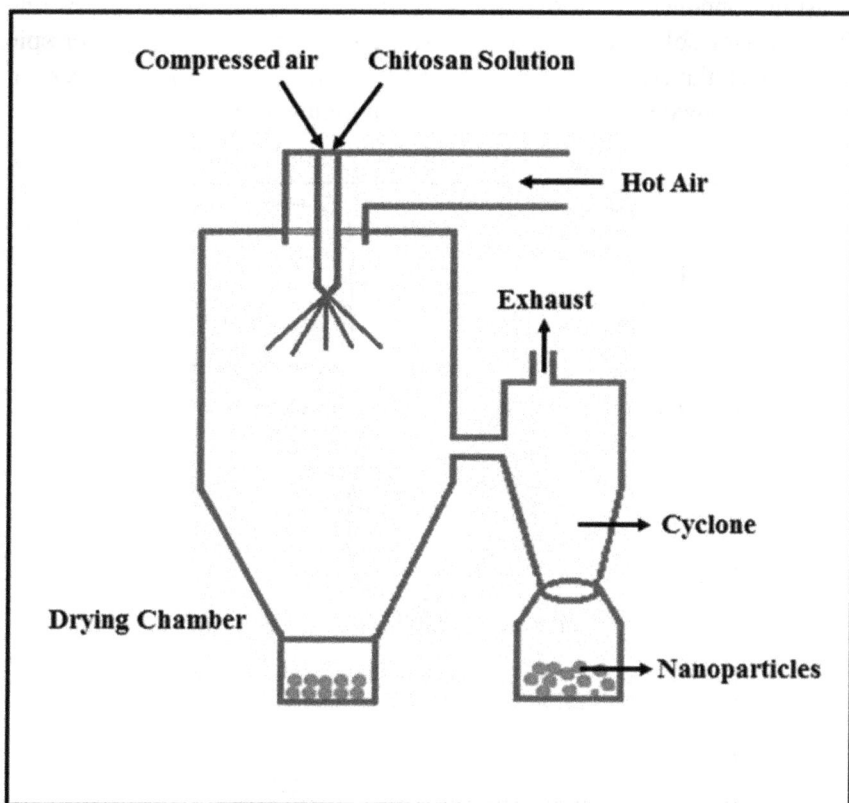

FIGURE 4.10 Spray drying technique.

The procedure involved in this technique is as followed: sol or colloidal solution is a solution where distribution of particles of the size ~ 0.1–1 μm takes place in a liquid in which the only suspending force is the Brownian

motion. Dispersion of each phase, i.e., solid phase into liquid phase leads
to the gel formation. In this technique, colloidal particles get dissolved in a
liquid which further forms a sol. Deposition of the sol develops the thin layer
on any substance by using various methods of spraying, spinning, or coating.
The particles in the sol are kept for the polymerization by eliminating the
stabilizing constituents which further produces a complex network gel. At
the end of the process, heat is applied to the residue of organic and inorganic
components so as to form the crystalline or amorphous layer coat. Hydrolysis
of alcoholic group and its condensation are the two main reactions which are
encompassed by solgel. The sol achieved by this process can be shaped by
a casting container. The formation of the film can be achieved by depositing
the precursor sol on the suitable substrate by using a dip coating or spin
coating techniques, and it is also used for synthesizing the microsphere or
nanosphere powders [109–112] as shown in Figure 4.11.

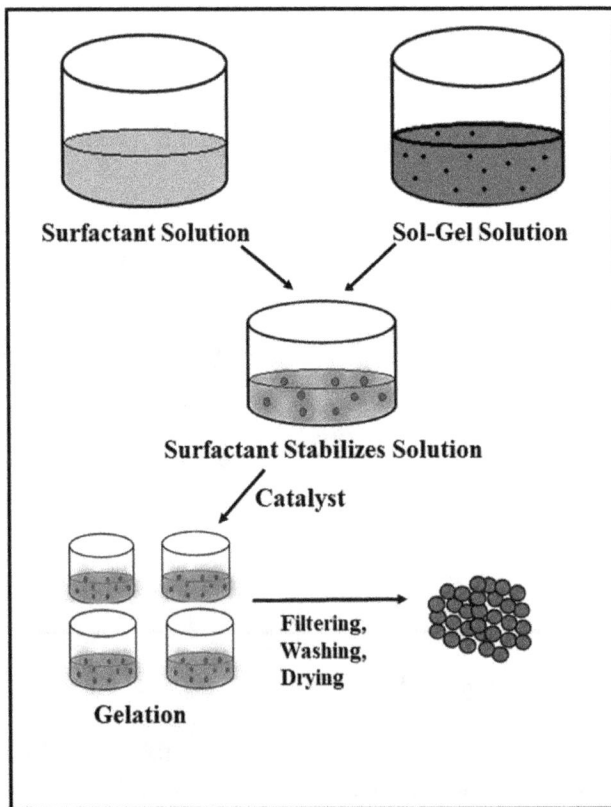

FIGURE 4.11   Sol-gel technique.

A distinctive benefit of the sol-gel method depends on the processability of the sols and gels, which is dependent on the processing step for powders, fibers, ceramics, and coatings. Nanomaterials with high permeability can be produced by this technique. During or after the formation of gel, the pores are filled, and the combination can be fabricated. During manufacturing of the nanomaterials, the temperature is lowered so as the substances can be embedded into gel formation; so, as they can be further stored or released in a controlled manner [113].

4.3.3 HIGH-PRESSURE HOMOGENIZATION (HPH)

Emulsions and suspensions are used to manufacture for many years through this technique. This technology has advantages such as it simplifies for scaling up, even to very volumes also is presently used in the pharmaceutical, chemical, and food production. Parenteral emulsions can be manufactured with this technology. Various homogenizer used in this method is established on the piston-gap principle. In piston-gap homogenizer the microsuspension is introduced through the container, containing the sample which is further required to pass through a minute gap such as 10 μm and the particle size reduction can be affected by sheer force, cavitation, and impaction. This force is sufficiently high to convert the drug microparticles into nanoparticles. Jet stream technology is an alternative for the piston gap principle. The micro-fluidizer is established on the principle of jet-stream. Two different liquid phases collide with each other, and due to the particle collision, the droplets or crystals size reduction are obtained, but the existence of cavitation must be measured. The fabrication of drug/APIs nanosuspensions can be attributed by this technique, as shown in Figure 4.12. The Microfluidizer processor possesses a continuous feed stream that gets processed by a fixed geometry which develops a high shear and break down the larger particles. This method gives accurate, repeated, and results and yields smaller particles with narrow particle size distribution [9, 114–116].

4.3.4 DESOLVATION OF MACROMOLECULES

Another technology is widely used for the formulation of polymeric nanoparticle is the desolvation process by adding the desolvating agent. Heat-sensitive drugs can be used as the main advantage of this technique is it requires minimum temperature for the synthesis. This method is used for the formulation of nanoparticles for proteins and polysaccharides. Different sizes of the particles are fabricated by the polymeric molecules using this technique. The different size of the particles depends on the various parameters like protein content, pH, ionic strength, amount of crosslinking agent, speed of agitation, desolvating agent concentration, etc. The aqueous phase containing the protein or polysaccharides can be desolvated by changes in pH and temperature by addition of a sufficient amount of counterions. Crosslinking affects instantaneously or resulting to the desolvation step [100, 101]. This technique includes three steps as followed: (i) protein dissolution; (ii) protein aggregation; and (iii) protein degradation. The aggregate nanoparticles are crosslinked using glutaraldehyde as shown in Figure 4.13. Sodium sulfate, acetone, alcohol, isopropanol, ethanol is used as a desolvating agent for preparing the nanoparticles. Nephelometer is used for the optimization of turbidity. Nanosphere, as the finished product can only be achieved by desolvation technique. Proteins get disaggregated which turns the suspension colloidal and hence it appears to be milky in nature. This technique can fabricate the nanoparticles by entrapping lipophilic as well as hydrophilic drugs [24, 117–121].

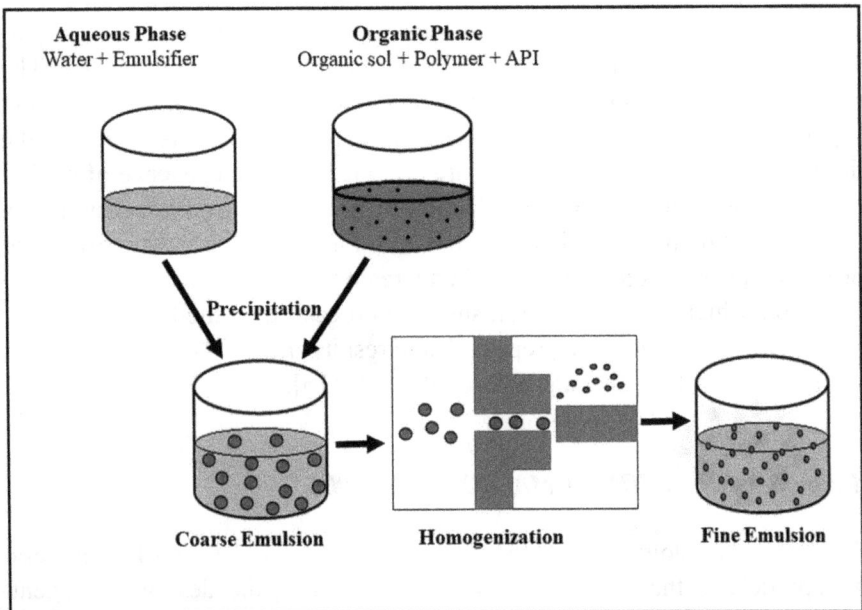

FIGURE 4.12   High-pressure homogenization technique.

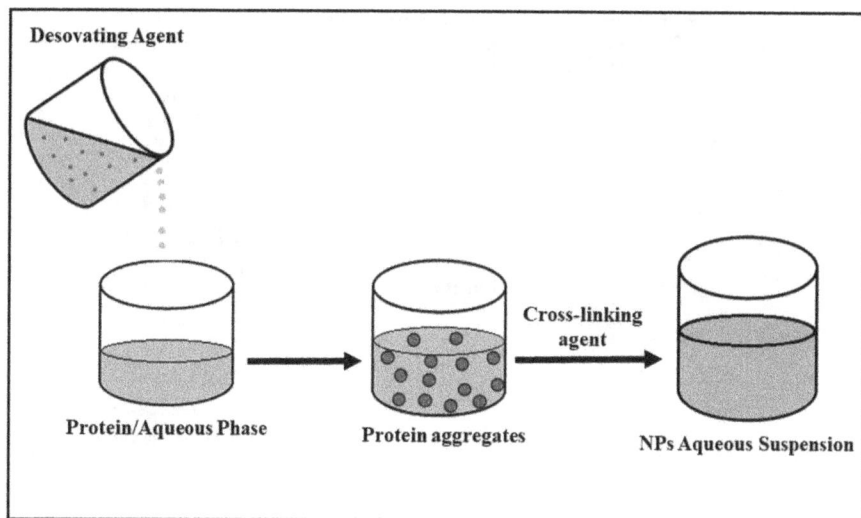

FIGURE 4.13   Desolvation technique.

4.3.5   *DIALYSIS*

Dialysis is a simple and effective technique used for the fabrication of polymeric nanoparticles with narrow distribution. In this method, the active ingredient and polymer are positioned on a dialysis tube/membrane after dissolving with water-miscible organic solvents with suitable molecular weight cutoff as shown in Figure 4.14. The organic phase disperses out through the dialysis tube/membrane into the aqueous phase, and hence decreases the interfacial tension between those phases. Later, the homogenous suspension of nanoparticles is formed in the membrane by the solvent displacement resulting in the progressive agglomeration of polymer due to the loss of solubility. The nanosuspension produced is freeze-dried using 5% mannitol as a cryoprotectant to attain a fine powder of nanoparticles (Table 4.3) [24, 122–124].

4.4   ROLE OF NANOPARTICLES IN NUTRACEUTICAL DRUG DELIVERY

Across the globe, enthusiastic researchers have worked exhaustively in delivering high bioavailable drug fractions through various nanoparticle systems. However, more interestingly, several nanoparticle systems have been reported such as Protein nanoparticles, Solid lipid nanoparticles

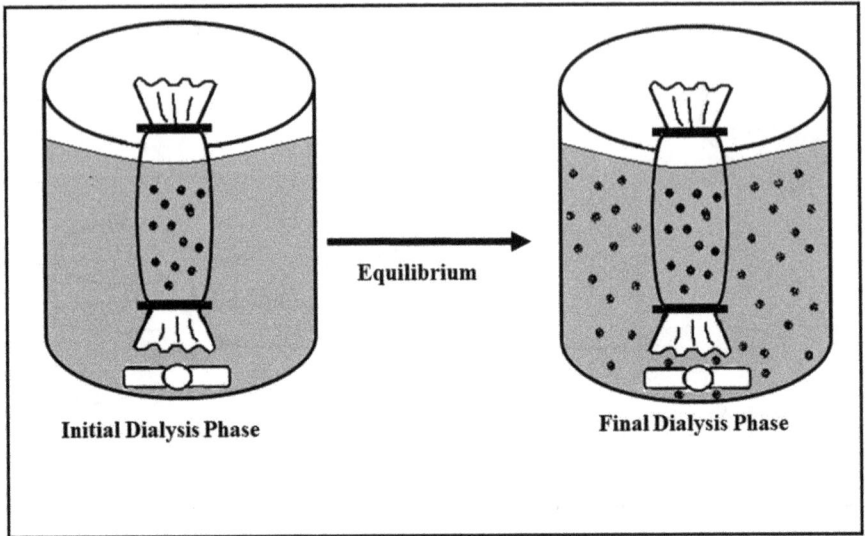

FIGURE 4.14   Dialysis technique.

TABLE 4.3   Fabrication of Various Drug and Polymer Nanoparticles by Using Advance Techniques

Advance Method	Drug	Material	References
Spray drying	Acetaminophen	Chitosan, tripolyphosphate	[125]
Sol-gel	Miramistin	Tetraethoxy silane, ammonium hydroxide	[126]
High-pressure homogenization	Efavirenz and Tenofovir disoproxil	Glyceryl tripalmitate (tripalmitin), glyceryl monostearate, glyceryl tristearate, Pluronic F68, Pluronic F127	[127]
Desolvation of macromolecules	5-Fluorouracil	Bovine serum albumin, glutaraldeyde	[128]
Dialysis	Acyclovir	Glyceryl monostearate (GMS) and lipoid S75	[129]

(SLNs), alginate nanoparticles, Milk protein nanoparticles, protein-lipid composite nanoparticles, CHT nanoparticles, biopolymer nanoparticles fabricated from whey protein isolate and beet pectin, Protein nanoparticles, Cationic β-Lactoglobulin nanoparticles, poly(lactic-co-glycolic acid nanoparticles, nanoparticles synthesized from soy protein, Sophorolipid-Coated Nanoparticles, CHT/β-lactoglobulin core-shell nanoparticles, Mesoporous Silica Nanoparticles, Core shell conjugate nanoparticles,

Lipid nanoparticles, Zein-carrageenan core-shell nanoparticles, Soybean β-Conglycinin nanoparticles, Omega-3 fatty acids based nanoparticles, Cationic beta-lactoglobulin nanoparticles, Carboxymethyl CHT-soy protein complex nanoparticles, Serum albumin Nanoparticles, poly-d,l-lactide (PLA) nanoparticles, Silver nanoparticles, Nanoparticles of oleoyl alginate ester, Protein-lipid composite nanoparticles, Barley protein nanoparticles, Zein/pectin core-shell nanoparticles, etc., which encapsulates several therapeutically privileged Hydrophilic as well as Hydrophobic Nutraceutical products such as Epigallocatechin-3-gallate, Resveratrol, Vitamins, Caesin, dextran, β-carotene, docosahexanoic acid, β-lactoglobulin, lactoferrin, Quercetrin, Afzelin, Anthocyanins, Vitamin D_3, Retinol, Avocado oil, Riboflavin, Probiotics, Fish oil, Lycopene, Tocopherol, Tea polyphenol, vitamin E, quercetin, curcumin, resveratrol, puerarin, red grape seed extract, theaflavin, Lycopene, rosmarinic acid, tangeretin, piperine, lutein, apigenin, gingerol, capsaicin, gossypin, diosgenin, β-carotene, quercitrin, etc. (Table 4.4) [130–163]. The above nanoparticle-based deliveries of the therapeutically active photochemicals resulted in an enhanced bioavailability (up to 85%) of the products by reducing the enzymatic (diverse classes of cytochrome P450 enzymes) attack, abridged metabolic processes by bypassing the first-pass metabolism, and reduction in the clearance process in the human body. Although, majority of these highly acclaimed nutraceutical delivery are experimentally reported recently and anxiously numerous researches are currently going on for their actual translation into the industrial-scale production.

4.5 CONCLUSION AND PERSPECTIVES

Nanotechnology has solved enormous difficulties of healthcare science by imposing the remarkable development of various drug delivery. Nanofabrication of nanoparticles can be achieved by novel techniques used for the fabrication. Nanoparticles have numerous challenges associated with and perhaps the most significant one in the change from lab-scale proof of research concept to reproducible with precisely physicochemical properties and high yielding production of useful nanomaterial. This key point is usually not addressed in the literature. Various technical challenges are developed for techniques in virus-like system for intracellular system, the architecting of biometric polymer, control of sensitive drug, nanochips for nanoparticles release, carriers for advanced polymers for the delivery of therapeutic peptide/protein. One promising path for the prevention of potential health hazards were proposed by a number of scientists to fabricate

TABLE 4.4 Nutraceutical Nano Drug Delivery Systems

Nutraceutical	Nanoparticle Drug Delivery System	References
Quercetin, afzelin	Silver nanoparticles	[130]
Vitamin D$_3$	Nanoparticles of oleoyl alginate ester	[131]
Anthocyanins	Biopolymer nanoparticles fabricated from whey protein isolate and beet pectin	[132]
Vitamins, probiotics, bioactive peptides, antioxidants	Chitosan nanoparticles	[133]
Epigallocatechin-3-gallate, resveratrol, vitamins, caesin, dextran, β-carotene, docosahexaenoic acid, β-lactoglobulin, lactoferrin	Milk protein nanoparticles	[134]
Retinol, avocado oil, riboflavin, probiotics, fish oil, lycopene, tocopherol	Protein nanoparticles	[135]
Epigallocatechin gallate, tea polyphenol, vitamin E, quercetin, curcumin, resveratrol, puerarin, red grape seed extract, theaflavin, lycopene, rosmarinic acid	Solid lipid nanoparticles	[136, 158, 161]
Curcumin	Nanoparticles synthesized from soy protein	[137]
Vitamins, hydrophobic phytochemicals, polyphenols	Chitosan/β-lactoglobulin core-shell nanoparticles	[138]
Apigenin, piperine, gingerol, capsaicin, gossypin, diosgenin	Poly(lactic-co-glycolic acid) nanoparticles	[139]
Vitamin B$_{12}$	Protein-lipid composite nanoparticles	[140]
Peppermint phenolic extract	Alginate nanoparticles	[141]
Vitamin D$_3$	Soybean β-conglycinin nanoparticles	[142]
Vitamin D$_3$	Carboxymethyl chitosan-soy protein complex nanoparticles	[143]
Curcumin	Soy β-conglycinin nanoparticles	[144]
Curcumin	Core-shell protein-polysaccharide nanoparticles	[145]
Resveratrol	Mesoporous silica nanoparticles	[146]
Resveratrol, curcumin	Core-shell conjugate nanoparticles	[147]

TABLE 4.4 *(Continued)*

Nutraceutical	Nanoparticle Drug Delivery System	References
Epigallocatechin-3-gallate	Serum albumin NPs	[148]
Hydrophilic nutraceuticals	Cationic β-lactoglobulin nanoparticles	[149]
Vitamin D_3	Alginate nanoparticles	[150]
Resveratrol	Lipid nanoparticles	[151]
Tangeretin	Protein nanoparticles	[152]
Curcumin, piperine	Zein-carrageenan core-shell nanoparticles	[153]
β-carotene	Barley protein nanoparticles	[154]
Vitamin B_{12}	Protein-lipid composite nanoparticles	[155]
Resveratrol	Zein/pectin core-shell nanoparticles	[156]
Curcumin	Polysaccharide-based nanoparticles	[157]
Lutein	Omega-3 fatty acids-based nanoparticles	[159]
Hydrophilic nutraceuticals	Cationic beta-lactoglobulin nanoparticles	[160]
Quercitrin	Poly-d,l-lactide (PLA) nanoparticles	[162]
Curcumin	Sophorolipid-coated nanoparticles	[163]

biodegradable particles. In addition, development, and regulatory concern arises when generic nano-products are presented for health authority approval with claims of equivalence to the innovator drug. Finally, health authorities who are paid with responsibilities for the endorsement of safe and effective medicines will need to respond to the various challenges posed by the emergence of products based on new technologies. Appropriate processes to develop definitions, quality standards, and requirements for development studies, including clinical trials, must be in place to proactively address rapid advances in drug development. Lastly, as Robert Langer said in 2003 in a publication entitled "Where a pill won't reach," we will still be looking for a day when any drug can be administered at the right time, at the right dose, for the correct duration, anywhere in the body with specificity and efficiency.

KEYWORDS

- **biodegradable polymers**
- **deoxyribonucleic acid**
- **drug delivery**
- nanofabrication
- nanoparticle
- nanotechnology

REFERENCES

1. Sarkar, S., & Sarkar, R., (2017). Sol-gel synthesis and meticulous characterization of zinc oxide nanoparticles. *Journal of Nanosciences: Current Research, 2*, 109.
2. Salata, O. V., (2004). Applications of nanoparticles in biology and medicine. *Journal of Nanobiotechnology, 2*(1), 3.
3. Konwar, R., & Ahmed, A. B., (2013). Nanoparticle: An overview of preparation and characterization and applications. *International Research Journal of Pharmacy, 4*(4). doi: 10.7897/2230/8407.04408.
4. Pal, S. L., Jana, U., Manna, P. K., Mohanta, G. P., & Manavalan, R. (2011). Nanoparticle: An overview of preparation and characterization. *Journal of Applied Pharmaceutical Science, 1*(6), 228–234.
5. Sailaja, A., Amareshwar, P., & Chakravarty, P., (2011). Different techniques used for the preparation of nanoparticles using natural polymers and their application. *Int. J. Pharm. Pharm. Sci., 3*(suppl 2), 45–50.

6. Shivshankara, V. S., Yogananda, R., & Bharati, D. R., (2012). A review on nanoparticles in different drug delivery system. *Am. J. Pharmatech. Res., 2*(6).

7. Bhatia, S., (2016). Nanoparticles types, classification, characterization, fabrication methods, and drug delivery applications. In: *Natural Polymer Drug Delivery Systems* (pp. 33–93). Springer International Publishing.

8. Jibowu, T., (2016). The formation of doxorubicin loaded targeted nanoparticles using nanoprecipitation, double emulsion and single emulsion for cancer treatment. *J. Nanomed. Nanotechnol., 7*(379), 2.

9. Gupta, R. B., & Kompella, U. B. (2006). *Nanoparticle Technology for Drug Delivery.* Taylor & Francis Group, LLC.

10. Jain, N. K. (1997). *Controlled and Novel Drug Delivery.* CBS Publisher.

11. Vila, A., Sanchez, A., Tobio, M., Calvo, P., & Alonso, M. J., (2002). Design of biodegradable particles for protein delivery. *Journal of Controlled Release, 78*(1), 15–24.

12. Mu, L., & Feng, S. S., (2003). A novel controlled release formulation for the anticancer drug paclitaxel (Taxol®): PLGA nanoparticles containing vitamin E TPGS. *Journal of Controlled Release, 86*(1), 33–48.

13. Guar, A., Minda, A., & Bhatiya, A. L., (2008). Nanotechnology in medical science. *Asian Journal of Pharmaceutics*, 80–85.

14. Sapra, P., Tyagi, P., & Allen, T. M., (2005). Ligand-targeted liposomes for cancer treatment. *Current Drug Delivery, 2*(4), 369–381.

15. Bertrand, N., Wu, J., Xu, X., Kamaly, N., & Farokhzad, O. C., (2014). Cancer nanotechnology: The impact of passive and active targeting in the era of modern cancer biology. *Advanced Drug Delivery Reviews, 66*, 2–25.

16. Desai, N., (2012). Challenges in the development of nanoparticle-based therapeutics. *The AAPS Journal, 14*(2), 282–295. doi: 10.1208/s12248-012-9339-4.

17. Manzoor, A. A., Lindner, L. H., Landon, C. D., Park, J. Y., Simnick, A. J., Dreher, M. R., & Koning, G. A., (2012). Overcoming limitations in nanoparticle drug delivery: Triggered, intravascular release to improve drug penetration into tumors. *Cancer Research, 72*(21), 5566–5575. doi: 10.1158/0008-5472.

18. Seynhaeve, A. L., Hoving, S., Schipper, D., Vermeulen, C. E., De Wiel-Ambagtsheer, G. A., Van, T. S. T., & Ten, H. T. L., (2007). Tumor necrosis factor α mediates homogeneous distribution of liposomes in murine melanoma that contributes to a better tumor response. *Cancer Research, 67*(19), 9455–9462. doi: 10.1158/0008-5472.

19. El-Kareh, A. W., & Secomb, T. W., (2000). A mathematical model for comparison of bolus injection, continuous infusion, and liposomal delivery of doxorubicin to tumor cells. *Neoplasia, 2*(4), 325–338.

20. Lauterwasser, C., (2005). *Small Sizes that Matter: Opportunities and Risks of Nanotechnologies: Report in Co-Operation with the OECD International Futures Program* (p. 45). Allianz AG. Munchen: Allianz Center for Technology-2006.

21. Sriharitha, (2014). A review on nanoparticles in targeted drug delivery system. *Research & Reviews: Journal of Material Science*, 28.doi: 10.4172/2321-6212.1000r003.

22. Ranade, V. V., & Hollinger, M. A., (2006). *Drug Delivery Systems* (p. 71). CRC press.

23. De Jong, W. H., & Borm, P. J., (2008). Drug delivery and nanoparticles: Applications and hazards. *International Journal of Nanomedicine, 3*(2), 133.

24. Mohanraj, V. J., & Chen, Y., (2006). Nanoparticles:a review. *Tropical Journal of Pharmaceutical Research, 5*(1), 561–573.

25. Lieberman, H. A., Rieger, M. M., & Banker, G. S., (1998). *Pharmaceutical Dosage Forms—Disperse Systems* (Vol. 2). M. Dekker.

26. Kompella, U. B., Bandi, N., & Ayalasomayajula, S. P., (2001). Poly (lactic acid) nanoparticles for sustained release of budesonide. *Drug Deliv. Technol., 1*(1), 7.

27. Kumar, M. R., Bakowsky, U., & Lehr, C. M., (2004). Preparation and characterization of cationic PLGA nanospheres as DNA carriers. *Biomaterials, 25*(10), 1771–1777. doi: 10.1016/j.biomaterials.2003.08.069.

28. Benita, S., Benoit, J. P., Puisieux, F., & Thies, C., (1984). Characterization of drug-loaded poly (d, l-lactide) microspheres. *Journal of Pharmaceutical Sciences, 73*(12), 1721–1724. doi: 10.1002/jps.2600731215.

29. Soppimath, K. S., Aminabhavi, T. M., Kulkarni, A. R., & Rudzinski, W. E., (2001). Biodegradable polymeric nanoparticles as drug delivery devices. *Journal of Controlled Release, 70*(1), 1–20. doi: 10.1016/S0168-3659(00)00339-4.

30. Scholes, P. D., Coombes, A. G. A., Illum, L., Daviz, S. S., Vert, M., & Davies, M. C., (1993). The preparation of sub-200 nm poly (lactide-co-glycolide) microspheres for site-specific drug delivery. *Journal of Controlled Release, 25*(1), 145–153. doi: 10.1016/0168-3659(93)90103-C.

31. Wang, Y., Li, P., Truong-Dinh, T. T., Zhang, J., & Kong, L., (2016). Manufacturing techniques and surface engineering of polymer based nanoparticles for targeted drug delivery to cancer. *Nanomaterials, 6*(2), 26. doi:10.3390/nano6020026.

32. Reis, C. P., Neufeld, R. J., Ribeiro, A. J., & Veiga, F., (2006). Nanoencapsulation I. Methods for preparation of drug-loaded polymeric nanoparticles. *Nanomedicine: Nanotechnology, Biology and Medicine, 2*(1), 8–21. doi: 10.1016/j.nano.2005.12.003.

33. Vauthier, C., & Bouchemal, K., (2009). Methods for the preparation and manufacture of polymeric nanoparticles. *Pharmaceutical Research, 26*(5), 1025–1058. doi: 10.1007/s11095-008-9800-3.

34. Quintanar-Guerrero, D., Allémann, E., Fessi, H., & Doelker, E., (1999). Pseudo latex preparation using a novel emulsion-diffusion process involving direct displacement of partially water-miscible solvents by distillation. *International Journal of Pharmaceutics, 188*(2), 155–164. doi: 10.1016/S0378-5173(99)00216-1.

35. McGinity, J. W., (1989). *Aqueous Polymeric Coating for Pharmaceutical Applications*. Marcel Dekker, New York.

36. Vays, S. P., & Khar, R. K., (2004). *Targeted & Controlled Drug Delivery*. CBC: New Delhi.

37. Quintanar-Guerrero, D., Allémann, E., Doelker, E., & Fessi, H., (1997). A mechanistic study of the formation of polymer nanoparticles by the emulsification-diffusion technique. *Colloid and Polymer Science, 275*(7), 640–647.

38. Quintanar-Guerrero, D., Fessi, H., Allémann, E., & Doelker, E., (1996). Influence of stabilizing agents and preparative variables on the formation of poly (D, L-lactic acid) nanoparticles by an emulsification-diffusion technique. *International Journal of Pharmaceutics, 143*(2), 133–141. doi.:10.1016/S0378-5173(96)04697-2.

39. Pawar, S. J., Pawar, P. S., Jadhav, S. B., Alkunte, A. S., & Patil, S. M., (2010). Nano-capsules as a novel drug delivery system. *Research Journal of Pharmaceutical Dosage Forms and Technology, 2*(2), 146–155.

40. Quintanar-Guerrero, D., Tamayo-Esquivel, D., Ganem-Quintanar, A., Allémann, E., & Doelker, E., (2005). Adaptation and optimization of the emulsification-diffusion technique to prepare lipidic nanospheres. *European Journal of Pharmaceutical Sciences, 26*(2), 211–218. doi: 10.1016/j.ejps.2005.06.001.

41. Trotta, M., Debernardi, F., & Caputo, O., (2003). Preparation of solid lipid nanoparticles by a solvent emulsification-diffusion technique. *International Journal of Pharmaceutics, 257*(1), 153–160. doi: 10.1016/S0378-5173(03)00135-2.

42. Battaglia, L., Trotta, M., Gallarate, M., Carlotti, M. E., Zara, G. P., & Bargoni, A., (2007). Solid lipid nanoparticles formed by solvent-in-water emulsion-diffusion technique: Development and influence on insulin stability. *Journal of Microencapsulation, 24*(7), 672–684. doi.org:10.1080/02652040701532981.

43. Quintanar-Guerrero, D., Ganem-Quintanar, A., Allémann, E., Fessi, H., & Doelker, E., (1998). Influence of the stabilizer coating layer on the purification and freeze-drying of poly (D, L-lactic acid) nanoparticles prepared by an emulsion-diffusion technique. *Journal of Microencapsulation, 15*(1), 107–119. doi: 10.3109/0265204980900684.

44. Win, K. Y., & Feng, S. S., (2005). Effects of particle size and surface coating on cellular uptake of polymeric nanoparticles for oral delivery of anticancer drugs. *Biomaterials, 26*(15), 2713–2722. doi: 10.1016/j.biomaterials.2004.07.050.

45. Banyal, S., Malik, P., Tuli, H. S., & Mukherjee, T. K., (2013). Advances in nanotechnology for diagnosis and treatment of tuberculosis. *Current Opinion in Pulmonary Medicine, 19*(3), 289–297.

46. Sahoo, S. K., Panyam, J., Prabha, S., & Labhasetwar, V., (2002). Residual polyvinyl alcohol associated with poly (D, L-lactide-co-glycolide) nanoparticles affects their physical properties and cellular uptake. *Journal of Controlled Release, 82*(1), 105–114. doi: 10.1016/S0168-3659(02)00127-X.

47. Xie, S., Wang, S., Zhao, B., Han, C., Wang, M., & Zhou, W., (2008). Effect of PLGA as a polymeric emulsifier on preparation of hydrophilic protein-loaded solid lipid nanoparticles. *Colloids and Surfaces B: Biointerfaces, 67*(2), 199–204. doi: 10.1016/j.colsurfb.2008.08.018.

48. Quintanar-Guerrero, D., Allémann, E., Fessi, H., & Doelker, E., (1998). Preparation techniques and mechanisms of formation of biodegradable nanoparticles from preformed polymers. *Drug Development and Industrial Pharmacy, 24*(12), 1113–1128. doi: 10.3109/03639049809108571.

49. Ibrahim, H., Bindschaedler, C., Doelker, E., Buri, P., & Gurny, R., (1992). Aqueous nano-dispersions prepared by a salting-out process. *International Journal of Pharmaceutics, 87*(1–3), 239–246. doi: 10.1016/0378-5173(92)90248-Z.

50. Allémann, E., Gurny, R., & Doelker, E., (1992). Preparation of aqueous polymeric nanodispersions by a reversible salting-out process: Influence of process parameters on particle size. *International Journal of Pharmaceutics, 87*(1–3), 247–253. doi: 10.1016/0378-5173(92)90249-2.

51. Shinde, A. J., & More, H. N., (2009). Nanoparticles: As carriers for drug delivery system. *Research Journal of Pharmaceutical Dosage Forms and Technology, 1*(2), 80–86.

52. Galindo-Rodriguez, S., Allémann, E., Fessi, H., & Doelker, E., (2004). Physicochemical parameters associated with nanoparticle formation in the salting-out, emulsification-diffusion, and nanoprecipitation methods. *Pharmaceutical Research, 21*(8), 1428–1439. doi: 10.1023/B:PHAM.000.

53. Balakrishanan, M. H., & Rajan, M., (2016). Size-controlled synthesis of biodegradable nanocarriers for targeted and controlled cancer drug delivery using salting out cation. *Bulletin of Materials Science, 39*(1), 69–77. doi: 10.1007/s12034-015-0946-4.

54. Jung, T., Kamm, W., Breitenbach, A., Kaiserling, E., Xiao, J. X., & Kissel, T., (2000). Biodegradable nanoparticles for oral delivery of peptides: Is there a role for polymers

to affect mucosal uptake?. *European Journal of Pharmaceutics and Biopharmaceutics, 50*(1), 147–160. doi :10.1016/S0939-6411(00)00084-9.

55. Ottenbrite, R. M., & Kim, S. W. (Eds.). (2019). *Polymeric Drugs and Drug Delivery Systems.* CRC Press.

56. Beck-Broichsitter, M., Rytting, E., Lebhardt, T., Wang, X., & Kissel, T., (2010). Preparation of nanoparticles by solvent displacement for drug delivery: A shift in the "ouzo region" upon drug loading. *European Journal of Pharmaceutical Sciences, 41*(2), 244–253.

57. Fessi, H. P. F. D., Puisieux, F., Devissaguet, J. P., Ammoury, N., & Benita, S., (1989). Nanocapsule formation by interfacial polymer deposition following solvent displacement. *International Journal of Pharmaceutics, 55*(1), R1–R4. doi: 10.1016/ 0378-5173(89)90281-0.

58. Crucho, C. I., & Barros, M. T., (2017). Polymeric nanoparticles: A study on the preparation variables and characterization methods. *Materials Science and Engineering: C.* doi: 10.1016/j.msec.2017.06.004.

59. Sternling, C. A., & Scriven, L. E., (1959). Interfacial turbulence: Hydrodynamic instability and the Marangoni effect. *AIChE Journal, 5*(4), 514–523. doi: 10.1002/aic. 690050421.

60. Ganachaud, F., & Katz, J. L., (2005). Nanoparticles and nanocapsules created using the ouzo effect: Spontaneous emulsification as an alternative to ultrasonic and high-shear devices. *ChemPhysChem, 6*(2), 209–216. doi: 10.1002/cphc.200400527.

61. Duclairoir, C., Nakache, E., Marchais, H., & Orecchioni, A. M., (1998). Formation of gliadin nanoparticles: Influence of the solubility parameter of the protein solvent. *Colloid & Polymer Science, 276*(4), 321–327. https://doi.org/10.1007/s003960050246.

62. Allouche, J., (2013). Synthesis of organic and bioorganic nanoparticles: An overview of the preparation methods. In: *Nanomaterials: A Danger or a Promise?* (pp. 27–74). Springer London. doi: 10.1007/978-1-4471-4213-3_2.

63. Lannibois-Drean, H., (1995). *Hydrophobic Molecules In Water: Manufacturing Nanoparticles by Precipitation (Doctoral Dissertation, Paris 6).*

64. Lannibois, H., Hasmy, A., Botet, R., Chariol, O. A., & Cabane, B., (1997). Surfactant limited aggregation of hydrophobic molecules in water. *Journal de Physique II, 7*(2), 319–342. doi: 10.1051/jp2:1997128.

65. Bilati, U., Allémann, E., & Doelker, E., (2005). Poly (D, L-lactide-co-glycolide) protein-loaded nanoparticles prepared by the double emulsion method—processing and formulation issues for enhanced entrapment efficiency. *Journal of Microencapsulation, 22*(2), 205–214. doi: 10.1080/02652040400026442.

66. Niwa, T., Takeuchi, H., Hino, T., Kunou, N., & Kawashima, Y., (1993). Preparations of biodegradable nanospheres of water-soluble and insoluble drugs with D, L-lactide/ glycolide copolymer by a novel spontaneous emulsification solvent diffusion method, and the drug release behavior. *Journal of Controlled Release, 25*(1, 2), 89–98. doi: 10.1016/0168-3659(93)90097-O.

67. Murakami, H., Kobayashi, M., Takeuchi, H., & Kawashima, Y., (2000). Further application of a modified spontaneous emulsification solvent diffusion method to various types of PLGA and PLA polymers for preparation of nanoparticles. *Powder Technology, 107*(1), 137–143. doi: 10.1016/S0378-5173(99)00187-8.

68. Peltonen, L., Aitta, J., Hyvönen, S., Karjalainen, M., & Hirvonen, J., (2004). Improved entrapment efficiency of hydrophilic drug substance during nanoprecipitation of poly (I) lactide nanoparticles. *AAPS Pharmscitech, 5*(1), 115. doi: 10.1208/pt050116.

69. Benita, S., (2005). *Microencapsulation: Methods and Industrial Applications*. CRC Press.
70. Remington, J. P., (2006). *Remington: The Science and Practice of Pharmacy* (Vol. 1). Lippincott Williams & Wilkins.
71. Gupta, R. B., & Kompella, U. B. (2009). Nanoparticle Technology for Drug Delivery. CRC Press. *Drugs and the Pharmaceutical Science* (Vol. 159, pp. 53–78). Chapter 3. Supercritical Fluid Technology for Particle Engineering.
72. Garg, A., Visht, S., Sharma, P. K., & Kumar, N., (2011). Formulation, characterization and application on nanoparticle: A review. *Der Pharmacia Sinica, 2*(2), 17–26.
73. Jung, J., & Perrut, M., (2001). Particle design using supercritical fluids: Literature and patent survey. *The Journal of Supercritical Fluids, 20*(3), 179–219. doi: 10.1016/S0896-8446(01)00064-X.
74. Montes, A., Gordillo, M. D., Pereyra, C., & De La Ossa, E. M., (2011). Particles formation using supercritical fluids. In: *Mass Transfer-Advanced Aspects*. InTech.
75. Thakkar, F. M. V., Soni, T. G., Gohel, M. C., & Gandhi, T. R. (2009). Supercritical fluid technology: a promising approach to enhance the drug solubility. *Journal of Pharmaceutical Sciences and Research, 1*(4), 1–14.
76. Kongsombut, B., Tsutsumi, A., Suankaew, N., & Charinpanitkul, T., (2009). Encapsulation of SiO_2 and TiO_2 fine powders with poly (DL-lactic-co-glycolic acid) by rapid expansion of supercritical CO_2 incorporated with ethanol cosolvent. *Industrial & Engineering Chemistry Research, 48*(24), 11230–11235. doi: 10.1021/ie900690v.
77. Wen, Z., Liu, B., Zheng, Z., You, X., Pu, Y., & Li, Q., (2010). Preparation of liposomes entrapping essential oil from *Atractylodes macrocephala* koidz by modified RESS technique. *Chemical Engineering Research and Design, 88*(8), 1102–1107. doi: 10.1016/j.cherd.2010.01.020.
78. Helfgen, B., Türk, M., & Schaber, K., (2003). Hydrodynamic and aerosol modelling of the rapid expansion of supercritical solutions (RESS-process). *The Journal of Supercritical Fluids, 26*(3), 225–242. doi: 10.1016/S0896-8446(02)00159-6.
79. Le, P. K., & Le, K. A., (2015). The effect of rapid expansion of supercritical solution (RESS) parameter on sub-micron ibuprofen particle forming. *Journal of Chemical Engineering & Process Technology, 6*(1), 1. doi: 10.4172/2157-7048.1000220.
80. Thies, J., & Müller, B. W., (1998). Size controlled production of biodegradable microparticles with supercritical gases. *European Journal of Pharmaceutics and Biopharmaceutics, 45*(1), 67–74. doi: 10.1016/S0939-6411(97)00124-0.
81. Choi, H. S., Liu, W., Liu, F., Nasr, K., Misra, P., Bawendi, M. G., & Frangioni, J. V., (2010). Design considerations for tumor-targeted nanoparticles. *Nature Nanotechnology, 5*(1), 42–47. doi: 10.1038/nnano.2009.314.
82. Zhang, Q., Shen, Z., & Nagai, T., (2001). Prolonged hypoglycemic effect of insulin-loaded polybutylcyanoacrylate nanoparticles after pulmonary administration to normal rats. *International Journal of Pharmaceutics, 218*(1), 75–80. Doi:0.1016/S0378-5173(01)00614-7.
83. Nagavarma, B. V. N., Yadav, H. K., Ayaz, A., Vasudha, L. S., & Shivakumar, H. G., (2012). Different techniques for preparation of polymeric nanoparticles: A review. *Asian J. Pharm. Clin. Res., 5*(3), 16–23.
84. Gaudin, F., & Sintes-Zydowicz, N., (2008). Core-shell biocompatible polyurethane nanocapsules obtained by interfacial step polymerization in miniemulsion. *Colloids and Surfaces A: Physicochemical and Engineering Aspects, 331*(1), 133–142. doi: 10.1016/j.colsurfa.2008.07.028.

85. Swati, T., & Vinay, K. P., (2016). Nanoparticles: An overview of preparation. *Research and Reviews: Journal of Pharmaceutics and Nanotechnology, 4*(2). Reviews on pharmaceutics and nanotechnology.

86. Medina, C., Santos-Martinez, M. J., Radomski, A., Corrigan, O. I., & Radomski, M. W., (2007). Nanoparticles: Pharmacological and toxicological significance. *British Journal of Pharmacology, 150*(5), 552–558. doi: 10.1038/sj.bjp.0707130.

87. Calvo, P., Vila-Jato, J. L., & Alonso, M. J., (1997). Evaluation of cationic polymer-coated nanocapsules as ocular drug carriers. *International Journal of Pharmaceutics, 153*(1), 41–50. doi: 10.1016/S0378-5173(97)00083-5.

88. Mainardes, R. M., & Evangelista, R. C., (2005). PLGA nanoparticles containing praziquantel: Effect of formulation variables on size distribution. *International Journal of Pharmaceutics, 290*(1), 137–144. doi: 10.1016/j.ijpharm.2004.11.027.

89. Budhian, A., Siegel, S. J., & Winey, K. I., (2007). Haloperidol-loaded PLGA nanoparticles: Systematic study of particle size and drug content. *International Journal of Pharmaceutics, 336*(2), 367–375. doi: 10.1016/j.ijpharm.2006.11.061.

90. Tewes, F., Munnier, E., Antoon, B., Okassa, L. N., Cohen-Jonathan, S., Marchais, H., & Chourpa, I., (2007). Comparative study of doxorubicin-loaded poly (lactide-co-glycolide) nanoparticles prepared by single and double emulsion methods. *European Journal of Pharmaceutics and Biopharmaceutics, 66*(3), 488–492. doi: 10.1016/j.ejpb.2007.02.016.

91. Lokhande, A. B., Mishra, S., Kulkarni, R. D., & Naik, J. B., (2013). Influence of different viscosity grade ethylcellulose polymers on encapsulation and *in vitro* release study of drug loaded nanoparticles. *Journal of Pharmacy Research, 7*(5), 414–420. doi/10.1016/j.jopr.2013.04.050.

92. Rafiei, P., & Haddadi, A., (2017). Pharmacokinetic consequences of PLGA nanoparticles in docetaxel drug delivery. *Pharmaceutical Nanotechnology, 5*(1), 3–23.

93. Qu, N., Lee, R. J., Sun, Y., Cai, G., Wang, J., Wang, M., & Teng, L., (2016). Cabazitaxel-loaded human serum albumin nanoparticles as a therapeutic agent against prostate cancer. *International Journal of Nanomedicine, 11*, 3451. doi: 10.2147/IJN.S105420.

94. Yadav, K. S., & Sawant, K. K., (2010). Modified nanoprecipitation method for preparation of cytarabine-loaded PLGA nanoparticles. *AAPS Pharmscitech, 11*(3), 1456–1465. doi: 10.1208/s12249-010-9519-4.

95. Betancourt, T., Brown, B., & Brannon-Peppas, L., (2007). Doxorubicin-loaded PLGA nanoparticles by nanoprecipitation: Preparation, characterization and *in vitro* evaluation. *Nanomedicine, 2*(2), 219–232. doi: 10.2217/17435889.2.2.219.

96. Akbari, Z., Amanlou, M., Karimi-Sabet, J., Golestani, A., & Shariaty, N. M., (2015). Production of ibuprofen-loaded solid lipid nanoparticles using rapid expansion of supercritical solution. In: *Journal of Nano Research* (Vol. 31, pp. 15–29). Trans Tech Publications. doi: 10.4028/www.scientific.net/JNanoR.31.15.

97. Akbari, Z., Amanlou, M., Karimi-Sabet, J., Golestani, A., & Niasar, M. S., (2014). Characterization of carbamazepine-loaded solid lipid nanoparticles prepared by rapid expansion of supercritical solution. *Tropical Journal of Pharmaceutical Research, 13*(12), 1955–1961. doi: 10.4314/tjpr.v13i12.1.

98. Oh, Y. S., Lee, S. Y., Ryu, J. H., & Lim, G. B., (2004). Preparation of drug loaded poly (L-lactide) nanoparticles using pure and modified supercritical CO_2. In: *Asian Pacific Confederation of Chemical Engineering Congress Program and Abstracts* (pp. 582–582). The Society of Chemical Engineers, Japan. doi.10.11491/apcche.2004.0.582.0.

99. Zhao, X., Zu, Y., Jiang, R., Wang, Y., Li, Y., Li, Q., & Zhang, X., (2011). Preparation and physicochemical properties of 10-hydroxycamptothecin (HCPT) nanoparticles by supercritical antisolvent (SAS) process. *International Journal of Molecular Sciences, 12*(4), 2678–2691. doi: 10.3390/ijms12042678.

100. Yang, S. C., Ge, H. X., Hu, Y., Jiang, X. Q., & Yang, C. Z., (2000). Doxorubicin-loaded poly (butyl cyanoacrylate) nanoparticles produced by emulsifier-free emulsion polymerization. *Journal of Applied Polymer Science, 78*(3), 517–526. doi: 10.1002/1097-4628 (20001017)78:3<517::AID-APP60>3.0.CO;2-3.

101. Krause, H. J., Schwarz, A., & Rohdewald, P., (1986). Interfacial polymerization, a useful method for the preparation of polymethyl cyanoacrylate nanoparticles. *Drug Development and Industrial Pharmacy, 12*(4), 527–552. doi: 10.3109/03639048609048026.

102. Mehrotra, A., & Pandit, J. K., (2015). Preparation and characterization and biodistribution Studies of lomustine loaded PLGA nanoparticles by interfacial deposition method. *Journal of Nanomedicine & Biotherapeutic Discovery, 5*(4), 1. doi: 10.4172/2155-983X.1000138.

103. Sun, L., Chen, Y., Zhou, Y., Guo, D., Fan, Y., Guo, F., & Chen, W., (2017). Preparation of 5-fluorouracil-loaded chitosan nanoparticles and study the sustained release *in vitro* and *in vivo*. *Asian Journal of Pharmaceutical Sciences*. doi.10.1016/j.ajps.2017.04.002.

104. Salar, R. K., & Kumar, N., (2016). Synthesis and characterization of vincristine loaded folic acid-chitosan conjugated nanoparticles. *Resource-Efficient Technologies, 2*(4), 199–214. doi: 10.1016/j.reffit.2016.10.006.

105. Eslamian, M., & Shekarriz, M., (2009). Recent advances in nanoparticle preparation by spray and microemulsion methods. *Recent Patents on Nanotechnology, 3*(2), 99–115.

106. Broadhead, J., Edmond, R. S. K., & Rhodes, C. T., (1992). The spray drying of pharmaceuticals. *Drug Development and Industrial Pharmacy, 18*(11, 12), 1169–1206. doi: 10.3109/03639049209046327.

107. Kumar, A., Yadav, N., Bhatt, M., Mishra, N. K., Chaudhary, P., & Singh, R., (2015). Sol-gel derived nanomaterials and it's applications: A review. *Research Journal of Chemical Sciences*.

108. Owens, G. J., Singh, R. K., Foroutan, F., Alqaysi, M., Han, C. M., Mahapatra, C., & Knowles, J. C., (2016). Sol-gel based materials for biomedical applications. *Progress in Materials Science, 77*, 1–79. doi: 10.1016/j.pmatsci.2015.12.001.

109. Singh, L. P., Bhattacharyya, S. K., Kumar, R., Mishra, G., Sharma, U., Singh, G., & Ahalawat, S., (2014). Sol-gel processing of silica nanoparticles and their applications. *Advances in Colloid and Interface Science, 214*, 17–37. doi: 10.1016/j.cis.2014.10.007.

110. *Introduction to Sol-Gel.* (2006). https://www.researchgate.net › download › sol++(1) (accessed on 30 July 2021).

111. Binns, C., (2010). *Introduction to Nanoscience and Nanotechnology* (Vol. 14). John Wiley & Sons. Binns C.

112. Gupta, V. K., Jain, R., Mittal, A., Saleh, T. A., Nayak, A., Agarwal, S., & Sikarwar, S., (2012). Photocatalytic degradation of toxic dye amaranth on TiO_2/UV in aqueous suspensions. *Materials Science and Engineering: C, 32*(1), 12–17. doi: 10.1016/j.msec.2011.08.018.

113. *Nanoparticle Production–How Nanoparticles are Made.* nanowerk. http://www.nanowerk.com/how_nanoparticles_are_made.php (accessed on 30 July 2021).

114. Nekkanti, V., Vabalaboina, V., & Pillai, R., (2012). Drug nanoparticles: An overview. In: *The Delivery of Nanoparticles*. InTech.

115. Gall, V., Runde, M., & Schuchmann, H. P., (2016). Extending applications of high-pressure homogenization by using simultaneous emulsification and mixing (SEM)—An overview. *Processes, 4*(4), 46. doi: 10.3390/pr4040046.

116. Aher, S. S., Malsane, S. T., & Saudagar, R. B., (2017). Nanosuspension: An overview. *Asian Journal of Research in Pharmaceutical Science, 7*(2), 81–86. doi: 10.5958/2231-5659.2017.00012.1.

117. Jahanshahi, M., & Babaei, Z., (2008). Protein nanoparticle: A unique system as drug delivery vehicles. *African Journal of Biotechnology, 7*(25).

118. Ashish, P., et al., (2017). Polymeric nanoparticles for tumor targeting: A review. *Int. J. Drug. Dev. & Res., 9*, 1.

119. Sailaja, A. K., & Amareshwar, P., (2012). Preparation of alginate nanoparticles by desolvation technique using acetone as desolvating agent. *Asian Journal of Pharmaceutical and Clinical Research, 5*(2), 132–134.

120. Coester, C. J., Langer, K., Von, B. H., & Kreuter, J., (2000). Gelatin nanoparticles by two-step desolvation a new preparation method, surface modifications and cell uptake. *Journal of Microencapsulation, 17*(2), 187–193. doi: 10.1080/026520400288427.

121. Sailaja, A. K., & Amareshwar, P., (2012). Preparation of BSA nanoparticles by desolvation technique using acetone as desolvating agent. *Int. J. Pharm. Sci. Nanotechnol., 5*, 1643–1647.

122. Krishnamoorthy, K., & Mahalingam, M., (2015). Selection of a suitable method for the preparation of polymeric nanoparticles: Multi-criteria decision making approach. *Advanced Pharmaceutical Bulletin, 5*(1), 57. doi: 10.5681%2Fapb.2015.008.

123. Liu, M., Zhou, Z., Wang, X., Xu, J., Yang, K., Cui, Q., & Zhang, Q., (2007). Formation of poly (L, D-lactide) spheres with controlled size by direct dialysis. *Polymer, 48*(19), 5767–5779. doi: 10.1016/j.polymer.2007.07.053.

124. Choi, S. W., & Kim, J. H., (2007). Design of surface-modified poly (D, L-lactide-co-glycolide) nanoparticles for targeted drug delivery to bone. *Journal of Controlled Release, 122*(1), 24–30. doi.10.1016/j.jconrel.2007.06.003.

125. Desai, K. G. H., & Park, H. J., (2005). Preparation and characterization of drug-loaded chitosan-tripolyphosphate microspheres by spray drying. *Drug Development Research, 64*(2), 114–128. doi: 10.1002/ddr.10416.

126. Dement'eva, O. V., Senchikhin, I. N., Kartseva, M. E., Ogarev, V. A., Zaitseva, A. V., Matushkina, N. N., & Rudoy, V. M., (2016). A new method for loading mesoporous silica nanoparticles with drugs: Sol-gel synthesis using drug micelles as a template. *Colloid Journal, 78*(5), 586–595. doi: 10.1134/S1061933X16050045.

127. Gupta, S., Kesarla, R., Chotai, N., Misra, A., & Omri, A., (2017). Systematic approach for the formulation and optimization of solid lipid nanoparticles of efavirenz by high pressure homogenization using design of experiments for brain targeting and enhanced bioavailability. *BioMed Research International, 2017*. doi: 10.1155/2017/5984014.

128. Maghsoudi, A., Shojaosadati, S. A., & Farahani, E. V., (2008). 5-Fluorouracil-loaded BSA nanoparticles: Formulation optimization and *in vitro* release study. *AAPS Pharmscitech, 9*(4), 1092–1096. doi: 10.1208/s12249-008-9146-5.

129. Newton, M. J., & Bhupinder, K., (2017). Acyclovir solid lipid nanoparticles for skin drug delivery: Fabrication, characterization and *in vitro* study. *Recent Patents on Drug Delivery & Formulation.*

130. Lotha, R., Sundaramoorthy, N. S., Shamprasad, B. R., Nagarajan, S., & Sivasubramanian, A., (2018). Plant nutraceuticals (Quercetin and Afzelin) capped silver nanoparticles exert

potent antibiofilm effect against foodborne pathogen *Salmonella enterica* serovar Typhi and curtail planktonic growth in zebrafish infection model. *Microbial Pathogenesis, 120*, 109–118.

131. Sun, F., Ju, C., Chen, J., Liu, S., Liu, N., Wang, K., & Liu, C., (2012). Nanoparticles based on hydrophobic alginate derivative as nutraceutical delivery vehicle: Vitamin D3 loading. *Artificial Cells, Blood Substitutes, and Biotechnology, 40*(1, 2), 113–119.

132. Arroyo-Maya, I. J., & McClements, D. J., (2015). Biopolymer nanoparticles as potential delivery systems for anthocyanins: Fabrication and properties. *Food Research International, 69*, 1–8.

133. Gomes, L. P., Paschoalin, V. M. F., & Del, A. E. M., (2017). Chitosan nanoparticles: Production, physicochemical characteristics and nutraceutical applications. *Rev. Virtual Quim., 9*(1), 387–409.

134. Abd El-Salam, M. H., & El-Shibiny, S., (2012). Formation and potential uses of milk proteins as nano delivery vehicles for nutraceuticals: A review. *International Journal of Dairy Technology, 65*(1), 13–21.

135. Chen, L., (2009). Protein micro/nanoparticles for controlled nutraceutical delivery in functional foods. In: *Designing Functional Foods* (pp. 572–600). Woodhead Publishing.

136. Nunes, S., Madureira, A. R., Campos, D., Sarmento, B., Gomes, A. M., Pintado, M., & Reis, F., (2017). Solid lipid nanoparticles as oral delivery systems of phenolic compounds: Overcoming pharmacokinetic limitations for nutraceutical applications. *Critical Reviews in Food Science and Nutrition, 57*(9), 1863–1873.

137. Teng, Z., Luo, Y., & Wang, Q., (2012). Nanoparticles synthesized from soy protein: Preparation, characterization, and application for nutraceutical encapsulation. *Journal of Agricultural and Food Chemistry, 60*(10), 2712–2720.

138. Chen, L., & Subirade, M., (2005). Chitosan/β-lactoglobulin core-shell nanoparticles as nutraceutical carriers. *Biomaterials, 26*(30), 6041–6053.

139. Nair, H. B., Sung, B., Yadav, V. R., Kannappan, R., Chaturvedi, M. M., & Aggarwal, B. B., (2010). Delivery of anti-inflammatory nutraceuticals by nanoparticles for the prevention and treatment of cancer. *Biochemical Pharmacology, 80*(12), 1833–1843.

140. Liu, G., Huang, W., Babii, O., Gong, X., Tian, Z., Yang, J., & Chen, L., (2018). Novel protein-lipid composite nanoparticles with an inner aqueous compartment as delivery systems of hydrophilic nutraceutical compounds. *Nanoscale, 10*(22), 10629–10640.

141. Mokhtari, S., Jafari, S. M., & Assadpour, E., (2017). Development of a nutraceutical nano-delivery system through emulsification/internal gelation of alginate. *Food Chemistry, 229*, 286–295.

142. Levinson, Y., Israeli-Lev, G., & Livney, Y. D., (2014). Soybean β-conglycinin nanoparticles for delivery of hydrophobic nutraceuticals. *Food Biophysics, 9*(4), 332–340.

143. Teng, Z., Luo, Y., & Wang, Q., (2013). Carboxymethyl chitosan-soy protein complex nanoparticles for the encapsulation and controlled release of vitamin D3. *Food Chemistry, 141*(1), 524–532.

144. Liu, L. L., Li, X. T., Zhang, N., & Tang, C. H., (2019). Novel soy β-conglycinin nanoparticles by ethanol-assisted disassembly and reassembly: Outstanding nanocarriers for hydrophobic nutraceuticals. *Food Hydrocolloids, 91*, 246–255.

145. Huang, X., Huang, X., Gong, Y., Xiao, H., McClements, D. J., & Hu, K., (2016). Enhancement of curcumin water dispersibility and antioxidant activity using core-shell protein-polysaccharide nanoparticles. *Food Research International, 87*, 1–9.

146. Summerlin, N., Qu, Z., Pujara, N., Sheng, Y., Jambhrunkar, S., McGuckin, M., & Popat, A., (2016). Colloidal mesoporous silica nanoparticles enhance the biological activity of resveratrol. *Colloids and Surfaces B: Biointerfaces, 144*, 1–7.

147. Liu, F., Ma, D., Luo, X., Zhang, Z., He, L., Gao, Y., & McClements, D. J., (2018). Fabrication and characterization of protein-phenolic conjugate nanoparticles for co-delivery of curcumin and resveratrol. *Food Hydrocolloids, 79*, 450–461.

148. Tyagi, N., De, R., Begun, J., & Popat, A., (2017). Cancer therapeutics with epigallo-catechin-3-gallate encapsulated in biopolymeric nanoparticles. *International Journal of Pharmaceutics, 518*(1, 2), 220–227.

149. Teng, Z., Li, Y., Luo, Y., Zhang, B., & Wang, Q., (2013). Cationic β-lactoglobulin nanoparticles as a bioavailability enhancer: Protein characterization and particle formation. *Biomacromolecules, 14*(8), 2848–2856.

150. Li, Q., Liu, C. G., Huang, Z. H., & Xue, F. F., (2011). Preparation and characterization of nanoparticles based on hydrophobic alginate derivative as carriers for sustained release of vitamin D3. *Journal of Agricultural and Food Chemistry, 59*(5), 1962–1967.

151. Neves, A. R., Lúcio, M., Martins, S., Lima, J. L. C., & Reis, S., (2013). Novel resveratrol nanodelivery systems based on lipid nanoparticles to enhance its oral bioavailability. *International Journal of Nanomedicine, 8*, 177.

152. Chen, J., Zheng, J., McClements, D. J., & Xiao, H., (2014). Tangeretin-loaded protein nanoparticles fabricated from zein/β-lactoglobulin: Preparation, characterization, and functional performance. *Food Chemistry, 158*, 466–472.

153. Chen, S., Li, Q., McClements, D. J., Han, Y., Dai, L., Mao, L., & Gao, Y., (2020). Co-delivery of curcumin and piperine in zein-carrageenan core-shell nanoparticles: Formation, structure, stability and *in vitro* gastrointestinal digestion. *Food Hydrocolloids, 99*, 105334.

154. Yang, J., Zhou, Y., & Chen, L., (2014). Elaboration and characterization of barley protein nanoparticles as an oral delivery system for lipophilic bioactive compounds. *Food & Function, 5*(1), 92–101.

155. Liu, G., Yang, J., Wang, Y., Liu, X., & Chen, L., (2019). Protein-lipid composite nanoparticles for the oral delivery of vitamin B12: Impact of protein succinylation on nanoparticle physicochemical and biological properties. *Food Hydrocolloids, 92*, 189–197.

156. Huang, X., Liu, Y., Zou, Y., Liang, X., Peng, Y., McClements, D. J., & Hu, K., (2019). Encapsulation of resveratrol in zein/pectin core-shell nanoparticles: Stability, bioaccessibility, and antioxidant capacity after simulated gastrointestinal digestion. *Food Hydrocolloids, 93*, 261–269.

157. Tan, C., Xie, J., Zhang, X., Cai, J., & Xia, S., (2016). Polysaccharide-based nanoparticles by chitosan and gum Arabic polyelectrolyte complexation as carriers for curcumin. *Food Hydrocolloids, 57*, 236–245.

158. Nazemiyeh, E., Eskandani, M., Sheikhloie, H., & Nazemiyeh, H., (2016). Formulation and physicochemical characterization of lycopene-loaded solid lipid nanoparticles. *Advanced Pharmaceutical Bulletin, 6*(2), 235.

159. Lacatusu, I., Mitrea, E., Badea, N., Stan, R., Oprea, O., & Meghea, A., (2013). Lipid nanoparticles based on omega-3 fatty acids as effective carriers for lutein delivery. Preparation and *in vitro* characterization studies. *Journal of Functional Foods, 5*(3), 1260–1269.

160. Teng, Z., Luo, Y., Li, Y., & Wang, Q., (2016). Cationic beta-lactoglobulin nanoparticles as a bioavailability enhancer: Effect of surface properties and size on the transport and delivery *in vitro. Food Chemistry, 204,* 391–399.

161. Campos, D. A., Madureira, A. R., Gomes, A. M., Sarmento, B., & Pintado, M. M., (2014). Optimization of the production of solid witepsol nanoparticles loaded with rosmarinic acid. *Colloids and Surfaces B: Biointerfaces, 115,* 109–117.

162. Kumari, A., Yadav, S. K., Pakade, Y. B., Kumar, V., Singh, B., Chaudhary, A., & Yadav, S. C., (2011). Nanoencapsulation and characterization of Albizia chinensis isolated antioxidant quercitrin on PLA nanoparticles. *Colloids and Surfaces B: Biointerfaces, 82*(1), 224–232.

163. Peng, S., Li, Z., Zou, L., Liu, W., Liu, C., & McClements, D. J., (2018). Enhancement of curcumin bioavailability by encapsulation in sophorolipid-coated nanoparticles: An *in vitro* and *in vivo* study. *Journal of Agricultural and Food Chemistry, 66*(6), 1488–1497.

CHAPTER 5

Polymeric Nanoparticles-Based Nutraceutical Delivery System

MAHESH P. MORE,[1,2] PRASHANT K. DESHMUKH,[2] PRAJAKTA JOSHI,[3] and PRASAD A. POFALI[4]

[1]Department of Pharmaceutics, SVKM's Institute of Pharmacy, Dhule, Maharashtra–424001, India

[2]Department of Pharmaceutics, H.R. Patel Institute of Pharmaceutical Education and Research, Shirpur, Maharashtra–425405, India

[3]Private Practitioner, VIBGYOR Pediatric and Family Dental Clinic, Mumbai–400024, Maharashtra, India

[4]National Institute of Immunohematology, Mumbai, Maharashtra, India, E-mail: prasad.pofali@gmail.com

ABSTRACT

Numerous nanotechnology-based initiatives for the delivery of nutraceuticals begun in early 2000. US market growth for delivery of nanocoatings on food beverages goes around $1 billion and is expected to increase up to $20 billion in the upcoming years. This is one of the fastest-growing industries after pharmaceuticals. Use of polymer or surfactant for encapsulation or enhancing the interaction with lipids, protein, or polysaccharides within formulation increases the stability of nutraceuticals. The applicability of polymers or surfactants to form a nanostructured material opens up new avenues in functional nanoparticulate delivery. Applicability of functional formulation enhances the delivery of nutraceuticals to desired site of absorption or action. The nanofabricated polymeric systems could engross the bioavailability of multiple nutraceuticals within formulations and dignify the underlying mechanism of delivery. The preparation of polymeric nanoparticulate delivery have two essential objectives, first to make a solid network and second to avoid aggregation by incorporating surfactant or emulsifier. Formulations containing Nutraceuticals like probioticsprobiotics and antioxidants are available into the market. These marketed formulations are considered safe and maybe act as substitute for prescription drugs. This chapter highlights the recent development of nanotechnological approaches for delivery of nutraceuticals. The nanotechnological approaches specifically include the use of polymers for modulating nutraceuticals, which helps in increasing the bioavailability, targetability, oral absorption, etc. The chapters also entitle the preparation methods and mechanism of stabilization of nutraceuticals for oral and targeted delivery, further emphasizes the FDA's current good manufacturing practices (GMPs) for nutraceutical formulations.

5.1 INTRODUCTION

Technological advancement in nanodelivery approaches reaches at the outfit of commercial markets for biomedical applications as well as enhancing the many areas of research. Nanotechnology is evident with the development of innovative solutions and availing the best product as per consumer needs. Heftily, the formulations designed in nutraceutical delivery using nanotechnological approaches, generally for the aim of enhancing the bioavailability and permeability. The emerging field of nanotechnology which was already been developed and utilized for enhancing bioavailability, dosing frequency, controlled release, targeted drug delivery, biodistribution, etc., for pharmaceuticals. Nutraceuticals are also dwelling with development to enhance the nutritional values and support the regulation of biocellular functions normally. Two categories of process generally used for preparation of nano-formulation, top-down and bottom-up methods. Top-down approaches specifically designed for converting larger solid particles into smaller portions by using milling or attrition, chemical methods, and volatilization of solid, etc. While in bottom-up approaches elaborates about condensation or polycondensation of atoms or molecules at liquid or gas phases to form a cluster. The mechanical approaches also underpin the fabrication of nanoparticles for active delivery of biomolecules.

From a couple of years, enormous development has been observed on dietary supplements (DS) and functional food ingredients. The food ingredient or fortified food ingredients which provide additional medical benefits other than food supplements helps in assisting in the treatment of disease or disorder is known as 'nutraceutical.' Nutritional and therapeutic value is a center point of evaluating the nutraceuticals. The customer demands are ever-increasing as the technological field developing. To drive customer focus, nutraceutical combined nutrition and pharmaceutical is emerging as one of the fastest-growing fields. It provides health benefits, nutrition, and therapeutic activity. Figure 5.1 shows the current necessity of nanonutraceuticals.

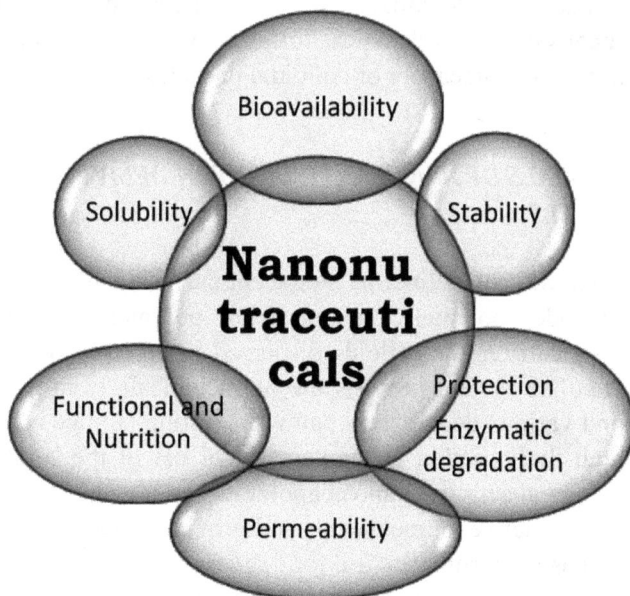

FIGURE 5.1 Potential attributes of nanonutraceuticals.

Bioactive nutraceutical preservation is an important goal to improve the functionality and maintaining the enrichment. The nutraceutical delivery provides a simplistic way of developing functional foods containing vitamins, probioticsprobiotics, bioactive peptides, antioxidants, etc., for physiological benefits with incurring side effects. Also, neutralize the abnormalities in human body, which beneficially reduces the risk of disease condition.

Generally, clear liquid oral formulations containing nutraceutical could be potentially delivering in market. With the round of possibilities, nutraceuticals generally extracted from agriproducts or its binary intermediates, are somehow contains a small amount of odor. Which can be potentially minimize during preparation of nanonutraceutical to enhance the customer acceptance. Clear beverages are another acceptance criterion of customer for nutraceutical formulation. The formulator must focus these issues to make market relevant product [1].

Nutraceutical formulation is classified into major categories: Nanocarriers for nutraceutical delivery, and functional packaging nanomaterials for nutraceutical protection. Manufacturers are applying nanotechnology in surveying food products via increasing the quality and durability of packaging materials. As far as concerned with the nanocarrier-based nutraceutical delivery, it can surely differentiate into nanoparticles containing nutraceuticals, nanoencapsulated nutraceutical formulation and clear liquid system containing dispersed nanocarrier or colloidal particles.

5.1.1 POTENTIALS OF NANOPARTICULATE IN DELIVERING NUTRACEUTICALS

The preferential way of delivering nutraceutical using nanotechnological approaches includes polymeric nanoparticles, polymeric clusters, conjugates, lipid nanocarriers, or colloids dispersed in an aqueous or oil base. The nanoparticulate system protects the nutraceuticals from autoxidation, hydrolysis, and various degradation pathways during storage and transportation, although the variation in temperature or pH of the solution might reduce the biological activity. Nanotechnological approaches can potentially encapsulate the bioactive nutraceuticals and provide sustained or controlled release effects based on substrate use for delivery.

They may help to enhance bioavailability, bioactivity, and stability of bioactive compounds along with shelf life, consumer acceptability, functionality, nutritional value, and safety of food systems. The nanocarrier-based nutraceuticals can be encapsulated or crosslinked or conjugated with carrier molecules which provides controlled release effect for encapsulated materials. Figure 5.2 elucidate the manufacturing, delivery, and storage attributes of the current process. This simply explains the necessity to develop nano-based approaches for nutraceutical delivery. Nutraceuticals processed using nanotechnological approaches could change the color and sensory characteristics. While the nanoformulations could improve the nutritional functionality as well as therapeutic value. It also stabilizes the nutraceutical nanoformulations by preventing bacterial attack or fungus/pathogenic growth [2].

Growing interest of nutraceutical use, availability from natural sources and high nutritional value with low side effects is enriching the lives of human being. As an isolated food ingredient or constituents, nutraceuticals have low bioavailability, solubility, and stability with limited delivery aspects hampers its usability and application arena. Photodegradation and lower systemic doses are another discriminating factor for formulation design. As these two parameters might not be focused during formulation design.

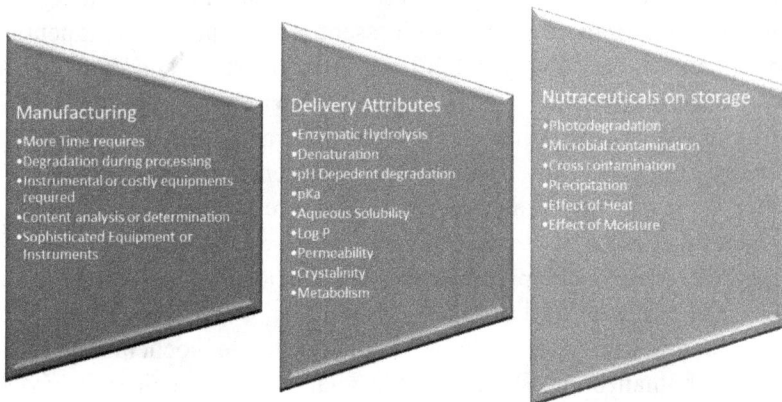

FIGURE 5.2   Current attributes of nutraceutical delivery.

Nanoencapsulation of nutraceuticals is a promising concept to encapsulate or protect the nutraceutical from degradation or environmental effects. Although nanoencapsulation also enhances the bioavailability and also endures the targeting specificity depends on surface modifier available [3].

Nanoprocessing can avoid degradation by free radicalization mechanism. The nanoformulations containing nutraceuticals possess better anti-aging properties. After encapsulated with nanocarrier, antimutagenic potential was likely enhanced with additionally provides increasing neurological function as well as endocrine and immunomodulatory functions. The nanoformulations containing nutraceuticals have better physical stability in solution or solid form, which also provides increasing absorption from cell surfaces. The nanocarrier as also avoids engulf by excretory proteins or enzymes.

Nutraceutical industry is an ever-increasing market due to enhanced potency and stability by the use of nanotechnological approaches. The nanoformulations of nutraceuticals include polymeric, lipid, bilayer lipid, micelles, phospholipids complexes, metal complexes, polymeric complexes, etc.

As nanotechnology governs the tuning the physical attributes of molecules, somehow chemical structure did not affect during nanoprocessing. With very low permeability, rapid metabolism and instability at physiological pH which is a problem encountered with some of the phytochemicals; are poorly absorbed in the human body [4].

In a recent business review written by Richard Kaufman on commercial nano-based nutraceuticals developed by nanosphere health sciences,

USA, a team of researchers has developed a gel-based formula containing nanonutraceutical. The gel formula does not contain fillers, binders, or other additives such as preservatives or plasticizers or stability enhancing agent. The nanoformulations embedded with essential nutrients and therapeutically active agent, which directly solubilized in mainstream and enables direct delivery into the system. The nanoformulations containing nutraceuticals avoid extensive destruction in the liver and GI tract [5].

Omega 3 Fatty acids, specifically α-Linolenic acid, eicosapentaenoic acid (EPA) and docosahexaenoic acid (DHA) are essential for human nutrition. Fish oil enriched with omega 3 fatty acid components, use to deliver using nanocarrier-based approaches to avoid oxidation and deterioration of physical properties as well as rancidity [6].

Lipid-soluble and water-soluble vitamins regulate biochemical reactions within the human body. Water-soluble vitamins are specifically prone to leaching during washing blanching and cooking stages, some of them may be prone to oxidation. Vitamin A and E oxidizes in the presence of light, metal ions, while vitamin K is prone to degrade in fluorescent light. These nutraceuticals can be protected using nanocarriers-based delivery systems [7]. Figure 5.3 describes the impact of nanocarrier or nano packaging materials that could potentially enhance the nutraceutical delivery system.

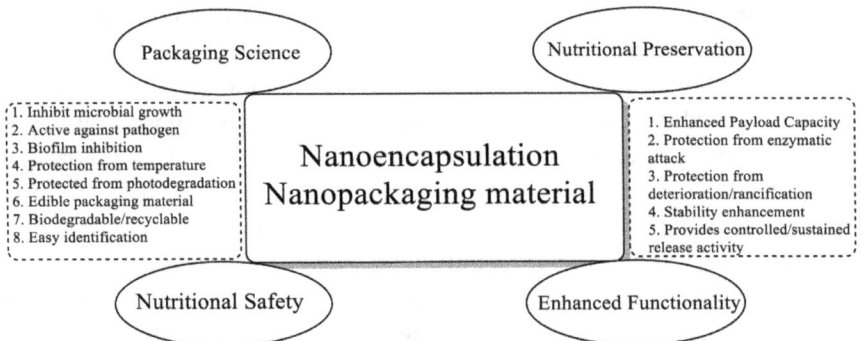

FIGURE 5.3   Implications of using nanocarrier or nanopackaging material for nutraceutical delivery.

5.1.2   *IMPLICATION AND TECHNIQUES FOR LARGE-SCALE PRODUCTIONS*

With the advent of numerous techniques and materials, researchers are working on potential techniques of commercialization for implementing nanotechnologies. By use of nanocarrier or asserted technique, one would improve the physicochemical character or stability concern over food ingredients. The nanotech industries from the US and other developed countries already have manufacturing units for food-based nanotechnologies at commercial scale, and few products are available in the market. Manipulating properties of substance at molecular scale sometimes shows beneficial effect or might become harmful, based on the use of processing conditions. Environmental Protection Agency (EPA) overseas on manufacturing criteria is the process harmful or produces toxic gases during manufacturing or not.

Molecular or atomic manipulation or tuning at lower level refers to nanotechnological processing, which helps in improving the processing capability of industry as well as reduces the manual efforts or physical energy required therein. The Nanoprocessing or nontechniques available or patented by researchers helps in improving the processing functionality, related to removing the odor or adding pertinent flavor to nanonutraceutical. It also improves traceability, shelf life, stability, etc. [8].

Critical processing parameters and critical attributes of food products, which is a major concern for transferring process from laboratory, level to commercial scale.

The industries are using statistical module for eliminating the potential defects during processing and validating the data. Few software packages like MATLAB, design of experiment (DoE) (Statease), Statgraphics, etc., were implemented for verification and validation of nanoprocessing approaches. The regulatory bodies are accepting such statistical-based analysis protocols and approving the dossiers for food manufacturers. Specificity to processing parameters are also underlie within these methodologies.

For commercial-scale production, many US-based nutraceutical manufacturers adopted the change and few products are available into the market.

5.2 TYPES OF POLYMERS USED IN DELIVERY OF NUTRACEUTICAL

Chitosan (CHT) is a golden macromolecule used as nanocarrier and itself is a nutraceutical agent. CHT is a marine polysaccharide containing acetyl D glucosamine crosslinked with D glucosamine via beta 1, 3 linkages. CHT is an acetylated derivate of chitin obtained from the exoskeleton of scribe or shellfish or marine organisms or extracted from fungi, etc. Storage conditions of many fruits was increased after CHT coating [9]. Recent findings on coacervates of CHT along with alpha and Beta-lactoglobulin forms polymers at isoelectric pH. Whey protein and CHT identified as nanocarriers for nutraceuticals delivery [10]. Tuning its structural configuration at nanoscale, researchers were consistently working on water-soluble CHT at nanoscale to enhance its effectiveness. Mucopolysaccharide already explored for pharmaceutical application and use in nanotechnological approaches nanocarriers for delivery of therapeutic agent. On the similar front marine CHT also has nutraceutical properties, like CHT itself act as antioxidant, lowers cholesterol level, antimicrobial, antifungal, anti-inflammatory properties. CHT inhibits the oxidation of substances via reactive oxygen species [11]. In an attempt to prove hypocholesterolemia, CHT efficiently entraps bile acid and decreases cholesterol absorption of the body. Due to the positive charge of CHT, it forms complex with bile acid, without absorption bile acid return to liver, which frequently decreases blood cholesterol level [12]. CHT shows prominent inhibitory potential against gram-positive and gram-negative bacteria [13].

Polyethylene glycol, polylactic acid, polylactideco-glycolide Polybeta benzyl aspartate, polycaprolactone, etc., synthetic versions of polymeric nanocarriers are reported for nutraceutical delivery. The casein polymeric core containing curcumin was delivered for better therapeutic potential [14].

Polycaprolactone-based nanocarrier delivers hydrophobic resveratrol into bloodstream. The Polyethylene coating enhances the systemic retention in the bloodstream. Although it also prevents sulfate and glucuronic metabolism after oral absorption [15].

Vitamin D 3 is more susceptible to light and temperature oleoyl alginate based nanocarrier efficiently protects from degradation. Noncovalent interaction between nanocarrier and Vitamin D3 provides burst release followed by controlled release [16].

Thymoquinone shows highest antioxidant potential after polylactide co glycolide nanoparticles (PLGA). PLGA nanoparticles show sustained release effect and improve bioavailability [17].

Dendrimer-based polymeric structure helps to enhance the payload capacity of nutraceuticals. Central core and hyper-branched macromolecules consist of hydrophobic core and hydrophilic branches. Nutraceutical loading on dendrimer follows passive loading or physical adsorption in which nutraceuticals directly are adsorbed on the branched structure via stearic hindrance. The active loading approach follows the crosslinking or conjugation in the presence of a specific crosslinking agent which forms appropriate covalent or hydrogen bonds in between them [18]. The curcumin also delivered via conjugate with PMMA (polymethyl methacrylate) shows 200-fold enhancement in solubility. The conjugated dendrimer demonstrates anticancer activity with the highest reactive oxygen species generation at intracellular level [19].

Milk protein or protein aggregates are another class of nanovehicles use for delivery of nutraceuticals, Casein, beta-casein, or whey proteins forms self-assembled structures either in the presence or in the absence of crosslinker in aqueous-organic environment. Milk proteins has the capability to bind or encapsulate hydrophobic substances via crosslinking or physical interactions. It mainly includes hydrogen bonds, hydrophobic interaction, and Van der Waals forces, governs through milk proteins. Unique structure and active binding sites on the surfaces have multiple payload capacity. Casein, whey protein, Lactoglobulin, Serum albumin, Immunoglobulin, fat globule membrane, etc., are major components found in milk proteins and use for delivery of nutraceuticals [20].

Lipid-based delivery system also shows proven nutraceutical delivery. As a critical aspect, nutraceuticals are measurably lipophilic in nature. Lipid-based delivery approaches amalgamate the process and encapsulate the maximum amount of nutrition converted into nanocarrier-based delivery. Due to enhanced lipid permeability at the cellular interface, an increased systemic concentration is observed. The lipid-based delivery system mainly includes solid lipid nanoparticles (SLNs), bilayer lipid membranes, liposomes, niosomes, phytosomes, etc. Phospholipid carriers can entrap the maximum amount of nutraceuticals based on the affinity towards to hydrophilic or hydrophobic end. Nature bixin encapsulated in SLN to enhance bioavailability. Trimyrisitin, glyceryl monostearate, soya, and egg lecithin were used to formulate bixin encapsulated SLN nanoparticles [21]. Curcumin activity also enhances after incorporating into SLN. Curcumin shows sustained-release effect at *in-vitro* effect [22].

The spherical bilayer of phospholipids encapsulates nutraceuticals at inner aqueous core or outer lipophilic shell. Prooxidant liposomes-based carotene was incorporated to prevent photo-oxidation. Lutine, beta Carotene, lycopene, and canthaxanthin individually form multilamellar vesicles (MLV), which increases the antioxidant property and provides a sustained release effect. Active delivery of Vitamin C is multilayered nanoliposome; desirable coating was achieved after simultaneous deposition of positive CHT negative sodium alginate. The multilayered nanoliposome vesicles applied to mandarin juice prevents peroxidation up to 90 days.

Polymeric hydrogel-based nutraceutical delivery increasing the arena and development of nutraceutical industries for therapeutic applications. The focus of simplistic approaches is to enhance the effectiveness. Certain topical approaches utilize polymeric hydrogel or aerogel for delivery of nutraceuticals. Physical entanglement and affinity of water deliver the nutraceutical in a sustained release manner [23].

Polyelectrolyte layer-by-layer technology is used to deliver multiple types of nutraceutical or therapeutic agents. Adsorption of oppositely charged layers on each other forms nanolaminated structures. The simplicity in techniques used to load multiple therapeutic in between the layers or inside the core. Multilayer nanolaminates containing folic acid-coated with simultaneous alginate and CHT show pH-dependent release of nutrients (Figure 5.4) [24].

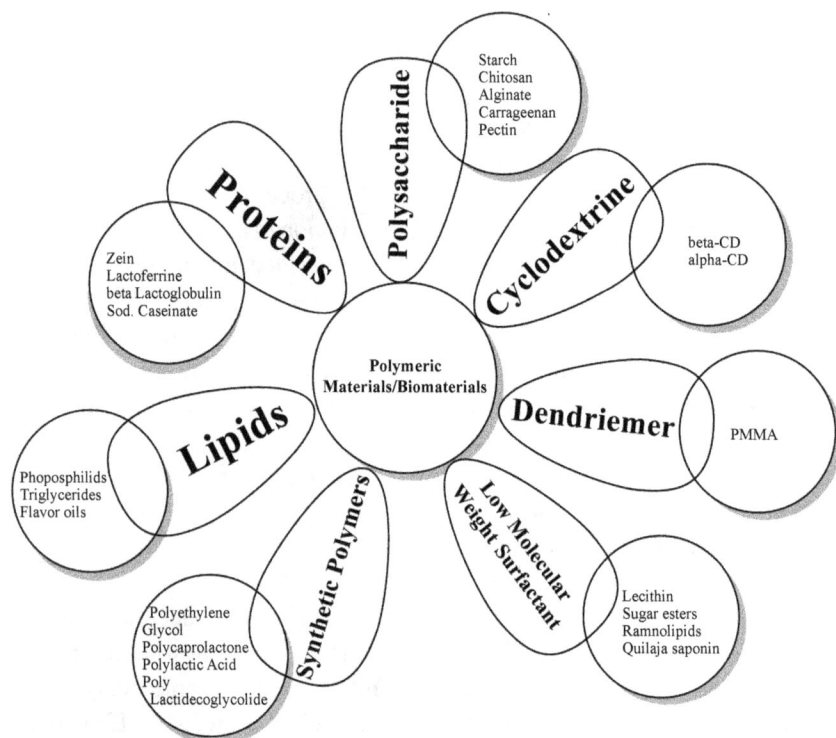

FIGURE 5.4   Different types of polymeric nanocarriers use for nutraceutical delivery.

5.3   MECHANISM OF NANOPARTICLE FORMATION AND ENTRAPMENT OF NUTRACEUTICALS

Nanoparticle formation is divided into top-down or bottom-up methodologies. Tuning of molecular or atom level could give a specific shape stabilized in the external environment. Shapes of nanomaterials might be spherical, cubes, tubes, etc., for pharmaceutical applications 1–100 nm particles have the highest acceptability due to stability and study available from a number of researchers. The mechanism behind polymeric nanoparticles formation is somewhat similar to the case use of drug entrapment and delivery approaches. Many sophisticated instruments or equipment are available for nanoencapsulation of bioactives. The encapsulated nanocarrier has a major function to protect the nutraceutical from degradation or detrimental effect during storage. Based on the interaction between nutraceutical and nanocarrier, it shows burst release, controlled or sustained release activity. The resultant nutraceutical is either entrapped inside the core of the nanocarrier or encapsulated within coated layer of nanomaterials.

Relatively polymers could form self-assembled structures or crosslinked in the presence or absence of crosslinking agent to get specific unique structure. The charged polymers such as CHT crosslinked with sodium tripolyphosphate using ionic gelation method. The CHT is cationic polymer activated at a lower pH range, while tripolyphosphate ions interact with tertiary amine of CHT and form noncovalent bonds. By using specialized techniques such as homogenization, ultrasonication, and vortexing forms a spherical structure. The CHT nanoparticles being potentially used for nutraceutical delivery as well as delivery of therapeutic agents [25].

Solvent evaporation is one of the useful techniques for PLGA and PLA nanocarriers' preparation. PLGA or PLA dissolved in dichloromethane (DCM), ethyl acetate, chloroform, or non-polar solvents. In the presence of surfactants such as polyvinyl alcohol or sodium lauryl sulfate (SLS), it forms solidified nanoparticles at reduced pressure [26].

Gelatin nanoparticles or nanodroplets were prepared after dissolving gelatin in warm water followed by fractionation in the presence of acetone or isopropyl alcohol. The gelatin was redissolved in water, after maintaining the isoelectric point of gelatin, subsequent addition or organic solvent nanoparticles starts to form. The nanodroplets further crosslinked with formaldehyde or glutaraldehyde [27]. Before the crosslinking with formaldehyde, one can add a nutraceutical agent for enhanced loading in gelatin nanoparticles.

Swellable water-soluble sodium alginate forms gel multivalent cation complex with calcium ions. At every drop of alginate, calcium chloride solution forms complex at the surfaces and regain particular shape for efficient delivery of nutraceuticals. For enhancing the encapsulation, nutraceutical dispersed in alginate solution and then followed crosslinking with calcium chloride solution [28].

Soy protein isolates dissolved in aqueous environment contain charged or polar groups. Upon desolvation in the presence of organic solvents, SPI hydrates and electrolysis of protein occurs. Attraction in between proteins starts to aggregate because of hydration of proteins and subsequent exposure of hydrophobic group at the surfaces. Resulting in increasing the particle size, the process can be reversed or stop at particular phased if starts to evaporate ethanol. In between these stages, nutraceuticals can be encapsulated efficiently. Curcumin dispersed in ethanol was slowly added to start encapsulation and hydration of proteins. Curcumin potentially interacts with hydrophobic surfaces of proteins and bound to their peripheral domains. Appropriate hardening of nanocarrier can be done via glutaraldehyde crosslinking with amide bond available on nanocarrier [29].

5.4 TECHNIQUES/METHODS FOR PREPARATION OF POLYMERIC NANOPARTICLES FOR NUTRACEUTICAL DELIVERY

Many approaches for the synthesis of polymeric nanoparticles to deliver nanonutrient in nutraceutical delivery have been studied so far. The use of nutraceuticals including polyphenols and antioxidants has been found to get significant potential in the treatment of neurodegenerative disorders and brain tumors [30]. We have described the recent approaches in Table 5.1.

Although various approaches have been invented, still there is enough scope with the advent of nanotechnology processes; nutraceuticals can be incorporated prior to nutrition-excipient compatibility studies.

5.5 BIOAVAILABILITY ASPECTS OF POLYMERIC NANOPARTICLES FOR NUTRACEUTICAL DELIVERY

The term bioavailability refers to the fraction of dose present at site of action [41]. Most of the nanoparticles have been found to increase the bioavailability since nanoparticles having smaller particle size with greater surface area. Conversion of food proteins into functional biomaterials has become a novel trend with loading and delivery of nutraceuticals at nanolevel. Poor bioavailability of nutraceuticals may be because of numerous physiological and/or physicochemical processes, low solubility in gastrointestinal tract (GIT), low permeability across epithelial cells or mucous layer and formation of insoluble complexes with other materials as well as biotransformation at molecular levels in GIT [42]. Nutraceutical bioavailability can be improved by controlling bioaccessibility (B*), absorption (A*) and transformation (T*) in GIT as compared to four classes of biopharmaceutical classification system (BCS) for drug. McClements et al. has described it in Table 5.2.

TABLE 5.1 Techniques Used for Synthesis of Nanonutraceuticals

SL. No.	Technique/Approach for Synthesis	Type of Nutraceutical/s	References
1.	Ultra-high-pressure homogenization was used to fabricate fermented soybean powder (FSP) and surfactants into an aqueous nanosuspension. homogenization pressure of 200 MPa and 15 cycles of homogenization produced the nanosuspension with desired particle size of 145.6 ± 1.5 nm and PDI 0.3 ± 1.1	Fermented soyabean nanonutraceutical	[31]
2.	Preparation process consisted of dispersion, desolvation, drug incorporation, crosslinking, and evaporation	Soy protein nanoparticles for drug encapsulation	[29]
3.	Use of enzymatically synthesized dextran nanoparticles to entrap a hydrophobic nutraceutical. Under optimal conditions (pH 5.2–6 and sucrose concentration >0.5 M), dextransucrase generated spherical dextran nanoparticles (100–450 nm).	The isoflavone genistein	[32]
4.	NPs were prepared by nanoprecipitation method and were characterized in terms of morphology and chemical properties	White tea extract-loaded NPs	[33]
5.	Nanoparticles were prepared by ionotropic crosslinking of two structurally different thiolated quaternary ammonium–chitosan conjugates. A hyaluronic acid solution, containing p-GSE or r-GSE, added to a stirred solution of each of the two–chitosan derivatives to obtain p- or r-GSE loaded nanoparticles (NP) of two types.	Polyphenol from red grape seed extract	[34]
6.	Nanoparticles fabricated using a hydrophobic protein (zein) as the core and a hydrophilic polysaccharide (pectin) as the shell. Particles were prepared by coating cationic zein nanoparticles with anionic pectin molecules using electrostatic deposition (pH 4).	Curcumin	[35]
7.	Biopolymer nanoparticles and caseinate-dextran conjugates were prepared using the Maillard reaction. Both the biopolymer nanoparticles and complexes protected trans-resveratrol from isomerization when exposed to UV light, with the nanoparticles being more effective.	Resveratrol	[36]
8.	Complex nanoparticles developed from carboxymethyl chitosan (CMCS) and soy protein isolate (SPI) by a simple ionic gelation method	Vitamin D3 (VD), a hydrophobic micronutrient	[37]

TABLE 5.1 *(Continued)*

SL. No.	Technique/Approach for Synthesis	Type of Nutraceutical/s	References
9.	Nonionic polymeric nanoparticles, poly(ethylene oxide)-poly(propylene oxide)-poly(ethylene oxide) (PEO-PPO-PEO) and poly(DL-lactic acid-co-glycolic acid) (PLGA) nanoparticles using	Kaempferol, a natural flavonoid	[38]
10.	Preparation of nanoemulsion using spontaneous emulsification process	Vitamin D	[39]
11.	Lipid polymer hybrid nanoparticles	Tartary buckwheat flavonoids	[40]

TABLE 5.2 The Nutraceutical Bioavailability Classification System based on Various Factors

Major Classes	Subclasses
B*	L-liberation
Bioaccessibility	S-solubilization
	I-interaction
A*	ML-mucous layer
Absorption	TJ-tight junction transport
	BP-bilayer permeability
	AT-active transporters
	ET-efflux transporters
T*	C-chemical degradation
Transformation	M-metabolism

5.6 CONCLUSION

The field of nutraceutical and food nanotechnology is showing significant growth due to higher interest of industry, academia, and industry. Major approaches have been taken for increasing the bioavailability of poorly water-soluble nutraceuticals however; very little efforts were taken on the improvement of soluble minerals and antioxidants such as calcium, iron, and isoflavones, respectively. Since the side effects of drugs are leading to cause more diseases, the future of organic sourced nutraceuticals has potential resulting into enhanced quality with nanotechnology advancement.

KEYWORDS

- biopharmaceutical classification system
- docosahexaenoic acid
- eicosapentaenoic acid
- Environmental Protection Agency
- gastrointestinal tract
- polymethyl methacrylate
- polylactide co glycolide nanoparticles

REFERENCES

1. Jampílek, J., & Kráľová, K., (2015). Application of nanotechnology in agriculture and food industry, its prospects and risks. *Ecological Chemistry and Engineering S., 22*(3), 321–361.

2. Chellaram, C., Murugaboopathi, G., John, A., Sivakumar, R., Ganesan, S., Krithika, S., et al., (2014). Significance of nanotechnology in the food industry. *APCBEE Procedia., 8*, 109–113.

3. Gopi, S., Amalraj, A., Haponiuk, J., & Thomas, S., (2016). Introduction of Nanotechnology in herbal drugs and nutraceutical: A review. *J. Nanomed. Biotherapeutic Discov., 6*, 2.

4. Kakkar, V., Modgill, N., & Kumar, M., (2016). From nutraceuticals to nanoceuticals. *Nanoscience in Food and Agriculture. 3*, 183–198. Springer.

5. (2019). *Future-proofing Nutraceuticals with Nanotechnology.* www.nutraceuticalbusiness review.com. Available from: https://www.nutraceuticalbusinessreview.com/technical/ article_page/Futureproofing_nutraceuticals_with_nanotechnology/103574 (accessed on 30 July 2021).

6. Ghorbanzade, T., Jafari, S. M., Akhavan, S., & Hadavi, R., (2017). Nano-encapsulation of fish oil in nano-liposomes and its application in fortification of yogurt. *Food Chemistry, 216*, 146–152.

7. Katouzian, I., & Jafari, S. M., (2016). Nano-encapsulation as a promising approach for targeted delivery and controlled release of vitamins. *Trends in Food Science & Technology, 53*, 34–48.

8. Weiss, J., Takhistov, P., & McClements, D. J., (2006). Functional materials in food nanotechnology. *Journal of Food Science, 71*(9), R107–R16.

9. Petriccione, M., De Sanctis, F., Pasquariello, M. S., Mastrobuoni, F., Rega, P., Scortichini, M., et al., (2015). The effect of chitosan coating on the quality and nutraceutical traits of sweet cherry during postharvest life. *Food and Bioprocess Technology, 8*(2), 394–408.

10. Lee, A. C., & Hong, Y. H., (2009). Coacervate formation of α-lactalbumin-chitosan and β-lactoglobulin-chitosan complexes. *Food Research International, 42*(5, 6), 733–738.

11. Park, P. J., Je, J. Y., & Kim, S. K., (2004). Free radical scavenging activities of differently deacetylated chitosans using an ESR spectrometer. *Carbohydrate Polymers, 55*(1), 17–22.

12. Liu, J. N., Xia, W. S., & Zhang, J. L., (2008). Effects of chitosans physicochemical properties on binding capacities of lipid and bile salts *in vitro* [J]. *Food Science, 1*.

13. Lim, S. H., & Hudson, S. M., (2003). Review of chitosan and its derivatives as antimicrobial agents and their uses as textile chemicals. *Journal of Macromolecular Science, Part C: Polymer Reviews, 43*(2), 223–269.

14. Sahu, A., Kasoju, N., & Bora, U., (2008). Fluorescence study of the curcumin- casein micelle complexation and its application as a drug nanocarrier to cancer cells. *Biomacromolecules, 9*(10), 2905–2912.

15. Lu, X., Ji, C., Xu, H., Li, X., Ding, H., Ye, M., et al., (2009). Resveratrol-loaded polymeric micelles protect cells from Aβ-induced oxidative stress. *International Journal of Pharmaceutics, 375*(1, 2), 89–96.

16. Li, Q., Liu, C. G., Huang, Z. H., & Xue, F. F., (2011). Preparation and characterization of nanoparticles based on hydrophobic alginate derivative as carriers for sustained release of vitamin D3. *Journal of Agricultural and Food Chemistry, 59*(5), 1962–1967.

17. Ganea, G. M., Fakayode, S. O., Losso, J. N., Van, N. C. F., Sabliov, C. M., & Warner, I. M., (2010). Delivery of phytochemical thymoquinone using molecular micelle modified poly (D, L lactide-co-glycolide)(PLGA) nanoparticles. *Nanotechnology, 21*(28), 285104.

18. Arora, D., & Jaglan, S., (2016). Nanocarriers based delivery of nutraceuticals for cancer prevention and treatment: A review of recent research developments. *Trends in Food Science & Technology, 54*, 114–126.

19. Wang, L., Xu, X., Zhang, Y., Zhang, Y., Zhu, Y., Shi, J., et al., (2013). Encapsulation of curcumin within poly (amidoamine) dendrimers for delivery to cancer cells. *Journal of Materials Science: Materials in Medicine, 24*(9), 2137–2144.

20. Kimpel, F., & Schmitt, J. J., (2015). Milk proteins as nanocarrier systems for hydrophobic nutraceuticals. *Journal of Food Science, 80*(11), R2361–R2366.

21. Rao, J., Decker, E. A., Xiao, H., & McClements, D. J., (2013). Nutraceutical nano-emulsions: Influence of carrier oil composition (digestible versus indigestible oil) on β-carotene bioavailability. *Journal of the Science of Food and Agriculture, 93*(13), 3175–3183.

22. Wang, P., Zhang, L., Peng, H., Li, Y., Xiong, J., & Xu, Z., (2013). The formulation and delivery of curcumin with solid lipid nanoparticles for the treatment of non-small cell lung cancer both *in vitro* and *in vivo. Materials Science and Engineering: C., 33*(8), 4802–4808.

23. Hoare, T. R., & Kohane, D. S., (2008). Hydrogels in drug delivery: Progress and challenges. *Polymer, 49*(8), 1993–2007.

24. Acevedo-Fani, A., Soliva-Fortuny, R., & Martín-Belloso, O., (2018). Photo-protection and controlled release of folic acid using edible alginate/chitosan nanolaminates. *Journal of Food Engineering, 229*, 72–82.

25. Fan, W., Yan, W., Xu, Z., & Ni, H., (2012). Formation mechanism of monodisperse, low molecular weight chitosan nanoparticles by ionic gelation technique. *Colloids and Surfaces B: Biointerfaces, 90*, 21–27.

26. Lemoine, D., & Préat, V., (1998). Polymeric nanoparticles as delivery system for influenza virus glycoproteins. *Journal of Controlled Release, 54*(1), 15–27.

27. Toshio, Y., Mitsuru, H., Shozo, M., & Hitoshi, S., (1981). Specific delivery of mitomycin c to the liver, spleen and lung: Nano-and m1crospherical carriers of gelatin. *International Journal of Pharmaceutics, 8*(2), 131–141.

28. Reis, C., Neufeld, R., Ribeiro, A., & Viega, F., (2005). Insulin-alginate nanospheres: Influence of calcium on polymer matrix properties. *Proceedings of the 13ᵗʰ International Workshop on Bioencapsulation Kingston.* Ontario, Canada: QueenTs University.

29. Teng, Z., Luo, Y., & Wang, Q., (2012). Nanoparticles synthesized from soy protein: Preparation, characterization, and application for nutraceutical encapsulation. *Journal of Agricultural and Food Chemistry, 60*(10), 2712–2720.

30. Squillaro, T., Schettino, C., Sampaolo, S., Galderisi, U., Di Iorio, G., Giordano, A., et al., (2018). Adult-onset brain tumors and neurodegeneration: Are polyphenols protective? *Journal of Cellular Physiology, 233*(5), 3955–3967.

31. Bhatt, P. C., Pathak, S., Kumar, V., & Panda, B. P., (2018). Attenuation of neurobehavioral and neurochemical abnormalities in animal model of cognitive deficits of Alzheimer's disease by fermented soybean nanonutraceutical. *Inflammopharmacology, 26*(1), 105–118.

32. Semyonov, D., Ramon, O., Shoham, Y., & Shimoni, E., (2014). Enzymatically synthe-sized dextran nanoparticles and their use as carriers for nutraceuticals. *Food & Function, 5*(10), 2463–2474.

33. Sanna, V., Lubinu, G., Madau, P., Pala, N., Nurra, S., Mariani, A., et al., (2015). Polymeric nanoparticles encapsulating white tea extract for nutraceutical application. *Journal of Agricultural and Food Chemistry, 63*(7), 2026–2032.

34. Felice, F., Zambito, Y., Belardinelli, E., D'onofrio, C., Fabiano, A., Balbarini, A., et al., (2013). Delivery of natural polyphenols by polymeric nanoparticles improves the resistance of endothelial progenitor cells to oxidative stress. *European Journal of Pharmaceutical Sciences, 50*(3, 4), 393–399.

35. Hu, K., Huang, X., Gao, Y., Huang, X., Xiao, H., & McClements, D. J., (2015). Core-shell biopolymer nanoparticle delivery systems: Synthesis and characterization of curcumin fortified zein-pectin nanoparticles. *Food Chemistry, 182,* 275–281.

36. Davidov-Pardo, G., Pérez-Ciordia, S., Marín-Arroyo, M. R., & McClements, D. J., (2015). Improving resveratrol bio-accessibility using biopolymer nanoparticles and complexes: Impact of protein-carbohydrate Maillard conjugation. *Journal of Agricultural and Food Chemistry, 63*(15), 3915–3923.

37. Teng, Z., Luo, Y., & Wang, Q., (2013). Carboxymethyl chitosan-soy protein complex nanoparticles for the encapsulation and controlled release of vitamin D3. *Food Chemistry, 141*(1), 524–532.

38. Luo, H., Jiang, B., Li, B., Li, Z., Jiang, B. H., & Chen, Y. C., (2012). Kaempferol nanoparticles achieve strong and selective inhibition of ovarian cancer cell viability. *International Journal of Nanomedicine, 7,* 3951.

39. Guttoff, M., Saberi, A. H., & McClements, D. J., (2015). Formation of vitamin D nanoemulsion-based delivery systems by spontaneous emulsification: Factors affecting particle size and stability. *Food Chemistry, 171,* 117–122.

40. Zhang, J., Wang, D., Wu, Y., Li, W., Hu, Y., Zhao, G., et al., (2018). Lipid-polymer hybrid nanoparticles for oral delivery of Tartary buckwheat flavonoids. *Journal of Agricultural and Food Chemistry, 66*(19), 4923–4932.

41. Acosta, E., (2009). Bioavailability of nanoparticles in nutrient and nutraceutical delivery. *Current Opinion in Colloid & Interface Science, 14*(1), 3–15.

42. McClements, D. J., Li, F., & Xiao, H., (2015). The nutraceutical bioavailability classification scheme: Classifying nutraceuticals according to factors limiting their oral bioavailability. *Annual Review of Food Science and Technology, 6,* 299–327.

PART III

Advances in Vesicular Delivery Systems for Nutraceutical Applications

CHAPTER 6

Phytosomes and Phytosomal Nanoparticles: A Promising Drug Delivery System for Flavonoids and Nutraceuticals

DARSHAN R. TELANGE,[1] SHIRISH P. JAIN,[2] ANIL M. PETHE,[1] and VIVEK S. DAVE[3]

[1]*Department of Pharmaceutics, Data Meghe College of Pharmacy, Wardha 442004, Maharashtra, India, Mobile: + 91-8698122949 E-mail: telange.darshan@gmail.com*

[1]*Datta Meghe College of Pharmacy, Datta Meghe Institute of Medical Sciences (Deemed to be University), Sawangi (Meghe), Wardha, Maharashtra, India.*

[2]*Rajarshi Shahu College of Pharmacy, Buldhana, Maharashtra. India*

[3]*St. John Fisher College, Wegmans School of Pharmacy, Rochester, New York, USA*

ABSTRACT

Phytosomes are lipid-compatible molecular complexes that can be successfully implemented for improving or enhancing the biopharmaceutical properties such as solubility, permeability, and bioavailability of phytoconstituents. Recently, many phytoconstituents have proven their potency *in vitro* as a potential candidate; however, its application to *in vivo* is restricted due to their large ring size, incompatibility with the passive diffusion process, and immiscibility with oils and lipids. Therefore, these plant actives have been made effective for *in vivo* by incorporating them into dietary phospholipids resulting in the formation of molecular complexes with acquiring amphiphilic properties. Phospholipids are one of the dietary components which demonstrates unique properties, i.e., compatibility with the biological membrane and inbuilt hepatoprotective properties. Moreover, it also displays a strong affinity for phytoconstituents leading to the formation of phyto-phospholipids complex, i.e., phytosomes. Till now, few methods have been explored by the researcher for the preparation of phytosomes such as solvent evaporation, mechanical dispersion, and nanoprecipitation, etc. Apart from this, the stability of phytosomes is an important issue that needs to be attained. The proposed chapter on phytosomes and phytosomal nanoparticles highlights regarding its concepts, formulation components, manufacturing, and characterization techniques and also its application towards targeted drug delivery system.

6.1   INTRODUCTION

The drugs obtained from plants have shown tremendous attractiveness due to its safety and efficacy over the synthetic medicines that caused a high level of complications to the human body. Approximately, 80% of the population all over the world is being satisfied by using plant-derived drugs. Because of this remarkable advantage, most of the life-saving drugs are procured from plant and natural sources [1, 2]. Moreover, the plant-based-formulations are generally prepared by extracting, isolating, and testing of phytoconstituents [3]. Among all phytoconstituents, the flavonoid acts as a promising active constituent, commonly available in many fruits, plants, vegetables, tea, chamomile, and wheat sprouts [4]. After oral administration, flavonoids produced many significant pharmacological activities such as antioxidant, [5] antimicrobial, [6] anti-inflammatory, [7] anti-proliferative, [8] antiviral, [9] antidiabetic, [10] and anticancer [11]. Regardless of flavonoid potential health benefits, its bioavailability is restricted by poor aqueous solubility, rapid metabolism, and fast elimination from the body. Abundant formulation techniques and strategies including liposomes, [12] nanocrystal gel, [13] SMEDDS [14] and phytosomes [15] have been developed by scientists to improve the biopharmaceutical and pharmacological potential of flavonoids.

Among all formulations, the phytosomes and phytosomal soft nanoparticles (P-SNP) create a significant reputation in the enhancement of solubility, permeability, and most important, the bioavailability of flavonoids [16, 17]. Phytosomes or flavonoids-phospholipids complexes (FPLC) are lipid compatible molecular complex, which forms micelles-like spherical structures [18]. This formulation technique encapsulates the phytoconstituents within the phosphatidylcholine-based phospholipids molecule for the formation of stable FPLC complex via involvement of polar and hydrogen-bonding interactions between the flavonoids and phosphate group of phospholipids [19]. Prepared amphiphilic phospholipids complex improves the transport facility of active constituents from aqueous to lipid environment via enhancing its solubility, membrane permeability, and water-oil partition coefficient [20, 21]. P-SNP, a modified form of phytosomes, also called self-assembled P-SNP. SNPs are prepared by nanoprecipitation technique with the involvement of four steps, i.e.: (a) formation of o/w suspension; (b) lowering of particle size of drug; (c) formation of soft nanoparticles; (d) precipitation of nanodroplets from an aqueous environment with the formation of SNP. Basically, SNPs are nanovesicle drug delivery system which shows remarkable advantages such as controlled delivery of drugs, maximizing efficiency, minimizing side effects and easy to fabricate [22, 23].

Phytosomes are patented technology, which was first developed in the year 1989, by Indena, Italy. Silybin phytosomes® is the first commercial phytosomes that significantly improves the biopharmaceutical properties of silybin. Keeping in view of phytosomes excellent benefits, many researchers and scientists have now shown their interest in this formulation strategy for improving biopharmaceutical as well as pharmacokinetic properties of flavonoid-based phytoconstituents. Therefore, based on the advantages and applications of phytosomes and self-assembled P-SNP, it can be suggested that both of these systems can be acting as a most preferable delivery system for phytoconstituents with poor biopharmaceutical and pharmacokinetic characteristics.

6.2 CONCEPT, DEFINITION, AND BASIC PROPERTIES OF PHYTOSOMES AND PHYTOSOMAL NANOPARTICLES

The concept of phytosomes is based on the complexation of water-insoluble phytoconstituents with the phospholipids carrier to improve its solubility and bioavailability. This concept was first introduced by Indena, an Italian-based pharmaceutical, and nutraceutical company. After the introduction of this concept, the Indena Company has patented this technology by the name of "Phytosomes®" [24].

Phytosomes are lipid-compatible molecular complex that shows more bioavailability compared to pure drug or phytoconstituents or herbal extracts, and this is attributed to the ability of the phytosomes to enter into the blood circulation via crossing the lipid-rich bio-membrane [24]. The phospholipids-based complex with phytoconstituents demonstrates numerous physical and chemical properties. These properties are discussed below:

- FPLC exhibits a lower melting point compared to pure drug or phyto-constituents [25].

- It shows maximum solubility in those solvents, i.e., (non-polar) where individual formulation components exhibit insolubility at the time of preparation.
- The amphiphilic nature of phytosomes improves the poor aqueous solubility, permeability, and bioavailability of phytoconstituents [26].
- FPLC shows a lower particle size and high zeta potential value and thus, shows its excellent suitability for oral as well as the transdermal route of administration [27].
- After preparation, FPLC, and P-SNP both displays the lowering of melting peak, shifting of the IR frequency to higher frequency signals and lowering of crystalline signals. This observed change in peaks/signals confirms the formation of a complex between active constituents and phospholipids [28].
- From a stability point of view, FPLC demonstrates more stable formulation compared to liposomes, and this is due to the involvement of strong ionic interactions such as hydrogen bonding, ion-dipole forces and van der Waals forces between plant drug and phospholipids [29].
- Compared to other formulations, the FPLC enhances the rate and extent of release for the longest period of time, and therefore it is employed as the most preferable drug delivery system.
- FPLC and P-SNP containing phytoconstituents show the multipurpose pharmacological activity [30].

6.3 MERITS OF PHYTOSOMES AND PHYTOSOMAL SOFT NANOPARTICLES (P-SNP) OVER CONVENTIONAL FORMULATIONS

1. FPLC and P-SNP are formed with the addition of only two components, i.e., flavonoid phytoconstituents and SP as compared to liposomes which required multiple numbers of formulation components.
2. Compared to liposomes and niosomes, the FPLC and P-SNP require less time for its preparation.
3. Phytosomes are more physically stable than liposomal formulations due to the establishment of strong intermolecular interactions between phytoconstituents and phospholipids [31].
4. Due to the involvement of amphiphilic phospholipids, FPLC can increase the biopharmaceutical properties of phytoconstituents as well as BCS II or IV drugs [32, 33].
5. FPLC and P-SNP bypasses the first-pass effect and thereby prevent the degradation of phytoconstituents [34].

6. Phytosomal formulations offer controlled release of flavonoids or BCS class II or IV in addition to minimization of adverse side effects.

7. Due to the unique characteristics of FPLC and phytosomal formulations, it can be successfully administered to the oral, transdermal, nasal, and most important, parenteral route [18].

6.4 FORMULATION COMPONENTS

6.4.1 FLAVONOIDS/EXTRACTS/DRUG (LOW SOLUBILITY OR LOW PERMEABILITY)

Flavonoids/extracts and BCS class II or IV drugs are most preferable candidates for the phytosomal formulations. *In vitro*, flavonoids show excellent pharmacological activity, however, following oral administration, this pharmacological activity is basically hindered by poor aqueous solubility, rapid metabolism, high molecular weight/ring size, low permeability, and bioavailability [35]. Herbal extracts also exhibit a similar problem by losing its active constituents in contact with gastric fluid when taken orally [36]. Moreover, the biopharmaceutical classification system (BCS) class II or IV drugs that show low solubility and high or low permeability can be employed as suitable and potential drug candidates for the preparation of FPLC and P-SNP.

6.4.2 PHOSPHOLIPIDS

Phospholipids are one of the key components of phytosomes. In this formulation, phospholipid acts as a carrier for improving the biopharmaceutical properties of flavonoids/extracts and BCS class II or IV drugs. Basically, phospholipids are amphiphilic in nature and show biocompatibility with the human plasma membrane. Due to these unique characteristics, phospholipid plays a significant role as a potential carrier for conveying hydrophobic as well as hydrophilic drugs across the biological membrane and thereby enhancing the oral bioavailability of drugs [20, 21]. Moreover, a phospholipids-based formulation offers many benefits to drugs such as easy to preparation, high drug loading capacity and long-term stability. Glycerolipids, sphingolipids, and sterols are their major classes of lipids. Out of these, glycerolipids are most preferred one over the others, because it contains a higher percentage of phosphatidylcholine (PC) and phosphatidylethanolamine (PE) involves in the formation of the lipid bilayer [37]. Earlier works of literature have shown that most of the phytosomes formulations were prepared by using soy phospholipids. Soya phospholipids (SP) are the lipids obtained from soybean, which contains more than 70% PC. The derived SP is usually accompanied by a higher concentration of polyunsaturated fatty acids (PUFAs) such as linoleic acid, linolenic acid, and oleic acid [38]. The studies based on phytosomes preparation and evaluation have shown that SP is free from teratogenic and carcinogenic effects, and consequently, SP-based phytosomes formulations not only improve the absorption rate (> 90%) of phytoconstituents but also reduces the mortality rate of laboratory animals. Moreover, the SP also demonstrates significant pharmacological activities like hepatoprotective and antihyperlipidemic [39].

6.5 MANUFACTURING TECHNIQUES OF PHYTOSOMES AND PHYTOSOMAL NANOPARTICLES

6.5.1 SOLVENT EVAPORATION

Solvent evaporation is the most widely used methods for the preparation of FPLC. Briefly, the flavonoid and phospholipids both are weighed in molar ratio and transferred into 100 mL round bottom flask. The weighed ingredients are then dissolved in sufficient quantity, i.e., 20 mL of absolute ethanol. The prepared solution is then heated at a controlled temperature range of 40°C to 60°C for the duration of 2 hours. The obtained liquid residue is then dissolved in the least amount of n-hexane, resulting in precipitation and formation of FPLC. Furthermore, the complex is dried and stored under vacuum desiccators to evaluate its detailed physicochemical characteristics. This method is successfully employed for complexation of apigenin, kaempferol, quercetin, and umbelliferone with phospholipids [40].

6.5.2 MECHANICAL DISPERSION

The mechanical dispersion method is another successful technique used for the formulation of marsupsin-phospholipids complex. Briefly, this method is initiated by dissolving an appropriate quantity of SP into diethyl ether and sonicated for a few minutes to dissolve it completely. Thereafter, an aqueous dispersion of marsupsin is then added dropwise to the above-prepared solution and left for 15 minutes, resulting in the formation of marsupsin-phospholipids complex dispersion. The prepared dispersion is further confirmed by scanning and transmission electron microscopy (TEM) studies [41, 42].

6.5.3 BULK CO-SONICATION

Bulk co-sonication method describes the process for the preparation of flavonosomes, i.e., multi flavonoids-phospholipids complex. Briefly, the three flavonoids; namely, kaempferol, apigenin, and quercetin are individually complexed with SP using dichloromethane (DCM) via thin-film hydration technique. Afterward, the individual complexes, i.e., quercetin, kaempferol, and apigenin-SP complex is combined together and subjected to sonication for a period of two hours. After sonication, the final dispersion resulting in the formation of multi flavonoids-phospholipids complex [43].

6.5.4 SERIALIZED CO-SONICATION

In this process, the quercetin and kaempferol-SP complex is initially mixed and then sonicated for up to two hours for the formation of the homogenous mixture. To this mixture, the third phospholipids complex, that is, apigenin-SP complex is added in a dropwise manner and again subjected to sonication for an additional two hours. This stepwise addition of individual phospholipids complexes into one another creates a stable complex between multi flavonoids and phospholipids [43].

6.5.5 BULK CO-LOADING

In bulk co-loading method, the three flavonoids are individually dissolved in a suitable solvent and then poured into SP solution. The prepared mixture is then sonicated for 30 minutes until the formation of a homogeneous solution. The obtained homogenous solution is refluxed at 40°C for a period of two hours. The refluxed solution is then added dropwise into a magnetically stirred aqueous solution, further resulting in the formation of flavonosomes with a high loading of quercetin, kaempferol, and apigenin [43].

6.5.6 SEQUENTIAL CO-LOADING

The sequential co-loading method is exactly similar to that of serialized co-sonication method. In this method, quercetin, and kaempferol solution is added into the already prepared SP solution and allowed to sonicate for the formation of a uniform solution. The uniform solution containing kaemp-ferol and quercetin is refluxed for 30 minutes. After 30 minutes, the apigenin solution is added into the above solution mixture and sonicated for an additional period of time. Thereafter, the final mixture is added dropwise into a beaker containing an aqueous solution and stirred overnight. The obtained final dispersion reports the high loading of flavonoids compared to bulk and serialized co-sonication method [43].

6.5.7 NANOPRECIPITATION

Nanoprecipitation method is employed to prepare the self-assembled P-SNP. The soft nanoparticles are produced by the addition of an optimized form of flavonoid-SP complex as a dispersed phase into magnetically stirred aqueous solution till to formation of uniform green colored dispersion. The dispersion is gradually evaporated to remove the organic solvent resulting in the formation of self-assembled P-SNP encapsulate with optimized phospholipids complex. Final dispersion is then lyophilized using a suitable cryoprotectant to improve the quality of the formulation as well as to prevent its unexpected decreasing of stability (Figure 6.1) [44, 45].

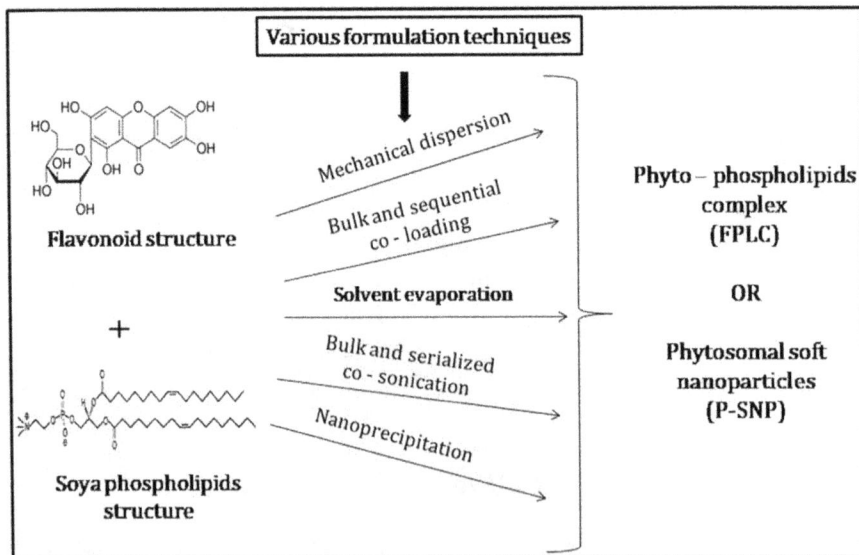

FIGURE 6.1   Schematic representations of phytosomes or phytosomal formulation techniques.

6.6 PHYSICOCHEMICAL AND FUNCTIONAL CHARACTERIZATION TECHNIQUE

6.6.1 COMPLEXATION RATE OR YIELD

UV-visible spectrophotometry-based method is generally used to estimate the complexation rate or yield of FPLC. Briefly, an approximate quantity of FPLC is weighed and dissolved in a sufficient volume of chloroform with the assistance of magnetic stirring. The obtained dispersion containing FPLC and SP is dissolved completely, whereas, the pure drug remains insoluble. The insoluble (non-complex part) drug is then dissolved in methanol and then measured its concentration using UV-visible spectroscopy. The complexation rate depends upon the successful complexation between flavonoids and SP. The non-polar solvent with low dielectric constant value helps to establish the stable complexation of flavonoid with SP. This characterization technique provides the basis for the selection of suitable formulation components [46].

6.6.2 ENCAPSULATION EFFICIENCY AND DRUG LOADING

The encapsulation efficiency and drug loading of flavonoids within the P-SNP are estimated by using ultracentrifugation method. In which, the P-SNP suspension is loaded into Eppendrof® Safe-Lock microcentrifuge tube (1.5 mL) and ultracentrifuged at a specified RPM for 40 minutes. The encapsulation efficiency provides the information regarding how much percentage drug/flavonoids is entrapped within the SNP, while drug loading gives information about how much amount of theoretical drug is loaded in the P-SNP after their separation from the medium. P-SNP with high encapsulation efficiency demonstrates the higher therapeutic efficacy of flavonoids. According to previous literature, the ideal value of encapsulation efficiency and drug loading in concern to SNP should be in the range of ~70 to 80% and ~10 to 15%, respectively. The P-SNP with this ideal value exhibits sustained drug release behavior without any sign of drug leakage [47].

6.6.3 PARTICLE SIZE AND ZETA POTENTIAL

Particle size and zeta potential of prepared FPLC are determined by using Photon Cross-Correlation Spectroscopy and NanoParticle Analyzer fitted with dynamic light scattering (DLS) technology. Briefly, the water-based

FPLC dispersion is loaded into sample analyzing the area and then recorded the particle size and zeta potential of FPLC within the optimized range of 1 to 10 nm and –200 to +200 mV, respectively. The behavior of submicron particles in the liquid medium is assessed by particle size distribution and zeta potential analysis. Detailed knowledge regarding these two indicators helps to understand the physical stability of formulation inside the biological system following oral administration. The small size colloidal nanoparticles containing drug play a significant role in the controlled release of drug as well as enhancing the passive target efficiency of the reticuloendothelial system. An optimal particle size and zeta potential value of FPLC also assists to decide its suitability either for the oral or transdermal route of administration [48–50].

6.6.4 PHOTOMICROSCOPY

The morphological assessment of FPLC is usually carried out by using Leica Microsystems AG. In this process, FPLC is diluted to 10-fold using double distilled water and then placed a single drop over the slide with a coverslip. The prepared slide of the formulation is observed under the microscope and captured the appropriate images at a magnification of 400×. The photomicroscopic images demonstrate that the phospholipids complex is a vesicle-like structure, which is made up of phospholipids and flavonoids molecule is added in the lipid layer. This photomicroscopic examination provides the preliminary confirmation about the formation of phospholipids complex and P-SNP [25].

6.6.5 SCANNING ELECTRON MICROSCOPY (SEM)

SEM is another valuable tool used for morphological characterization of FPLC and P-SNP. Briefly, the testing FPLC and P-SNP sample are spread over the double-sided carbon tape and then introduced into the sample testing area. Afterward, a thin layer of gold/palladium coating (approximately 400°) is applied over the sample and then captured the images at a suitable magnification using SEM. The captured image is interpreted by accompanying the software. SEM displays that prepared FPLC is a sphere-like structure with a smooth surface. This formation confirms that crystalline shape particles of flavonoids are disappeared, and this is attributed to the formation of a complex between flavonoids and SP. Many times, SEM is used as a noteworthy indicator for the establishment of comparison among crystalline flavonoids, amorphous SP, and prepared FPLC [51].

6.6.6   FOURIER TRANSFORM-INFRARED SPECTROSCOPY (FT-IR)

The physicochemical interaction among the formulation components at the molecular level is evaluated by using FT-IR spectrophotometer. Briefly, the FT-IR spectrum of samples is determined by preparing the homogenous mixture with FT-IR grade KBr and then compressed into thin transparent discs using Mini Hand Press Machine. The transparent disc is scanned between the wavelength ranges of 4,000 to 400 cm^{-1}. The scanned spectrum of each sample is interpreted by software supplied with the FT-IR instrument. The FT-IR spectrum of flavonoids shows the presence of multiple numbers of functional groups such as phenolic O-H, C-H, C=O and C=C stretching groups. The presence of these groups indicates that flavonoids are the most preferable molecule for making of the complex with SP. The SP FT-IR spectrum displays that there is an existence of long-chain fatty acid and ester group with C-H and C=O stretching vibration frequencies. Compared to flavonoids and SP spectrum, the FT-IR of FPLC completely shows different spectrum characteristics with the shifting of absorption frequencies from lower to higher and this is possibly due to the formation of weak intermolecular interaction, i.e., hydrogen bonding, van der Waals forces, ion-dipole forces between the flavonoids and SP. This strong interaction confirms the formation of FPLC [52].

6.6.7   DIFFERENTIAL SCANNING CALORIMETRY (DSC)

The thermal behavior of formulation components such as flavonoids, SP, and FPLC under the influence of controlled increasing temperature is analyzed by using a differential scanning calorimeter. In the sample analyzing area, an approximate amount (~ 2 mg) of testing samples is heated in the temperature range of 40°C to 400°C at a heating rate of 10°C/min. Gained DSC spectra for each sample is further understood and interpreted by using accompanying DSC software. Flavonoid thermograms exhibit the presence of a strong melting peak and this is corresponding to the purity and crystalline nature of flavonoids. Under the influence of controlled increasing temperature, SP demonstrates more than five small and diffused melting peak indicates that SP is amorphous in nature with somewhat crystalline characteristics. However,

FPLC exhibits a single melting peak with completely new characteristics. Formation of a single peak compared to flavonoid and SP indicates that hydrogen bonding, van der Waals forces, and ion-dipole forces are predominantly involved between the polar segment of flavonoids and SP, which in turn, resulting in the formation of FPLC with amorphous characteristics. Moreover, the changes in peak shape, surface area, shifting of peak position in DSC thermograms also suggest that there is a formation of FPLC [52].

6.6.8   POWDER X-RAY DIFFRACTOMETRY (PXRD)

PXRD measures the comparative crystalline nature among flavonoids, SP, and FPLC. In this method, a definite amount ($\sim$ 1 g) of samples is placed into the sample holder and then irradiated with installed monochromatic Cukβ radiation at a wavelength of (λ = 1.5406 A°). The irradiated each sample is scanned with the diffraction angle increasing from 3° to 60° on the 2θ scale. At the time of scanning, the angular spin is fixed at 360°. PXRD spectrum of pure flavonoids shows the sharp and intense peak on the 2θ scale indicates the high crystalline state of flavonoids, whereas, PXRD spectrum of SP exhibits a less number of intense and sharp peaks with small intensity indicates the amorphous nature of SP. In contrast to this, FPLC showed the single SP-dominated peaks with the lowest number of flavonoid peaks demonstrates that SP reduces the crystalline nature of flavonoids with the conversion of multiple sharp peaks to a single peak that corresponds to SP. Moreover, while complexation; there is a dispersion of crystalline flavonoid into amorphous SP, further resulting in the formation of FPLC via physicochemical modification and weak intermolecular interactions between flavonoid and SP [53].

6.6.9   PROTON NUCLEAR MAGNETIC RESONANCE SPECTROSCOPY (¹H-NMR)

¹H-NMR determines the carbon-hydrogen framework within the formulation components. This is determined by using 400 MHz FT-NMR spectrophotometers. The ¹H-NMR spectrum of flavonoids shows the chemical shift values on δ scale that usually matches to protons attached to C-5, C-6, and C-8, respectively. Flavonoids also show doublet signals and this is corresponding to protons attaches to C-3 and C-4 positions. The ¹H-NMR values for FPLC are shifted significantly to higher frequencies, and this might be attributable to the involvement of flavonoid protons of C-5 and

C-4 positions with polar part of SP. This formed the basis for the formation and confirmation of FPLC [52].

6.6.10 SOLUBILITY STUDIES

The solubility studies are carried out to analyze the aqueous and non-aqueous solubilities of flavonoids and prepared FPLC formulations. Briefly, the excess quantity of flavonoids and FPLC formulations are dispersed in sufficient amount of water or *n*-octanol. The prepared dispersion is then centrifuged and filtered using a membrane filter. Subsequently, a small aliquot of the filtered solution with suitable dilutions is used to record the absorbance either on spectrophotometry or high-performance liquid chromatography (HPLC). Solubility studies are carried out at ambient temperature (25°C). The flavonoid, due to its lipophilic nature and larger ring size displays the poor aqueous solubility, and thus, it is classified as BCS II or IV drugs. The FPLC enhances the aqueous solubility of flavonoids, and this completely depends upon the amorphization and physicochemical modifications of flavonoids while complexation with SP. P-SNP containing flavonoid also improves the aqueous solubility via converting the entire formulation into nano-vesicle drug delivery system with reduced crystalline properties of flavonoids [54].

6.6.11 DISSOLUTION STUDIES

The dialysis membrane-based dissolution method is used to determine the *in vitro* dissolution behavior of FPLC or P-SNP. In this method, the prepared dispersion of FPLC or P-SNP is filled into the prepared dialysis bag and tied with the thread. The phosphate buffer saline (PBS) solution (PBS, pH 7.4) is used as dissolution media for the entire study. Later on, at a designated time interval, the smaller aliquot of the sample is removed and analyzed for drug concentration using either spectrophotometry or HPLC. The dissolution studies are carried out to understand the drug release performance in the dissolution media. FPLC increases the rate and extent of release of drug through increasing it is the solubility and wettability in PBS (pH 7.4), resulting in the formation of uniform dispersion, which in turn, shows sustained drug release behavior. During dissolution, the P-SNP exhibits biphasic release behavior, i.e., burst and sustained drug release. The biphasic release performance offers significant and synergistic advantages to the phytosomes and nanoformulations (Figure 6.2) [55].

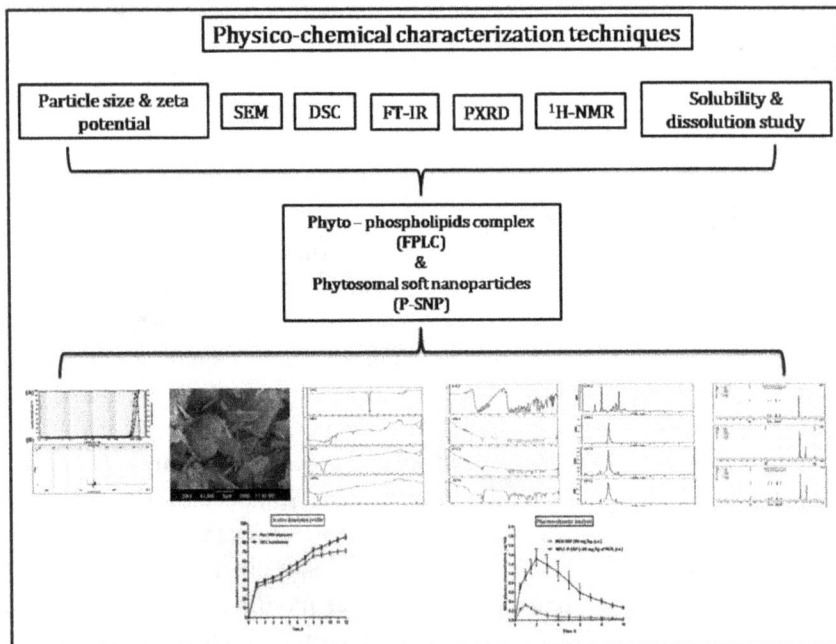

FIGURE 6.2   Schematic representations of physicochemical characterization techniques for analysis of phytosomes or phytosomal formulations.

6.6.12   *BIOAVAILABILITY STUDIES*

Either sex of Wister Albino rats with weight approximately 200–250 g is specifically used to study the *in vivo* bioavailability of FPLC or P-SNP. This study is started with the administration of respective formulations to animals via the oral route. Thereafter, blood samples (around 0.5 to 1 mL) are collected from the retro-orbital plexus and centrifuged. The supernatant samples are then extracted by liquid-liquid extraction, solid-liquid extraction or protein precipitation and then analyzed using HPLC. On the basis of HPLC results, the C_{max} and T_{max} are calculated from the plasma concentration-time profile curve. Remaining pharmacokinetic parameters are obtained by using a program-based software. FPLC or P-SNP both increases the *in vivo* bioavailability of flavonoids and BCS class II or IV drugs. Both these formulations enhance the biopharmaceutical and absorption of properties of drugs via increasing their pharmacokinetic properties. Additionally, the drug extraction technique from FPLC or P-SNP also significantly influences the bioavailability [47, 52].

6.7 CONCLUSION

The present chapter describes that phytosomes/FPLC or P-SNP is an excellent formulation system for delivering the phytoconstituents as well as BCS class II or IV drugs that demonstrate poor biopharmaceutical and pharmacokinetic attributes. Compared to all phospholipids, the SP containing a higher percentage of PC showed a most preferred carrier system for manufacturing of phytosomal formulations. FPLC or P-SNP formulations are most successfully prepared by easy to prepare, solvent evaporation and nanoprecipitation methods by showing high drug entrapment efficiency (EE), compared to other reported methods. Physicochemical characterization by DSC, FT-IR, PXRD, and ^{1}H-NMR confirms that FPLC or P-SNP are formed with the involvement of weak intermolecular forces of interactions, for instance, hydrogen bonding, van der Waals and ion-dipole forces between the flavonoids/drug and SP. FPLC or P-SNP enhances the aqueous solubility as well as the release rate in an excellent manner as compared to conventional dosage forms containing the same drug candidate. From the bioavailability study, it has been demonstrated that phytosomal formulations improve the bioavailability of flavonoids phytoconstituents by raising the pharmacokinetic parameters compared to other reported nanoformulations. However, there is a scope of exploration on phytosomal formulations with respect to its design and manufacturing process so that it can be targeted to different types of cancer diseases. In conclusion, the phytosomal formulations with support of worthy manufacturing process can be employed as a successful and effective nanovesicle delivery system for flavonoids with improving biopharmaceutical and pharmacological attributes.

KEYWORDS

- chemical characterization
- flavonoids-phospholipids complexes
- formulations
- phosphatidylcholine
- phosphatidylethanolamine
- physical characterization
- phytosomal soft nanoparticles
- phytosomes

REFERENCES

1. WHO, (2004). *Guidelines on Developing Consumer Information on Proper Use of Traditional, Complementary and Alternative Medicine.* World Health Organization.
2. Barnes, P. M., Powell-Griner, E., McFann, K., & Nahin, R. L., (2004). *Complementary and Alternative Medicine use Among Adults: United* States (pp. 1–19). Adv. Data.
3. Sasidharan, S., Chen, Y., Saravanan, D., Sundram, K. M., & Yoga, L. L., (2011). Extraction, isolation and characterization of bioactive compounds from plants' extracts. *Afr. J. Tradit. Complement. Altern. Med., 8,* 1–10.
4. Shukla, S., & Gupta, S., (2010). Apigenin: A promising molecule for cancer prevention. *Pharm. Res., 27,* 962–978.
5. Stanojević, L., Stanković, M., Nikolić, V., Nikolić, L., Ristić, D., Čanadanovic-Brunet, J., & Tumbas, V., (2009). Antioxidant activity and total phenolic and flavonoid contents of *Hieracium pilosella* L. extracts. *Sensors, 9,* 5702–5714.
6. Taleb-Contini, S. H., Salvador, M. J., Watanabe, E., Ito, I. Y., & Oliveira, D. C. R. D., (2003). Antimicrobial activity of flavonoids and steroids isolated from two *Chromolaena* species. *Rev. Bras. Cienc. Farm., 39,* 403–408.
7. Rithidech, K. N., Tungjai, M., Reungpatthanaphong, P., Honikel, L., & Simon, S. R., (2012). Attenuation of oxidative damage and inflammatory responses by apigenin given to mice after irradiation. *Mutat. Res. Genet. Toxicol. Environ. Mutagen., 749,* 29–38.
8. Johnson, J. L., & Gonzalez De, M. E., (2013). Interactions between dietary flavonoids apigenin or luteolin and chemotherapeutic drugs to potentiate antiproliferative effect on human pancreatic cancer cells, *in vitro. Food Chem. Toxicol., 60,* 83–91.
9. Shibata, C., Ohno, M., Otsuka, M., Kishikawa, T., Goto, K., Muroyama, R., Kato, N., et al., (2014). The flavonoid apigenin inhibits hepatitis C virus replication by decreasing mature microRNA122 levels. *Virology, 462, 463,* 42–48.
10. Choi, J. S., Nurul, I. M., Yousof, A. M., Kim, E. J., Kim, Y. M., & Jung, H. A., (2014). Effects of C-glycosylation on anti-diabetic, anti-Alzheimer's disease and anti-inflammatory potential of apigenin. *Food Chem. Toxicol., 64,* 27–33.
11. Choudhury, D., Ganguli, A., Dastidar, D. G., Acharya, B. R., Das, A., & Chakrabarti, G., (2013). Apigenin shows synergistic anticancer activity with curcumin by binding at different sites of tubulin. *Biochimie., 95,* 1297–1309.
12. Arsić, I., Tadić, V., Vlaović, D., Homšek, I., Vesić, S., Isailović, G., & Vuleta, G., (2011). Preparation of novel apigenin-enriched, liposomal and non-liposomal, anti-inflammatory topical formulations as substitutes for corticosteroid therapy. *Phytother. Res., 25,* 228–233.
13. Al Shaal, L., Shegokar, R., & Müller, R. H., (2011). Production and characterization of antioxidant apigenin nanocrystals as a novel UV skin protective formulation. *Int. J. Pharm., 420,* 133–140.
14. Zhao, L., Zhang, L., Meng, L., Wang, J., & Zhai, G., (2013). Design and evaluation of a self micro emulsifying drug delivery system for apigenin. *Drug Dev. Ind. Pharm., 39,* 662–669.
15. Hou, Z., Li, Y., Huang, Y., Zhou, C., Lin, J., Wang, Y., Cui, F., et al., (2013). Phytosomes loaded with mitomycin C-soybean phosphatidylcholine complex developed for drug delivery. *Mol. Pharm., 10,* 90–101.
16. Bhattacharyya, S., Ahmmed, S. M., Saha, B. P., & Mukherjee, P. K., (2014). Soya phospholipid complex of mangiferin enhances its hepatoprotectivity by improving its bioavailability and pharmacokinetics. *J. Sci. Food Agric., 94,* 1380–1388.

17. Freag, M. S., Elnaggar, Y. S. R., & Abdallah, O. Y., (2013). Lyophilized phytosomal nanocarriers as platforms for enhanced diosmin delivery: Optimization and *ex vivo* permeation. *Int. J. Nanomedicine, 8*, 2385–2397.

18. Semalty, A., Semalty, M., & Rawat, M. S. M., (2007). The Phyto-phospholipid complexes- phytosomes: A potential therapeutic approach for herbal hepatoprotective drug delivery. *Pharmacog. Rew., 1*(2), 369–374.

19. Telange, D. R., Patil, A. T., Pethe, A. M., Tatode, A. A., Anand, S., & Dave, V. S., (2016). Kaempferol-phospholipid complex: Formulation, and evaluation of improved solubility, *in vivo* bioavailability, and antioxidant potential of kaempferol. *J. Excipients Food Chem., 7*, 89–112.

20. Renukuntla, J., Vadlapudi, A. D., Patel, A., Boddu, S. H. S., & Mitra, A. K., (2013). Approaches for enhancing oral bioavailability of peptides and proteins. *Int. J. Pharm., 447*, 75–93.

21. Pichot, R., Watson, R. L., & Norton, I. T., (2013). Phospholipids at the interface: Current trends and challenges. *Int. J. Mol. Sci., 14*, 11767–11794.

22. Minelli, C., Lowe, S. B., & Stevens, M. M., (2010). Engineering nanocomposite materials for cancer therapy. *Small., 6*(21), 2336–2357.

23. Rozhkova, E. A., (2011). Nanoscale materials for tackling brain cancer: Recent progress and outlook. *Adv. Mater., 23*(24), 136–150.

24. Semalty, A., Semalty, M., Rawat, M. S. M., & Franceschi, F., (2010). Supramolecular phospholipids-polyphenolics interactions: The PHYTOSOME® strategy to improve the bioavailability of phytochemicals. *Fitoterapia, 81*, 306–314.

25. Maiti, K., Mukherjee, K., Saha, B. P., Murugan, V., & Mukherjee, P. K., (2009). Exploring the effect of hesperetin–HSPC complex—a novel drug delivery system on the *in vitro* release, therapeutic efficacy and pharmacokinetics. *AAPS PharmSciTech., 10*(3), 943–950.

26. Singh, D., Rawat, M. S. M., Semalty, A., & Semalty, M., (2012). Chrysophanol-phospholipid complex. *J. Therm. Anal. Calorim., 111*, 2069–2077.

27. Telange, D. R., Wavare, K., Patil, A., Umekar, M., Anand, S., & Dave, V., (2018). Drug-phospholipid complex-loaded matrix film formulation for the enhanced transdermal delivery of quercetin. *J. Excipients Food Chem., 9*, 31–50.

28. Zhang, J., Tang, Q., Xu, X., & Li, N., (2013). Development and evaluation of a novel phytosome-loaded chitosan microsphere system for curcumin delivery. *Int. J. Pharm., 448*, 168–174.

29. Ruan, J., Liu, J., Zhu, D., Gong, T., Yang, F., Hao, X., & Zhang, Z., (2010). Preparation and evaluation of self-nanoemulsified drug delivery systems (SNEDDSs) of matrine based on drug-phospholipid complex technique. *Int. J. Pharm., 386*, 282–290.

30. Khan, J., Alexander, A., Ajazuddin, Saraf, S., & Saraf, S., (2013). Recent advances and future prospects of phyto-phospholipid complexation technique for improving pharmacokinetic profile of plant actives. *J. Cont. Release, 168*, 50–60.

31. Lasonder, E., & Weringa, W. D., (1990). An NMR and DSC study of the interaction of phospholipid vesicles with some anti-inflammatory agents, *J. Colloid Interface Sci., 139*, 469–478.

32. Venkatesh, M., Mukherjee, K., Maiti, K., & Mukherjee, P. K., (2009). Enhanced oral bioavailability and antioxidant profile of ellagic acid by phospholipids. *J. Agric. Food Chem., 57*, 4559–4565.

33. Saoji, S. D., Belgamwar, V. S., Dharashivkar, S. S., Rode, A. A., Mack, C., & Dave, V. S., (2016). The study of the influence of formulation and process variables on the

functional attributes of simvastatin-phospholipid complex. *J. Pharm. Innov., 11*(3), 264–278.

34. Maiti, K., Mukherjee, K., Gantait, A., Saha, B. P., & Mukherjee, P. K., (2007). Curcumin-phospholipid complex: Preparation, therapeutic evaluation and pharmacokinetic study in rats. *Int. J. Pharm., 330*, 155–163.

35. Panche, A. N., Diwan, A. D., & Chandra, S. R., (2016). Flavonoids: An overview. *J. of Nut. Sci., 5*(47), 1–15.

36. Bhattacharyya, S., (2009). Phytosomes: The new technology for enhancement of bioavailability of botanicals and nutraceuticals. *Int. J. Health Res., 2*, 225–232.

37. Meer, G. V., & Kroon, A. I. P. M., (2011). Lipid map of the mammalian cell. *J. of Cell Sci., 124*, 5–8.

38. Scholfield, C. R., (1981). Composition of soybean lecithin, *J. Am. Oil Chem. Soc., 58*, 889–892.

39. Schmahl, D., (1980). *Comment on Carcinogenicity of Phosphatidylcholine.* Res. Report No. 0061/80.

40. Telange, D. R., Patil, A. T., Pethe, A. M., Anand, S., Fegade, H., & Dave, V. S., (2016). Formulation and characterization of an apigenin-phospholipid phytosome (APLC) for improved solubility, *in vivo* bioavailability, and antioxidant potential. *Eur. J. Pharm. Sci., 108*, 36–49.

41. Sikarwar, M. S., Sharma, S., Jain, A. K., & Parial, S. D., (2008). Preparation, characterization and evaluation of marsupsin-phospholipid complex. *AAPS PharmSciTech, 9*(1), 129–137.

42. Pathan, R. A., & Bhandari, U., (2011). Gymnemic acid-phospholipid complex: Preparation and characterization. *J. Disp. Sci. and Tech., 32*, 1165–1172.

43. Karthivashan, G., Masarudin, M. J., Kura, A. U., Abas, F., & Fakurazi, S., (2016). Optimization, formulation, and characterization of multiflavonoids-loaded flavanosome by bulk or sequential technique. *Int. J. Nanomedicine, 11*, 3417–3434.

44. Zhang, Z., Huang, Y., Gao, F., Bu, H., Gu, W., & Li, Y., (2011). Daidzein-phospholipid complex loaded lipid nanocarriers improved oral absorption: *In vitro* characteristics and *in vivo* behavior in rats. *Nanoscale, 3*, 1780–1787.

45. Yang, X., Xu, L., Zhou, J., Ge, Y., Wu, S., Huang, J., Li, Y., et al., (2019). Integration of phospholipid-complex nanocarrier assembly with endogenous N-oleoylethanolamine for efficient stroke therapy. *J Nanobiotechnol., 17*(8), 2–14.

46. Bombardelli, E., & Patri, G. F., (1991). *Complex Compounds of Bioflavonoids with Phospholipids, Their Preparation and Use, and Pharmaceutical and Cosmetic Composition Containing Them.* U.S. Patent: 5,043,323.

47. Yu, F., Li, Y., Chen, Q., He, Y., Wang, H., Yang, L., Guo, S., Meng, Z., Cui, J., Xue, M., & Chen, X. D., (2016). Monodisperse microparticles loaded with the self-assembled berberine-phospholipid complex-based phytosomes for improving oral bioavailability and enhancing hypoglycemic efficiency. *Euro. J. Biopharm. Pharmacokinetics, 103*, 136–148.

48. Zhang, L., Yang, M., Wang, Q., Li, Y., Guo, R., & Jiang, X., (2007). 10-hydroxycamptothecin loaded nanoparticles: Preparation and antitumor activity in mice. *J. Controlled Release, 119*(2), 153–162.

49. Soma, C. E., Dubernet, C., Barratt, G., Benita, S., & Couvreur, P., (2000). Investigation of the role of macrophages on the cytotoxicity of doxorubicin and doxorubicin-loaded nanoparticles on M5076 cells *in vitro. J. Controlled Release, 68*(2), 283–289.

50. Xu, Z., Chen, L., Gu, W., Gao, Y., Lin, L., Zhang, Z., et al., (2009). The performance of docetaxel-loaded solid lipid nanoparticles targeted to hepatocellular carcinoma. *Biomaterials, 30*(2), 226–232.
51. Zhang, J., Xiong, H., Wang, H., Chen, X., Wu, M., Yin, H., Liu, S., Tan, Q., & He, D., (2012). Design and evaluation of a novel evodiamine-phospholipid complex for improved oral bioavailability. *AAPS PharmSciTech., 13*, 534–547.
52. Telange, D. R., Nirgulkar, S. B., Umekar, M. J., Patil, A. T., Pethe, A. M., & Bali, N. R., (2019). Enhanced transdermal permeation and anti-inflammatory potential of phospholipids complex-loaded matrix film of umbelliferone: Formulation development, physicochemical and functional characterization. *Eur. J. Pharm. Sci., 131*, 23–38.
53. Pathan, R. A., & Bhandari, U., (2011). Preparation & characterization of embelin-phospholipid complex as effective drug delivery tool. *J. Incl. Phenom. Macrocycl. Chem., 69*, 139–147.
54. Singh, D., Rawat, M. S. M., Semalty, A., & Semalty, M., (2012). Rutin-phospholipid complex: An innovative technique in novel drug delivery system-NDDS. *Curr. Drug Deliv., 9*, 305–314.
55. Perrut, M., Jung, J., & Leboeuf, F., (2004). Enhancement of dissolution rate of poorly soluble active ingredients by supercritical fluid processes. *Int. J. Pharm., 288*, 3–10.

CHAPTER 7

Liposomal Delivery System for the Effective Delivery of Nutraceuticals and Functional Foods

PRANESH KUMAR,[1] DEBARSHI KAR MAHAPATRA,[2] DILEEP KUMAR,[3] MOHAMAD TALEUZZAMAN,[4] SACHIN BORIKAR,[5] VISHAL S. GULECHA,[6] AMAR G. ZALTE,[6] KANHAIYA M. DADURE,[7] MANISHA PURANIK,[8] MANIK DAS,[9] and TOMY MURINGAYIL JOSEPH[10]

[1]*Department of Pharmacology, Aryakul College of Pharmacy & Research, Lucknow, Uttar Pradesh, India*

[2]*Department of Pharmaceutical Chemistry, Dadasaheb Balpande College of Pharmacy, Nagpur, Maharashtra, India, E-mail: mahapatradebarshi@gmail.com*

[3]*Department of Pharmaceutical Chemistry, Poona College of Pharmacy, Bharati Vidyapeeth (A Deemed to be University), Pune, Maharashtra, India*

[4]*Department of Pharmaceutical Chemistry, Faculty of Pharmacy, Maulana Azad University, Jodhpur, Rajasthan, India*

[5]*Department of Pharmacology, Rajarshi Shahu College of Pharmacy, Buldhana, Maharashtra. India*

[6]*School of Pharmaceutical Sciences, Sandip University, Nashik, Maharashtra, India*

[7]*Department of Chemistry, J. B. College of Science, Wardha–442001, Maharashtra, India*

[8]*Institute of Pharmaceutical Education and Research, Borgaon (Meghe), Wardha, Maharashtra, India*

[9]*Department of Pharmaceutical Chemistry, Gokaraju Rangaraju College of Pharmacy, Hyderabad, Telangana, India*

[10]*Chemical Faculty, Polymers Technology Department, Gdansk University of Technology, Gdansk–80233, Poland*

ABSTRACT

Liposome was discovered earliest in the year 1961 by Dr. Alec Bangham, a British hematologist who tried this delivery system for transporting bioactive substances (hydrophobic therapeutic agents and hydrophilic therapeutic agents) into the human body in a biocompatible manner. The system is well known for decades in effectually delivering the pharmacotherapeutically privileged molecules from natural sources or synthetic drug classes (anti-cancer, anti-inflammatory, anti-infective, analgesic, etc.). But, the use of this carrier system for delivering the nutraceutical products and functional food is a relatively new concept, and very limited work has been done so far. The present book chapter successfully highlighted the history, background, classification, production, characterization, stability, role, composition function, beneficial functions, objective, advantages, disadvantages, etc., of the liposomes and their role in delivering the bioactive nutraceutical compounds.

7.1 INTRODUCTION

Liposome was discovered earliest in the year 1961 by Dr. Alec Bangham, a British hematologist who tried this delivery system for transporting bioactive substances (hydrophobic therapeutic agents and hydrophilic therapeutic agents) into the human body in a biocompatible manner [1]. This brilliant delivery system prevents the bioactive components from the acid present in the stomach, promotes direct absorption in the buccal cavity, reduced the risk of any toxic effect or facilitates limited side effects, and has considerable concern for chemotherapeutics [2].

7.1.1 DEVELOPMENTAL JOURNEY

In a broad manner, Liposomes are the lipid-based deliveries of colloidal nature, let us talk about the developmental journey. The most common form is a simple emulsion (water and oil are stabilized for a limited period) which exists in a skin cream or food products like mayonnaise [3]. Emulsions (W/O emulsion or O/W emulsion) are stabilized by the application of natural surfactants (lecithin) and synthetic surfactants (polyethylene glycols) [4]. The utilization of high-shear processes like homogenization and sonication leads to the formation of small globules of size 10 nm to 200 nm range

[5]. This progressive journey leads to the concept of micelles formation, nanoemulsions, solid lipid nanoparticles, and nanostructured lipid carriers (NLCs) [6]. These sub-100 nm particles have been known to exhibit Brownian movement which results in the movement of oils to the top by exceeding the force of gravity which leads to longer shelf life, higher stability, and exhibits characteristic clarity [7]. While looking at liposomes, several appealing features were seen: the phospholipids are thoroughly assembled into the spherical cellular membrane (hydrophilic heads arrange in aqueous medium and hydrophobic tails pushes toward each other), instead of the presence of surfactant that stabilizes the oil drops in the water [8]. Liposomes create a cavity where aqueous components (containing bioactive compounds) are entrapped and further protect from harsh GIT environment and promote higher absorption [9]. The most distinct feature of liposome is that both hydrophobic and hydrophilic components can be delivered where the bilayers host the lipid-dissolving drugs [10]. The system is taken up by the endosomal mechanisms after interaction with the cell membranes [11]. Successful liposome carrier technologies arrived in the late 90s and productive commercial products (injectable and oral) containing nystatin, doxorubicin, vincristine, and amphotericin B [12]. At present, superior grade phospholipids and better size reduction techniques afford quality liposomal formulations [13].

7.2 PRODUCTION

When the lipid (lecithin) was aqueously dispersed by the first creator, spherical multilayered structures were created impulsively. With the timely progress, it was observed that *"the smaller the system, the more benefits will be obtained"* [14]. Researchers have applied numerous methods such as high-pressure homogenization, rotor-stator dispersion, extrusion, freeze-thaw cycles, and sonication to obtain uniform and non-sized formulation that facilitated enhancement of circulation time and augmentation in the absorption kinetics [15].

7.3 CLASSIFICATION

On the basis of layering and size dimension, the liposomes are generally classified. Small unilamellar vesicles (SUV) of size less than 100 nm, large unilamellar vesicles (LUV) where the size of each layer is greater than 100 nm, and multilamellar vesicles (MLV) have concentric lipid bilayers of 100–500 nm diameter where aqueous interlayers lie [16]. In general, these MLV structures are initially formed when the phospholipids come in contact with the aqueous environment [17].

7.4 INGREDIENTS

Commercially, Phospholipids are obtained from the lecithin that is procured from sunflower seed oil, soy seed oil, and canola seed oil as well as from milk and egg yolks [18]. Phosphatidylcholine (PC) obtained from the fractions of raw lecithin and purified lecithin ranges from 15% to 95% [19]. PC is a multi-application-oriented component having therapeutic as well as excipient roles and is the most useful form of phospholipids. The application of soy phospholipids is known for centuries and a high source of PC [20]. Very recently, soya PC is replaced by sunflower PC and is into application by commercial companies.

Phospholipid, particularly PC, is not only regarded as a carrier but they hold several beneficial therapeutic effects (used as functional medicine) and is situated in the cellular constitution (cell membranes) [21]. In general, flexible membranes are produced by the unsaturated phospholipid, obtained from sunflower or soya that facilitates high intraoral absorption. In contrast, stiffer membranes are produced by the saturated phospholipid, obtained from hydrogenated phospholipids that facilitate high GI absorption [22]. Although, traditionally, the phospholipids, oils (medium-chain triglycerides), membrane stiffeners (cholesterol), and surface coating agents (chitosan (CHT), alginates, hyaluronic acid, etc.), play critical role in the formation of the bilayer membrane of the liposome, but at present, non-surfactant lipid molecules and surfactant lipid molecules are employed to produce stable absorbable formulations [23].

7.5 CHARACTERIZATION

Photon correlation spectrometry, also known as dynamic light scattering (DLS), is the primary laser-based tool for recognizing the exact mean size, size population distribution, and dimensions of the formed vesicular system. Electron spectroscopy is the subsequent tool for the judgment of morphology and absolute size [24].

7.6   STABILITY

DLS unit is exclusively used for studying the stability of the liposome formulations. Long duration stability of these formulations is extremely challenging, and instability is usually observed in the surfactant system where sedimentation (insoluble compounds fall out and settle) and creaming (free fats rise up to the top) are seen predominantly [25]. Under both the above instability conditions, the potency of the system decreases considerably. An ideally stable formulation demonstrates an incessant single phase in a beaker, and small-sized formulations are the best to visually evaluate the degree of flaws or quality [26].

7.7   BENEFICIAL CHARACTERISTICS

The reticuloendothelial system (RES), also known as the mononuclear phagocyte system (MPS), is responsible for the clearance of liposomes and lipid particles from the blood. MPS is a macrophage or monocyte-based system that exists in lymph nodes, spleen, and liver [27]. The smaller the size of the liposome, the higher will be the clearance. The longest circulation of the liposomal form is found to be unilamellar vesicles which have the best size distribution and small mean diameter [28]. Even though all the factors remain uniformly fair, large volume of the product lies in the non-ideal range of vesicle size. Recently, liposomal formulations intended for the nutritional drug delivery, produced through high lecithin content and medium shear methods, have shown milky products in a size range of 200 nm–400 nm [29]. The encapsulated component in small-sized liposomes expressed the highest efficacy. Narrow-sized range liposomes have been found to enhance the cellular uptake by 9-folds at 97 nm and 34-folds at 64 nm. When the surface of the liposomes is coated with PEGs (having hydrophilic chains), the formulation escapes (stealth property) the RES cells and protects them from getting metabolized or gets cleared, thereby enhancing the circulatory time [30].

7.7.1   ADVANTAGES OF LIPOSOMAL DELIVERY [31]

1.   As compared to miscellaneous types of oral delivery systems, a very high bioavailability is seen.

2. Non-injectable form helps avoiding pain that occurs with traditional injections and further reduces the risk of contamination.
3. Encapsulation of liposomes prevents GIT degradation and augments oral uptake and absorption.
4. Enhanced intracellular delivery of the bioactive compounds.
5. Both hydrophobic molecules as well as hydrophilic molecules can be delivered.
6. It can be recommended for those patients whom oral administration is not possible.
7. Incremental and incremental dosing is possible for both adults and children.
8. Lower doses offer higher response that is an economic approach.

7.7.2 POTENTIAL DISADVANTAGES OF LIPOSOMAL DELIVERY [32]

1. At present, the initial cost of therapy is high.
2. High formulation variability or quality issues.
3. Stability issues are high.
4. Amplified intracellular delivery.

7.8 USE IN NUTRACEUTICAL INDUSTRY

There is no hesitation that the utilization of liposomes in functional food industries is developing swiftly in the last five years. With the espousal of high yield production procedures, good quality assurance techniques, evaluation methods, pharmaceutical excellence (stability, size, and effectiveness), etc., several liposomal products containing nutraceuticals have been developed [33].

7.8.1 ENZYMES AND PROTEINS

The appliance of the liposome encapsulating active enzyme forms as nutritional supplements or processing (such as cheese ripening) has been recently studied. Various researchers have studied the therapeutic, non-pharmaceutical, and pharmaceutical roles of numerous enzymes. Alkhalaf et al. developed the proteolytic enzyme-loaded charged (negatively, positively, and neutral) liposomal system; Larivière et al. developed the trypsin-loaded liposomal system and applied for the cheese ripening; Laloy et al. developed the trypsin-loaded liposomal system and determined the release of the enzyme in the cheese matrix; Kheadr et al. developed the fungal protease-, lipase-, and bacterial protease-loaded liposomal system and reported the enhancement in the flavor intensity and mature texture; Yoshimoto et al. developed the yeast alcohol dehydrogenase-loaded liposomal system and established the stabilized quaternary structures and tertiary structures of the enzyme; Li et al. developed the covalently coupled cellulose-based liposome system and reported that this system exhibited better delivery of the loaded content as compared to the free form; et al. developed nisin-loaded liposomal system and reported the better anti-food borne pathogen (anti-bacterial) activity which leads to better cheese preservation; Huang et al. developed bovine lactoferrin-loaded liposomal system and studied the antioxidant potentials at pH of 6.6; Huang et al. also developed the casein hydrolysate-loaded liposomal system and reported the decrease in the bitterness and hydrophobicity of the hydrolysates [34].

7.8.2 ENERGETIC SUBSTRATES

The newly fabricated liposomal formulations have unique encapsulation of energetic substrates (ATP: adenosine triphosphate, fatty acids, etc.), that facilitated better delivery of the constituents in the biological system. Researchers developed ATP-loaded liposome system and reported to play function as an effectual exogenous resource in mediating cardioprotective action on is chemically damaged hearts. These ATP-loaded liposome systems have also demonstrated tremendous recovery of the energy state in cold-stored rat livers. Similarly, medium-chain fatty acids-loaded liposome system was reported that has capabilities to supply energy (through fast metabolism) to the weight-loaded swimming mice by providing them with non-storage fat. Co-enzyme Q10 (CoQ10)-loaded liposome system has been prepared by the researcher and reported their bioenergetic application such as elevated energy phosphate formation and enhanced deployment of oxygen [35].

7.8.3 FLAVOR

The quality and acceptability of the food are enhanced several folds due to the flavor (essential oils, peptides, fatty acids, and aromatic esters).

However, low volatility and low stability limit their appliance during transportation, manufacturing, and storage. The encapsulation technology through liposome is an emerging approach for overcoming these limitations by encapsulating the flavors and protecting against environmental conditions, and slowly releasing the flavor. Liolios et al. developed phosphatidylcholine-based liposomes containing thymol and carvacrol, isolated from *Origanum dictamnus* L. This encapsulation technique facilitated the antioxidant potency and antimicrobial attributes of the product. Yoshida et al. developed phosphatidylcholine-based multilamellar liposomes containing essential oils, isolated from Brazilian cherry leaves for better flavoring utility [36].

7.8.4   VITAMINS

Polymer encapsulation, Emulsion, Surfactant systems, and solid lipid nanoparticles (SLNs) are the reported and prevalent technologies for the delivery of vitamins. Recently, liposome encapsulation is employed for improving the vitamin bioavailability and better shelf life. Marsanasco et al. developed soy-phosphatidylcholine-based liposomes containing vitamin-C (Ascorbic acid) and vitamin-E (alpha-Tocopherol) and applied for fortifying the orange juice. The researchers found that the encapsulated liposomes exhibited sufficient protective effect and preserving the antioxidant activity of the present vitamins. Reports have been reviewed where improved stability of vitamin A-loaded liposomal system under light, pH, temperature, etc., have been seen. Additionally, folic-acid-targeted liposomal system for delivering peptides has been fabricated for enhancing the GIT absorption and accumulation at the target site [37].

7.8.5   MINERALS

Xia and Zu developed ferrous sulfate-loaded liposomes from the reverse-phase evaporation method that, when fortified with milk leads to higher heat stabilization and freshness for 7 days at 4°C. Toyran and Severcan fabricated liposomes encapsulating magnesium and vitamin D_2. The study revealed that liposomes delivered the nutrients in a much better way that interacted successfully with the biological membranes, facilitating higher absorption. Similar studies have been done so far with zinc liposomes as supplementary component in fortified foods [38]. Table 7.1 highlights the various liposomal Nutraceutical systems that are reported across the globe by researchers.

TABLE 7.1 Examples of Reported Liposomal Nutraceutical

Nutraceutical	Benefits	Diameter (nm)
Curcumin	Higher oral absorption	263
Green tea (Catechin)	Higher antioxidants	182
Ascorbic acid	Prevents oxidation of molecule	173
Ferrous sulfate	Nutraceutical applications	200
Calcein	Nutraceutical applications	84
Retinol	Slows retinol degradation	251
Medium-chain fatty acids	Prevents body fat accumulation	77
Carotene	Better peroxide radical scavenging	166
Thyme leaf polyphenols	Better free radical scavenging	174
Cholecalciferol	Increase concentration in skin	233
Trypsin	Rapid cheese ripening	110
Rosemary extract	Antioxidant principles delivery	223
Debitrase DBP20	Food grade pro-liposome	40
Tocopherol	Nutraceutical applications	212
Beef loin	Higher fat content delivery	294

7.9 CONCLUSION

The book chapter highlights the pharmacotheraputic applications, pharmaceutical approaches, and futuristic perspectives of the liposomes and their application as a carrier for delivering the nutraceuticals and functional foods like curcumin, enzymes, meat components, etc., with higher bioavailability, reduced hepatic metabolism through stealth characteristics, and reduced clearance level which affords both protective (free-radical scavenger, hepatoprotective, etc.), as well as therapeutic effects.

KEYWORDS

- delivery
- drug
- functional food
- large unilamellar vesicles
- liposome
- mononuclear phagocyte system
- nutraceutical
- phospholipid

REFERENCES

1. Samad, A., Sultana, Y., & Aqil, M., (2007). Liposomal drug delivery systems: An updated review. *Current Drug Delivery, 4*(4), 297–305.
2. Mansoori, M. A., Agrawal, S., Jawade, S., & Khan, M. I., (2012). A review on liposome. *International Journal Advanced Research Pharmaceutical and Bio-Sciences, 2*(4), 453–464.
3. Xiangqian, P., & Jian, Z., (2005). Review on the research progress of liposomes as carriers for topical and transdermal delivery [J]. *Chinese Pharmaceutical Affairs, 6.*
4. Loveleenpreet, K., Prabhjot, K., & Khan, M. U., (2013). Liposome as a drug carrier: A review. *Int. J. Res. Pharm. Chem., 3,* 121–128.
5. Mufamadi, M. S., Pillay, V., Choonara, Y. E., Du Toit, L. C., Modi, G., Naidoo, D., & Ndesendo, V. M., (2011). A review on composite liposomal technologies for specialized drug delivery. *Journal of Drug Delivery, 2011.*
6. Patel, N., & Panda, S., (2012). Liposome drug delivery system: A critic review. *JPSBR, 2*(4), 169–175.
7. Vemuri, S., & Rhodes, C. T., (1995). Preparation and characterization of liposomes as therapeutic delivery systems: A review. *Pharmaceutica Acta Helvetiae, 70*(2), 95–111.
8. ElBayoumi, T. A., & Torchilin, V. P., (2010). Current trends in liposome research. In: *Liposomes* (pp. 1–27). Humana Press.
9. Sercombe, L., Veerati, T., Moheimani, F., Wu, S. Y., Sood, A. K., & Hua, S., (2015). Advances and challenges of liposome assisted drug delivery. *Frontiers in* pharmacology, *6,* 286.
10. Singh, R., (2015). A Review on Liposome. *Research Journal of Pharmaceutical Dosage Forms and Technology, 7*(3), 226–231.
11. Uhumwangho, M. U., & Okor, R. S., (2005). *Current trends in the Production and Biomedical Applications of Liposomes: A Review. 4*(1), 9–21.
12. Karimi, N., Ghanbarzadeh, B., Hamishehkar, H., Keyvani, F., Pezeshki, A., & Gholian, M. M., (2015). *Phytosome and Liposome: The Beneficial Encapsulation Systems in Drug Delivery and Food Application. 2*(3), 17–27.

13. Dua, J. S., Rana, A. C., & Bhandari, A. K., (2012). Liposome: Methods of preparation and applications. *Int. J. Pharm. Stud. Res., 3*(2), 14–20.
14. Chauhan, T., Arora, S., Parashar, B., & Chandel, A., (2012). Liposome drug delivery: A review. *Int. J. Pharmaceutical and Chem. Sci., 3*, 754–764.
15. Tikshdeep, C., Sonia, A., Bharat, P., & Abhishek, C., (2012). Liposome drug delivery: A review. *Int. J. Pharm. Chem. Sci., 1*(3), 754–764.
16. Thulasiramaraju, T. V., Babu, A. S., Arunachalam, A., Prathap, M., Srikanth, S., & Sivaiah, P., (2012). Liposome: A novel drug delivery system. *International Journal of Biopharmaceutics, 2229*, 7499.
17. Agrawal, M. M., Jawade, S., & Khan, S., (2012). A review on liposome. *International Journal of Advanced Research in Pharmaceutical & BioSciences, 2*(1), 453–465.
18. Langner, M., & Kral, T. E., (1999). Liposome-based drug delivery systems. *Polish Journal of Pharmacology, 51*(3), 211–222.
19. Barenholz, Y., (2001). Liposome application: Problems and prospects. *Current Opinion in Colloid & Interface Science, 6*(1), 66–77.
20. Mali, A. D., & Bathe, R. S., (2015). An updated review on liposome drug delivery system. *Asian Journal of Pharmaceutical Research, 5*(3), 151–157.
21. Kaur, L., Kaur, P., & Khan, M. U., (2013). Liposome as a drug carrier—a review. *International Journal of Research in Pharmacy and Chemistry, 3*(1), 121–128.
22. Schwendener, R. A., (2014). Liposomes as vaccine delivery systems: A review of the recent advances. *Therapeutic Advances in Vaccines, 2*(6), 159–182.
23. Wasankar, S. R., Deshmukh, A. D., Ughade, M. A., Burghat, R. M., Gandech, D. P., Meghwani, R. R., & Faizi, S. M., (2012). Liposome as a drug delivery system: A review. *Research Journal of Pharmaceutical Dosage Forms and Technology, 4*(2), 104–112.
24. Pradhan, B., Kumar, N., Saha, S., & Roy, A., (2015). Liposome: Method of preparation, advantages, evaluation and its application. *Journal of Applied Pharmaceutical Research, 3*(3), 01–08.
25. Lokhande, S. S., (2018). Liposome drug delivery: An updated review. *Pharma Science Monitor, 9*(1).
26. Zylberberg, C., & Matosevic, S., (2016). Pharmaceutical liposomal drug delivery: A review of new delivery systems and a look at the regulatory landscape. *Drug Delivery, 23*(9), 3319–3329.
27. Van, R. N., & Sanders, A., (1994). Liposome mediated depletion of macrophages: Mechanism of action, preparation of liposomes and applications. *Journal of Immunological Methods, 174*(1, 2), 83–93.
28. Gao, W., Hu, C. M. J., Fang, R. H., & Zhang, L., (2013). Liposome-like nanostructures for drug delivery. *Journal of Materials Chemistry B, 1*(48), 6569–6585.
29. Akbarzadeh, A., Rezaei-Sadabady, R., Davaran, S., Joo, S. W., Zarghami, N., Hanifehpour, Y., & Nejati-Koshki, K., (2013). Liposome: Classification, preparation, and applications. *Nanoscale Research Letters, 8*(1), 102.
30. Immordino, M. L., Dosio, F., & Cattel, L., (2006). Stealth liposomes: Review of the basic science, rationale, and clinical applications, existing and potential. *International Journal of Nanomedicine, 1*(3), 297.
31. Ahmed, K. S., Hussein, S. A., Ali, A. H., Korma, S. A., Lipeng, Q., & Jinghua, C., (2019). Liposome: Composition, characterization, preparation, and recent innovation in clinical applications. *Journal of Drug Targeting, 27*(7), 742–761.

32. Maherani, B., Arab-Tehrany, E., R Mozafari, M., Gaiani, C., & Linder, M., (2011). Liposomes: A review of manufacturing techniques and targeting strategies. *Current Nanoscience, 7*(3), 436–452.

33. Liu, W., Ye, A., & Singh, H., (2015). Progress in applications of liposomes in food systems. In: *Microencapsulation and Microspheres for Food Applications* (pp. 151–170). Academic Press.

34. Kumar, P., & Shariff, R., (2011). Development of nutraceutical carriers for functional food applications. *Nutrition and Food Science*.

35. Liu, W., Ye, A., Liu, W., Liu, C., & Singh, H., (2013). Liposomes as food ingredients and nutraceutical delivery systems. *Agro. Food Industry Hi-Tech, 24*(2), 68–71.

36. Singh, H., Thompson, A., Liu, W., & Corredig, M., (2012). Liposomes as food ingredients and nutraceutical delivery systems. In: *Encapsulation Technologies and Delivery Systems for Food Ingredients and Nutraceuticals* (pp. 287–318). Woodhead Publishing.

37. Garti, N., & McClements, D. J., (2012). *Encapsulation Technologies and Delivery Systems for Food Ingredients and Nutraceuticals*. Elsevier.

38. Shade, C. W., (2016). Liposomes as advanced delivery systems for nutraceuticals. *Integrative Medicine: A Clinician's Journal, 15*(1), 33.

PART IV

Biphasic Systems for Delivering Nutraceutical Products

Self-Emulsifying Drug Delivery System for Potential Nutraceuticals: Solidification Techniques and Quality by Design (QbD)

SHAILESH S. CHALIKWAR,[1] PANKAJ V. DANGRE,[2] POORVA P. DUSAD,[1] and SANJAY J. SURANA[1]

[1]*Department of Pharmaceutical Quality Assurance,*
R.C. Patel Institute of Pharmaceutical Education and Research, Shirpur,
Dhule, Maharashtra, India

[2]*Department of Pharmaceutics, Data Meghe College of Pharmacy,*
Wardha 442004, Maharashtra, India

ABSTRACT

The newly innovated medications have extraordinary lipophilicity and lowest water solubility (biopharmaceutics classification system class IV and II), which consequences in reduced oral bioavailability, lack of dosage proportionality, and high intra- and inter-subject variability. For a better course of therapy, solubility is the utmost commanding standard to accomplish the preferred concentration of remedy in the systemic circulation. Self-micro emulsifying drug delivery system (SMEDDS) is an exclusive technique that helps in solving problems related to the transport of medications having the lowest aqueous solubility. SMEDDS are an isotropic mixture of oils, co-surfactant, and surfactants and are highly explored in resolving the bioavailability problem of drugs having low solubility. In recent times, nutraceuticals loaded SMEDDS has attracted to the researchers of medical sciences and industries lasting to their physical constancy, simple development approaches, and can be occupied in soft gelatin capsules after solidification. On oral administration of SMEDDS, it produces a medication comprising microemulsion with a great surface area upon distribution in the gastric tract. The micro-emulsion helps in the transport of drugs through the gut lymphatic pathway. The present chapter deals with nutraceuticals and its categorization, therapeutic applications, flavonoids, and citrus flavonoids, SEEDS, and its classifications, mechanism of self-emulsification, the formulation components in SMEDDS, solidification techniques of SMEDDS, QbD, critical quality attributes (CQAs), risk assessment and some genuine examples related with nutraceuticals.

8.1 INTRODUCTION

The oral drug delivery system is most commonly used for medication treatment due to its suitability of administration, patient comforts, economical, and simple enterprise of dosage form [1]. Though, oral administration of 50% of drug molecules is delayed because of their high lipophilicity [2]. Approximately, 40% of newly established new chemical entities (NCEs) show low water solubility, which results in poor bioavailability [3]. The absorption of such molecules from the GIT is typically controlled by the rate of dissolution [4]. Numerous research works have been implemented for emerging appropriate preparations to progress the bioavailability and solubility of BCS class II or IV drugs.

Oral route is popular and patient-convenient means of remedy management. Most of the drugs are being taken in the form of tablets and capsules by almost all patients. Though, nearby 26 to 50% of patients finds difficult to administered tablets and hard gelatin capsule orally [5]. These patients mostly comprise, aged (who have problems captivating conventional oral medications due to hand tremors and dysphasia), pediatric patients (who are often terrible at taking solid oral medicines, remaining to their immature muscular and nervous systems) [6] and others which include the psychologically ill, developmentally immobilized, patients who are unhelpful, on reduced liquid-intake plans or nauseous, and tourists who may not have access to aquatic medium [7, 8].

8.1.1 NUTRACEUTICALS

Nutraceuticals are the combination of 'nutrition' and 'pharmaceutical.' Nutraceuticals can be considered as the health assuring natural drug delivery systems which are foods or parts of food that maintains and alters the overall functions of the body that keeps the promising approach to regulate the healthy lifestyle of humans [9]. The global nutraceutical market is developing rapidly because of the healthy trends of the current population. The nutraceuticals are divided into different categories, which are dietary fibers (DFs), prebiotic, probiotic, polyunsaturated fatty acids (PUFA), antioxidants, and other various classifications of nutritive sources. These nutraceuticals are called dietary supplements (DS), which constitute the various phytochemicals as well as the nutritional ingredients like minerals, fibers, proteins, and vitamins. Nutraceuticals are intended to provide in the treatments of the various pathophysiological manifestations likewise, cardiovascular diseases (CVDs), cancer, obesity, diabetes, arthritis, and osteoporosis, etc. Nutraceuticals contribute versatile functions such as to interrupt the process of aging, improves health, and enhances life expectancy [10]. Particularly, the nutriment business is rising as per the exploration leaning zone owing to the DS which are prominent to the adapted period of remedy and fitness [11].

In the last few decades, various plant-based bioactive agents have been investigated as functional foods, nutraceuticals, and also in treatments of numerous critical disorders. Unfortunately, the herbal bioactive molecules often represent their inherent problems such as sensitivity to moisture, temperature, oxygen, pH, enzymes, etc., and lead to decreased pharmacological effects [12].

8.1.2   CLASSIFICATION OF NUTRACEUTICALS [9]

Nutraceuticals can be schematized in numerous approaches reliant on its effortless acceptance and use, i.e., for speculative education, proven experimental strategy, purposeful nutrition improvement or nutritional suggestions. Certain, greatest shared habits of classifying nutraceuticals can be grounded on diet bases, mechanism of action, biochemical environment, etc. The healthful basics used as DS can be categorized as:

1. **Polyphenols:** These form a great collection of phytochemicals, which are created by plants as subordinate metabolites to safeguard them from photosynthetic trauma, reactive oxygen classes. There are nearly 8,000 altered categories of polyphenols, the significant being anthocyanins, flavonols, flavanones, flavones, and flavan-3-ols. The exceedingly divided phenyl-propionic pathway synthesizes bulk of polyphenols. The most frequently happening polyphenols in food contain flavonoids and phenolic acids. Nutritive polyphenols are of existing attention because substantial proof *in vitro* have recommended that they can disturb abundant cellular procedures like, gene expression, apoptosis, platelet combination,

intercellular signaling, that can have anticancer-causing and anti-atherogenic suggestions.

These distant, polyphenols also have antioxidant, anti-inflammatory, antimicrobial, cardioprotective actions and play a role in the anticipation of neurodegenerative diseases and diabetes mellitus. Polyphenols are typically acknowledged for their antioxidant accomplishments on the basis of their fundamental chemistry. As compared to the vitamin E and Vitamin C, polyphenols are considered to be better antioxidant. The bioavailability of polyphenols is a significant dynamic defining their biological action.

2. **Probiotics:** A probiotic can be well-defined as a live microbial food supplement, when organized in acceptable quantities and helpfully marks the host animal by purifying its gastric bacterial stability.

3. **Polyunsaturated Fatty Acids (PUFAs):** These are also called "essential fatty acids" as these are fundamental to the body's role and are introduced rapidly via the nourishment. It is divided into two parts: omega-6-(n-6) fatty acids and omega-3-(n-3) fatty acids. Studies recommend that omega-3-fatty acids have three key special effects as cardiovascular syndromes, anti-arrhythmic.

4. **Prebiotics:** These are dietary ingredients that helpfully affect the host by selectively fluctuating the composition or metabolism of the gut microbiota. The prebiotic ingestion usually arouses the Lactobacillus and Bifid bacterial development in the gut, therefore assisting in breakdown. Some examples of these oligosaccharides are stachyose and raffinose found in peas and beans.

5. **Dietary Fiber (DF):** It is the food material, more specifically the plant material that is not hydrolyzed by enzymes concealed by the digestive tract, however, integrated by enzymes in the gastric tract. Foods rich in soluble fiber include fruits, oats, barley, and beans. Chemically DF resources include carbohydrate polymers with a degree of polymerization not lesser than 3, which are neither spent nor immersed in the small intestine. Built on their water solubility, DFs may be distinguished into two forms:

    i.   Insoluble dietary fiber (IDF), which involves celluloses, hemi-celluloses, and lignin which is enflamed to a limited range in the colon.

    ii. Soluble dietary fiber (SDF), which includes mucilage, pectin, gums, β-glycan, and hemicelluloses that are fermented in the colon.

6. **Antioxidant Vitamins:** Vitamins like vitamin E, vitamin C, and carotenoids are jointly known as antioxidant vitamins. These vitamins turn both separately as well as synergistically for the avoidance of oxidative reactions prominent to quite a lot of deteriorating syndromes counting malignancy and cardiac syndromes. These vitamins are abundant in numerous green veggies and fruits and use their protective action by free-radical scavenging tools. Vitamin E embraces of tocopherols and tocotrienols together with transmission of hydrogen atom and scavenge singlet oxygen and other over sensitive species thus shielding the per-oxidation of PUFA within the biological membrane and LDL. Tocotrienols are more mobile within the biological sheath than tocopherols because of the occurrence of the unsaturated side-chain and hence enters tissues with soaked fatty layers, i.e., in brain and liver more proficiently. They have extra reprocessing capacity and are a well inhibitor of liver oxidation.

7. **Spices:** These are esoteric nutrition attachments that are recycled for thousands of years to improve the sensory excellence of foods. The capability and the variability of the spices expended in the hot kingdoms are chiefly wide. These include distinctive aroma, flavor, and color to foodstuffs, motivating our hunger as well as alter the consistency of nutrients. New research discloses that nutritional spices in their little quantities has a huge impact on the human fitness by their chemopreventive, anti-oxidative, anti-inflammatory, ant mutagenic, immune-modulatory effects on cells and a wide range of beneficial effects on human health by the action of gastrointestinal (GI), cardiovascular, respiratory, metabolic, reproductive, neural another system.

8.1.3 FLAVONOIDS

Flavonoids are a class of polyphenolic molecules, existent in foodstuffs such as fruits, vegetables, and plant derivative juices comprising tea, coffee, and wine. There are many categories of flavonoids, counting flavonols, flavanones, flavones, anthocyanins, flavan-3-ols, and iso-flavones, which explain these molecules fabricated on their carbon structure and level of oxidation. Some studies have verified a relationship between the ingestion of flavonoid-rich régimes and the inhibition of human sickness containing cancer, type 2 diabetes, neurodegenerative syndromes, and osteoporosis. A latest potential study shown that depletion of citrus flavanones from orange and grapefruit juice was associated with a compact threat (19%) of ischemic stroke in women, indicating a cardio-protective outcome of these particles [13].

8.1.4 CITRUS FLAVONOIDS

Citrus flavonoids include numerous subcategories of flavonoids including O-polymethoxylated flavones (tangeretin and nobiletin) and flavanones (Hesperidin and naringin) and the bioactivity of these molecules depend on their structure and subsequent metabolism; naringin and hesperidin require hydrolysis to their active aglycone forms naringenin (NRG) and hesperidin, while nobiletin and tangeretin absence a glycoside moiety and are extra effortlessly fascinated by the intestine. In humans, following the ingestion of 200 mg of NRG as grapefruit juice, plasma levels reached 6 mmol/L, whereas plasma concentrations of hesperetin reached 1.3–2.2 mmol/L after absorption of 130–220 mg of hesperetin as orange juice. Though, these results are reported on flavonoid consumption from nutrition sources, and are consequently affected by the plenty food [13].

8.2 THERAPEUTIC APPLICATIONS OF NUTRACEUTICALS

8.2.1 DIABETES AND NUTRACEUTICALS

The utmost joint form of diabetes is type 2 diabetes with 95% dominance and is connected with obesity. Although countless medicines for hindrance and cure of diabetes have been announced, however, worldwide the total integer of individuals with diabetes with innumerable roots is enhancing diabetes, not only executes extensive financial problems on specific patients and their families but also places substantial economic burdens on society.

Iso-flavones have been premeditated most and their feasting has been accompanying with lower occurrence and mortality rate of type II diabetes, heart syndrome, osteoporosis, and assured malignances. Omega-3 fatty acids have been recommended to diminish glucose tolerance in patients susceptible to diabetes. For the synthesis of long-chain $n - 3$ fatty acids, insulin is mandatory; the heart may thus be mainly predisposed to their fading in diabetes. Ethyl esters of $n - 3$ fatty acids may be prospective favorable in diabetic patients. A lot of plants extract such as Toucriumpolium, cinnamon, and bitter melon have been presented to stop or cure diabetes [10].

8.2.2 INFLAMMATION AND NUTRACEUTICALS

Inflammation is characterized by puffiness, aching, inflammation, and warmth, and is the response of body muscles to annoyance or wound. Nutraceuticals that their regulation on osteoarthritis has been established are ginger, soybean, unsaponifiable, glucosamine, chondroitin, S-adeno-sylmethionine. Although they are harmless and healthy endured, however, the results are troubled by heterogeneity of the trainings and inconsistent results. Vitamins D and C are micronutrients for which sign of profit survives [14].

8.2.3 CARDIAC SYNDROMES AND NUTRACEUTICALS

Globally, the dominance of CVD and the investigation in this zone is developing [15–19]. CVD is a term which is utilized for syndromes of the heart and blood vessels and consists of coronary heart disease (heart attack), heart failure, hypertension, exterior vascular diseases, etc. CVD can be deserted by ingestion of root vegetables and fruitlets [20]. Many studies have described a defending part for a diet rich in vegetables and fruits in contrast to CVD [21–23]. The molecules such as polyphenols modify cellular metabolism and signaling, which is supposed to decrease arterial syndrome [24, 25].

8.2.4 CANCER AND NUTRACEUTICALS

Cancer has appeared as a chief community healthiness trouble in increasing kingdoms. A strong standard of living and diet can comfort in inhibition of tumor [19]. Carotenoids are a crowd of phytochemicals accountable for dissimilar shades of the diets. They have antioxidant actions and operational on cancer anticipation. Latest awareness in carotenoids has motivated on the part of lycopene in human fitness, exclusively in cancer disease [26]. Plants ironic in daidzein, biochanin, isoflavones, and genistein, also obstruct prostate cancer cell development [27]. Because of the unsaturated environment of lycopene, it is reflected to be a powerful antioxidant and a singlet oxygen quencher. Lycopene reflects in the testes, prostate, and skin, where it protects counter to malignancy [26, 27].

8.3   SELF-EMULSIFYING DRUG DELIVERY SYSTEMS [28]

Self-emulsifying drug transport classifications are composite lipid-based drug transport classifications constituted of a blend of oils (lipids), co-surfactants, and surfactants and These organizations are classically self-emulsifying, thus having the capability to produce satisfactory microemulsions upon minor stirring subsequent watering with an aqueous phase or mild stirring delivered by intestinal indication *in vivo*. To allow distinction amongst several lipid classifications Pouton presented the lipid formulation classification system (LFCS), which compromises a well clarification and contrast of conveyed documents according to LFCS; self-emulsifying classifications fit into class II and IIIA.

8.3.1   MECHANISM FOR SELF-EMULSIFICATION [29]

Conservative emulsions are established by collaborating two non-miscible liquors precisely water and oil developed steady by use of an emulsifier. When an emulsion is prepared surface area enlargement is produced amongst the two stages. The emulsion is steadied by the surfactant molecules that form a film nearby the internal stage droplet. In conventional emulsion materialization, the surplus surface free energy is reliant on the droplet size and the interfacial pressure. If the emulsion is not soothed using surfactants, the two segments will detach decreasing the interfacial tension and the free energy. In the case of SMEDDS, the free energy of establishment is exact little and progressive or even undesirable which results in thermodynamic spontaneous emulsification. It has been advocated that self-emulsification occurs due to dispersion of water into the liquid crystalline (LC) stage that is designed at the oil/surfactant-water boundary in which liquid can penetrate facilitated by mild stirring throughout self-emulsification. After water enters to a definite level, there is interference of the interface and a droplet development. This LC phase is deliberated to be in authority for the extraordinary stability of the ensuing nanoemulsion compared to coalescence.

SEDDS are categorized as follows:

i.   Self-micro emulsifying drug delivery systems; and
ii. Self-nano emulsifying drug delivery systems.

8.3.1.1   SELF-MICRO EMULSIFYING DRUG DELIVERY SYSTEMS (SMEDDS) [30]

Self-micro-emulsifying drug delivery system (SMEDDS) is an incredible approach for improving the solubility of the compounds having the lowest aqueous solubility. SMEDDS are an isotropic mixture of surfactants, co-surfactant, and oils that produces microemulsion, upon mild agitation followed by dilutions in aqueous medium, such as GI liquids. The gastric motility of the stomach results in the production of microemulsion into the GIT. SMEDDS displays the systems creating clear microemulsions with oil drops fluctuating between 100 and 250 nm.

8.3.1.1.1   Advantages of SMEDDS

1. **Improvement in Oral Bioavailability:** Dissolution ratio reliant on absorption is the main aspect that bounds the bioavailability of many ailing aqueous solvable medicines. The ability of SMEDDS to surviving the medication into the gut in dispersed and micro emulsified custom and subsequent growth in fixed posturing area permit additional well-organized medication passage through the intestinal aqueous border layer and through the absorptive brush boundary sheath resulting to enriched bioavailability [26].

2. **Ease of Manufacture and Scale-Up:** Ease of production and scale-up is one of the greatest significant benefits that mark SMEDDS exceptional when paralleled to former drug delivery systems like liposomes, nanoparticles, solid dispersions (SDs), etc. It deals with development of bioavailability. SMEDDS requisite very modest and cost-effective production accommodations like a simple mixer with agitator and volumetric liquid filling equipment for extensive manufacturing. This clarifies the attention of industry in the SMEDDS [27].

3. **Decrease in Inter-Subject and Intra-Subject Inconsistency and Food Effects:** Nearby abundant drugs are there which shows

enormous inter-subject and intra-subject alteration in captivation prominent to declined routine of medication and long-suffering non-compliance. Food is a key feature moving the healing routine of the drug in the patient body. SMEDDS are a detriment for such medications [31, 32].

4. **Ability to Deliver Peptides That are Prone to Enzymatic Hydrolysis in GIT:** One unique possession that sorts SMEDDS grander as associated to the other drug delivery systems is their skill to distribute macromolecules like enzyme substrates, hormones, peptides, and inhibitors and their capability to agree defense from enzymatic hydrolysis.

8.3.1.1.2   Disadvantages of SMEDDS [1]

1. High concentrations of surfactants and storage temperature, etc.;
2. Interaction of fill with the capsule shell;
3. At low temperatures there might be precipitation of APIs and/or some excipients, which can be dissolved again when warmed to room temperature;
4. Low medication filling capability.

8.3.1.1.3   Components in the SMEDDS Formulation [1]

1. **Oils:** This is deliberated as the important component in SEDDS. It has the skill to solubilize the mandatory dose of the hydrophobic drug and helps self-emulsification as well as progress the lymphatic transportation of lipophilic medicine which increases the fascination of the medication from micro gut flora. The saturated fatty oils (medium-chain or long-chain) and hydrolyzed vegetable oils have been extensively employed in the formulation of SMEDDS due to their formulation compatibility and physical advantages. Conversely, the SMEDDS comprises together unsaturated and saturated lipids. The choice of oil depends on their properties, composition, application, and HLB. The myristic, capric, caprylic, caproic, and lauric acid are highly employed oils in the formulation of SEDDS (Figure 8.1).

2. **Surfactant:** It is the greatest vital constituent of SMEDDS formulation. Surfactant imparts the crucial emulsifying features to the

SMEDDS. Surfactants of the usual source are preferred because they are harmless than the synthetic surfactants. The assortment of a particular surfactant for formulation depends upon its HLB value and safety concern. The widely utilized are the nonionic surfactants with a moderately higher HLB value. The frequently utilized nonionic surfactant consists of Tween 80 and Pluronic F-127. Surfactant has the capability to dissolve fairly huge quantity of hydrophobic drug molecules and thus stop the precipitation of the drug inside the GIT.

3. **Co-Surfactant:** The co-surfactant in SMEDDS formulation enables the dispersion procedure and expands the dispersion rate. Co-surfactant is regularly active to dissolve greater quantities of either the hydrophilic surfactant or the drug in the lipid base. The innovative co-solvents such as Transcutol™ and Glycofurol™ have several pluses over the outdated ones, including superior stability and less impulsiveness.

4. **Drug:** Medications belonging to BCS class II and Class IV have perfect characteristics that satisfy all the necessities of drug selection standards for SMEDDS preparations.

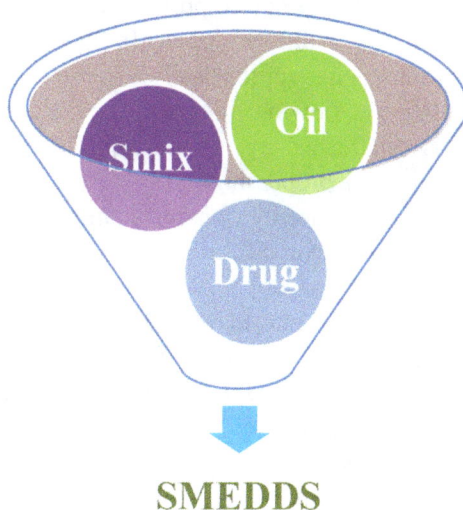

SMEDDS

FIGURE 8.1 Components in the SMEDDS formulation.

8.3.1.1.4 *Solidification Techniques for Liquid SMEDDS [1]*

Normally, the formulated SMEDDS is liquid in state, but sometimes it could be in a semisolid state depending on the physical state of excipients used.

Solid SMEDDS also offers added versatility in terms of possible dosage forms. The following description elaborates various liquid to solid SMEDDS transformation techniques [1]:

1. **Melt Granulation:** In this process, the agglomerates of the powder blend containing SMEDDS are formed. The process employed a moldable polymer and melting is performed at a relatively low temperature. An extensive series of solid and semisolid lipids can be active as moldable polymers. Amongst these, Gelucire is usually utilized. It also helps in the improvement in the dissolution rate. The melt granulation process is commonly employed for adsorbing SMEDDS onto inert solid carriers.

2. **Spray Drying:** The procedure includes the solubilization of the medication in the liquid constituents so as to produce a uniform combination. The same liquid blend is then atomized in the arrangement of a spray of drops. The droplets are carried into a drying compartment, so as to vaporize water confined in the liquid fusion ensuing in the creation of dry constituents. The cautious assessments are approved out to come across the preferred provisions of the residue.

3. **Adsorption to the Solid Support:** In this approach, the liquid SMEDDS formulation is appropriately adsorbed on inert solid support so as to acquire free-flowing fine particles. The method is relatively simple and is established by mixing liquid SMEDDS formulation with solid carrier in a proper mixer.

   The procedure is used extensively and has plentiful benefits, that is, drug content, drug uniformity, and outstanding drug-loading capability (up to 70% w/w).

4. **Alginate Beads Loaded Liquid SMEDDS:** Alginate beads comprising liquid SMEDDS are the admirable formulation to boost the gastric steadiness of the liquid SMEDDs by transforming them into SMEDDS loaded sodium alginate beads [33, 34]. It is the auspicious methodology for accurate drug targeting at its position; as the alginate beads loaded SMEDDS act as transporters for drug targeting in numerous cures of syndromes. SMEDDS loaded alginate beads are formulated by the Inotropic gelation technique by which preparation filling (SMEDDS loading) into beads carried out [35]. The Sodium alginate is the biopolymer which is harmless, harmonious, and risk-free in nature and the calcium chloride acts as the dispersion medium liable for the crosslinking method of the alginate beads comprehending SMEDDS [36]. Additional beads formulations are also offered to have tactics towards

firmness and drug pointing such as; floating alginate beads [37] and entrapment of peptides and proteins in hydrogel beads [38].

8.3.1.2   SELF-NANO EMULSIFYING DRUG DELIVERY SYSTEMS (SNEDDS)

SNEDDS are anhydrous isotropic liquid blends of co-surfactant, oils, and surfactant which instantaneously produce o/w nanoemulsions upon dispersion in the aqueous phase with mild stirring. The simple modification between SMEDDS and SNEDDS is between the dimensions of the oil globules produced afterward the emulsification. The dimensions of SMEDDS signify the globule size between 100 and 250 nm, whereas in the circumstances with the SNEDDS, the size globule is deliberated less than 100 nm. Both SMEDDS and SNEDDS have been displayed to be the greatest prosperous methodologies in the enrichment of solubility and bioavailability of the BCS class IV and II medications.

8.4   QUALITY BY DESIGN (QBD)

Quality by design (QbD) is an innovative methodology where product provisions, development process, and unsafe parameters are comprised in order to have the final endorsement and continuing quality control (QC) of new medication [39].

QbD is all-inclusive tactics to enlarge those newcomers with predefined intentions, and impactful on product and manner sympathetic and procedure regulator, based on sound science and quality risk supervision. The use of QbD philosophies has established plenty of curiosity in pharmaceutical production. Design of experiment (DoE) is a subdivision of functional statistics, broadly executed in critical systems to learn the sound effects of numerous elements and their collaboration on system reply and enhance the situations for the preferred outcome with lowest trials. The application of DOE is actually resourceful and noticeably rarer efforts areas linked with the outdated methodology. Statistical software such as Design Expert and JMP, etc., is supportive in designing and optimization of the experiments with compulsory screening prototypes. The screening models are associated in accepting the influence of variables. The full factorial design is usually exploited into screening models in the pharmaceutical industry, and it is careful the most proficient in scrutinizing the result of separable variables along with the communicating product of every variable on required responses [40, 41].

8.4.1   CRITICAL QUALITY ATTRIBUTES (CQAS)

The relevant critical quality attributes (CQAs) of the SMEDDS formulation can be justified by quality risk management system and experimentation. The general CQAs of the SMEDDS formulation should be considered during the product development. Hereinafter, are described some of the critical common quality attributes that should be considered during the SMEDDS development:

1. **Physical Attributes:** The liquid and solid SMEDDS formulation after preparation are generally packaged either in the capsule or transferred into another suitable dosage form. Therefore, the physical attributes, namely, color, odor, and appearance of the formulation are not considered as critical attributes. Furthermore, these attributes are not associated with efficacy and safety of the patient.

2. **Assay and Drug Content:** The SMEDDS formulation being the homogeneous dispersion should contain the appropriate amount of the drug to ensure the desired therapeutic effect. The variability in the drug assay and content uniformity is likely to influence the drug safety and efficacy [42]. Therefore, these attributes are considered moderately critical.

3. **Self-Emulsification Time:** It is a time taken by SMEDDS to get emulsified in the aqueous medium. The fading of the SMEDDS in the mediocre provides a signal for emulsification. The emulsification is prime essential for the SMEDDS and hence is considered highly critical. The time of emulsification varies with the composition of the SMEDDS, as the more amount of oil in the formulation requires more time for emulsification [39]. However, less time for emulsification indicates the maximum efficiency of the formulation.

4. **Globule Size:** The globule size of SMEDDS is also considered highly critical since the smaller globule size allows better penetration through GI epithelial lining and para-cellular pathways [43]. The size of the globule depends upon the amount and chemical nature of the surfactant and co-surfactant in the SEDDS formulation.

5. **Thermodynamic Stability:** The thermodynamic stability of SMEDDS is considered a critical attribute as the SMEDDS should withstand the variation in temperature, mainly throughout the storing time. For this study, the SMEDDS formulation is exposed to different stress conditions through freeze-thaw cycle (–21 and +25°C) and heating-cooling cycle (4 and 45°C) with the storage at each temperature of not less than 48 h [44].

6. **Permeability:** The permeation of the drug molecule is highly desirable for achieving the therapeutically effective concentration in plasma blood concentration. SMEDDS is notably employed for enhancing the permeation characteristics of the drug, and therefore this parameter is considered a critical attribute.
7. **Bioavailability:** This is regarded as the amount of the drug that enters into the systemic circulation. The SMEDDS is commonly employed to improve the bioavailability of lipophilic drugs or those drugs which have less bioavailability. The efficiency of the SMEDDS formulation depends upon its ability to improve the bioabsorption of the drug, and therefore s considered highly critical.
8. **Dissolution Efficiency:** Dissolution profile of the SMEDDS formulation provides information about the drug release pattern as well as the solubilization of the drug in the dissolution medium. The performance of the SMEDDS formulation completely depends upon its dissolution efficiency and hence is considered a critical attribute.

8.4.2   RISK ASSESSMENT

Failure mode effect analysis (FMEA) was employed in the risk analysis studies for identification of potential CMAs/or CPPs of SMEDDS. In this, each potential failure mode was ranked on the basis of anticipated frequency of occurrence, i.e., probability (P); severity (S) indicates impact of potential failure mode on final dosage form, and detectability (D) indicates finding of potential failure mode during manufacturing. Failure risk was estimated by risk priority number (RPN) representing the overall magnitude of the risk [45].

8.4.2.1   PROSPECTIVE ZONES OF UTILIZATION FOR FAILURE MODE EFFECTIVE ANALYSIS (FMEA) [46]

- The productivity/outcomes of FMEA can be recycled as an origin for design or additional investigation or to monitor reserve exploitation.
- FMEA can be functional to tools and conveniences and might be used to evaluate the production process and its outcome on invention or development.

8.5 SMEDDS CONTAINING PROMINENT NUTRACEUTICALS

Some prominent examples of SEDDS, SMEDDS, and SNEDDS loaded with nutraceuticals are explored herewith. These explored formulations have given special emphasis on improvement in solubility, better drug dissolution, enhancement of pharmacological efficacy, ease in oral administration, and likewise so many objectives were accomplished. Herein, the prominent nutraceuticals incorporated in the self-emulsifying formulations are detailed as follows;

8.5.1 CURCUMIN

An oral colon-targeted impermeable capsule medication was developed for Curcumin (Cur) encompassing SMEDDS in alginate beads. The presented SMEEDS technique leads to solubility enhancement of Cur. Here, the prepared liquid SMEDDS-Cur was then incorporated into alginate beads. An impermeable capsule body was employed to deliver Cur and tablet plug (konjac glucomannan (KG), lactose (Lac), and hydroxypropyl methylcellulose (HPMC) were used to form tablet plug) was placed in mouth of capsule body to avoid the drug release. Finally, the capsule body was enclosed with enteric cap. The tablet plug cannot be hydrolyzed in the upper gastrointestinal tract (GIT), however, in the small intestine, KG gels get swelled and blocked the mouth of the capsule. In the colon, the microbial enzymes degraded the KG and disintegrated the designed tablet plug. This impermeable capsule has shown potential for use in colon-targeted drug delivery and also exhibited a sustained-release of Cur [35].

8.5.2 AQUEOUS INSOLUBLE NUTRACEUTICALS

In the present study, five bioactive compounds such as quercetin, vitamin K2, trans-resveratrol, vitamin A, and coenzyme Q10 were chosen as model nutraceuticals as they represent major bioavailability problem because of their poor water solubility. The SMEDDS components used were Capmul MCM NF, Captex 355 EP/NF, and Tween 80, which belongs GRAS (Generally regarded as safe) category. The tried lipids and tween 80 showed good solubilization capacity for above nutraceuticals. The prepared formulations were filled into a hard gelatin capsule. All bioactive compounds showed enhanced solubility with SMEEDS formulations. Therefore, presented report provides a simple and organic solvent free SMEDDS (lipid-based) for the oral delivery of poorly water-soluble nutraceuticals [47].

8.5.3 ORIDONIN

A pharmacologically active oridonin, an *ent*-kaurane diterpenoid compound is isolated from the Chinese herb *Raddosia rubescens* (*Hamsl.*) *Hara* and chosen as a model drug for development of SMEEDS. Screening of oil and surfactants was done by considering the solubility and loading capacity of oridonin. The TEM study on oridonin SMEDDS reveled spherical micro-emulsion droplets. In SMEDDS, more than 85% of oridonin was released during the first 6 h followed by 100.2% at the end of 12 h, indicating complete drug release. *In vivo* pharmacokinetic study was conducted in Sprague Dawley (SD) rats. The relative bioavailability of the SMEDDS was determined and found to be 220.21% in comparison to suspension of pure oridonin. These results suggested the potential use of SMEDDS for oral administration of oridonin [48].

8.5.4 TOTAL FLAVONES OF HIPPOPHAE RHAMNOIDES L.

The kind of literature revealed that total flavones extracted from sea buckthorn (*Hippophae rhamnoides* L.) (TFH) are well known as herbal medicines and DS. TFH exhibited therapeutically significant effects in the treatment of cardiovascular and cerebrovascular diseases. Oral SMEEDS was developed using a central composite design to overcome the inherent drawbacks of TFH. SMEEDS drastically increased solubility of TFH. Author conducted *in vitro* and *in vivo* studies for TFH SMEEDS and TFH suspension. The *in vitro* drug release (TFH) from SMEDDS was quicker and more complete than that from suspension. *In vivo* pharmacokinetic study was for TFH-SMEDDS in Sprague-Dawley (SD) rats to determine the relative bioavailability of TFH. It was spectacularly increased for SMEEDS, i.e., 3.09 folds as compared with the CMC-Na suspension of TFH. This research indicated the prospective application of SMEDDS as a vehicle to increase the oral bioavailability of poorly soluble functional food ingredient, i.e., TFH [49].

8.5.5   *NARINGENIN (NRG)*

In the present days, epidemiological experiments and nutritional studies have recommended that increased consumption of fruits and vegetables rich in antioxidants to defend against chronic disorders such as CVDs and cancer. NRG, dominant flavanone obtained from grapefruits has anti-inflammatory, anti-cancer, hepato-protective, and anti-lipid peroxidation effects. As it is poorly water-soluble that leads to slow dissolution and thereby yield low oral bioavailability, which restricts its therapeutic application. Thus, in the current investigation, an attempt has been made to enhance solubility and thereby oral bioavailability of NRG by employing SNEEDS. Crucially the components of SNEEDS such as oil, surfactant, and co-surfactant were selected and developed SNEEDS were evaluated thoroughly. The NRG SNEEDS under the TEM was spherical and oil globules ranging diameters from 40 to 55 nm. *In vitro* release of NRG from SNEDDS was significantly higher ($p<0.005$) than pure drug. *In vivo* pharmacokinetic studies were performed in male Albino Wistar rats. The area under curve (AUC_{0-24}) of NRG from SNEDDS formulation revealed a significant increase ($p<0.005$) in NRG absorption compared to native NRG suspension (0.5% w/v of CMC). Thus, the developed system could be used as an effective approach for enhancing the solubility and bioavailability of poorly water-soluble grapefruit flavonoid like NRG [50].

8.5.6   *APIGENIN*

Flavonoids have a several potential pharmacological activities such as antioxidant, anti-tumor, anti-inflammatory, anti-viral, anti-bacterial, and anti-anxiety. Apigenin is widely distributed in fruits and vegetables, such as onions, orange, tea, chamomile, and wheat sprouts. The poor water solubility of apigenin has restricts its exploration of medical applications. Thus, the author developed apigenin loaded SMEEDS formulation and optimized by using a simplex lattice experiment design. In preliminary work, ternary phase diagrams were constructed in order to obtain an appropriate concentration range of components. The equilibrium solubility of apigenin in the optimized SMEDDS formulation was found to be enhanced. TEM picture of the apigenin microemulsion droplets appeared as spherical in shape. *In vitro* dissolution studies showed about 95% of apigenin was released within 10 min. The promising results of SMEDDS would be a potential carrier to ameliorate the oral absorption of apigenin and other likely flavonoids [51].

8.5.7 LIMONENE

Today worldwide extensive investigation is going on to study the functional ingredients obtained from edible plants for exploring their potential applications in food engineering and clinical use. The favorable health effects of the functional ingredient exhibited relatively fair toxicity along with side effects than synthetic drugs used to eventually treat similar disorders. Limonene, one of them, seems to be a classic representative. It is a functional compound and represents poor dissolution as the main obstacle in the effectual development of oral formulations. Thus, to improve solubility and low oral bioavailability, limonene-loaded SMEDDS were formulated and thoroughly characterized. TEM analysis of limonene-loaded SMEEDS revealed discrete and spherical shapes. *In vitro* drug release study was performed to confirm the enhanced solubility of limonene SMEEDS. A pharmacokinetic study was conducted in male SD rats. Oral bioavailability of limonene SMEDDS was found to be 3.71-fold greater than pure limonene. Furthermore, the biodistribution studies in Kunming mice suggested that the limonene SMEDDS predominantly accumulated in various tissues, particularly in the liver, kidney, and brain when compared to limonene alone. The current research further indicated that SMEDDS could act as a promising alternative platform for improving oral bioavailability of functional but poorly soluble compound to that of commercially available capsules of limonene [52].

8.5.8 RESVERATROL

Polyphenolic phytoconstituents are well known for their diverse health promoting effects. Among flavonoids, resveratrol not only as a food supplement but also as a drug in human medicine and rich in grapes, and peanuts. It has antioxidant, anti-cancer, anti-inflammatory, and phytoestrogenic activities. As it belongs to BCS class II and undergo extensive first-pass intestinal and hepatic metabolism, which resulted in poor oral bioavailability. Thus, to exploit the health benefits of resveratrol an effectual, SMEDDS was employed. The dissolution study of pure resveratrol and SMEDDS containing resveratrol was performed using hydrochloric acid solution (pH 1.2) and phosphate buffer solution (pH 6.8) as dissolution medium. As expected, dissolution of pure resveratrol was low as compared to resveratrol in SMEDDS. The *in vitro* cell vitality and integrity performance of resveratrol-loaded SMEDDS were assessed with rat intestine and Caco-2 cells. The result suggested that SMEDDS would be a promising approach for resveratrol to overcome its biopharmaceutical, pharmacokinetic, and toxicological issues, leading to explore resveratrol as a food supplement having potential pharmacological activity [53].

8.5.9 METHOXYFLAVONES IN KAEMPFERIA PARVIFLORA (KP)

Kaempferia parviflora (KP) plant belongs to the family of Zingiberaceae found especially in the north of Thailand and widely used as herbal medicine for long back. Its reported extract has anti-inflammatory, antimicrobial, anti-peptic ulcer, aphrodisiac, anti-allergic, anti-cancer, anti-obesity, cardioprotection, anticholinesterase, antimutagenicity, and antidepressant action/activity. Methoxyflavones such as 5,7-dimethoxyflavone (DMF), 5,7,4′-trimethoxyflavone (TMF), and 3,5,7,3′,4′-pentamethoxyflavone (PMF) are reported as the major and active components. Methoxyflavones are lipophilic, thus yield poor oral bioavailability (1–4%) and limits its potent utility. Accordingly oral SMEDDS and cyclodextrin (CD) complex formulations were employed to enhance the absorption of KP. The prepared formulations were then characterized for *in vitro* dissolution study, permeability through Caco-2 cells, and *in vivo* oral absorption in male SD rats. The results showed remarkable change in the dissolution of methoxyflavones from KP-SMEDDS and KP-2-HP-β-CD complex in both media (0.1 N HCl and phosphate buffer saline (PBS) pH 6.8). For both (KP-SMEDDS and KP-2-HP-β-CD complex), oral bioavailability values were greater than those of pure KP. Developed new strategic KP-SMEDDS and KP-2-HP-β-CD complex formulations stood successfully to ameliorate oral bioavailability of methoxyflavones [54].

8.5.10 SILYBIN

Silybin, a natural flavonoid extracted from plant seeds and fruits of milk thistle (Silybum marianum (L.) Gaertn) used to treat several disorders of liver, spleen, and gallbladder. Especially as a heaptoprotectants, silybin was found clinically effective in the treatment of a variety of liver disorders such as acute and chronic viral hepatitis, toxin-, and drug-induced hepatitis and cirrhosis, and alcoholic liver disease. Silybin is poorly water-soluble (0.4 mg/mL) bioactive ingredient in turn results in poor oral absorption and bioavailability. Thus, the author has planned in the current investigation to explore a high payload supersaturable self-emulsifying drug delivery system (S-SEDDS) for enhancement of oral bioavailability of silybin. Herein,

HPMC was used as a precipitation inhibitor. *In vitro* dilution of the S-SEDDS formulation resulted in the formation of a microemulsion, followed by a slow precipitation of silybin, but in the traditional SEDDS formulation, silybin undergoes rapid precipitation. This yield low silybin solution concentration. The *in vivo* pharmacokinetic study conducted in male Sprague-Dawley (SD) rats indicated that the relative bioavailability of the silybin-S-SEDDS increased by 3.02-fold than those of the conventional SEDDS. This research investigation clearly demonstrated that the oral bioavailability of silybin has significantly enhanced by employing supersaturable S-SEDDS formulation technique [55].

8.5.11 PUERARIN

Puerarin (4,7-dihydroxy-8_-d-glucosyl isoflavone) is insoluble in water and derived from the roots of *Pueraria lobata* belonging to the family Fabaceae. Literature reports revealed certain beneficial properties related to puerarin such as hypertension, hyperlipidemia, hemicrania, coronary heart disease, myocardial infarction, and angina pectoris. It also improves micro-circulation, dilation of coronary artery, and can increase the blood flow in the brain along with anti-thromboxane, antispam, and anti-platelet aggregation properties. In spite of these activities, it has poor bioavailability. Thus, the author planned to develop puerarin SMEEDS for sustained release in the form of pellet. Extrusion-spheronization technique was employed for the production of pellets. Particle size distribution was studied using SEM and TEM analysis. *In vivo* study was carried out using beagle dogs to explore the pharmacokinetic parameters of puerarin-SMEDDS sustained-release pellets. Relative bioavailability was increased by 2.6-fold for puerarin-SMEDDS sustained-release pellets when compared with puerarin tablets. Stability studies of puerarin-SMEDDS sustained-release pellets proved their robustness when conducted at $30 \pm 2°C$ along with $65 \pm 5\%$ RH for three months. The results demonstrated that the formulated puerarin-SMEDDS sustained-release pellets could be a noteworthy approach for enhancement of oral bioavailability of puerarin [56].

8.5.12 GINGEROL

Ginger (*Zingiber officinale*) belonging to the family Zingiberaceae, one of the most pharmacological important spices. Ginger is accepted worldwide as it contains so many potent biologically active moieties which include gingerols, shogaols, parasols, and zingerone. These compounds are producing the "hot" sensation in the mouth and consist of [6]-Gingerol [5-hydroxy-1-(4-hydroxy-3methoxy phenyl) decan-3-one] as the main bioactive constituent. It appears as white powder with the bitter taste and routinely referred to as spice. It is slightly soluble in water, thus limiting its therapeutic benefits. Thus, the purpose of the current research was to employ the SMEEDS as effectual drug delivery system for loading of [6]-Gingerol. The [6]-Gingerol-SMEDDS consists of ethyl oleate as oil, Cremophor EL35 as surfactant, and 1,2-propanediol as co-surfactant. The TEM study on [6]-Gingerol SMEDDS revealed spherical, homogenous, and well dispersed particles. The three different media such as HCl (pH 1.2); Double distilled water (pH 7.0), and phosphate buffer solution (pH 7.4) were used for *in vitro* release study. It was significantly higher than in SMEEDS formulations as that of the free [6]-Gingerol, which further confirmed with*in vivo* pharmacokinetic study. Oral bioavailability of [6]-Gingerol SMEEDS was found to be 6.58-fold greater than the free [6]-Gingerol. Therefore, to explore therapeutic potentials, [6]-Gingerol-SMEDDS could be a promising alternative [57].

8.5.13 ASTILBIN

Astilbin, flavonoid obtained from Chinese herb *Rhizoma smilacis Glabrae.* It is widely used in traditional Chinese medicine because of its potential therapeutic activities, such as antioxidant, antihypertensive, anti-inflammatory, and selective immunosuppressant activity. However, its low water solubility and bioavailability restricts its clinical use. Thus, authors developed SMEDDS for astilbin. Pseudoternary phase diagrams were constructed to screen the components along with their ranges based on the micro-emulsification area. Furthermore, central composite design was implemented for the production of astilbin SMEDDS formulation batches. Spherical shape astilbin microemulsion was confirmed by using a transmission electron microscope. Astilbin loaded SMEEDS was subjected for *in vitro* drug release study by using the reverse dialysis method. *In vivo* pharmacokinetic study was conducted in beagle dogs and astilbin analysis from plasma samples were carried out using LC-MS technique. The relative bioavailability of the astilbin SMEDDS was found to be 5.59-fold greater than that of raw astilbin suspension. Therefore, *in vitro,* and *in vivo* results demonstrated the SMEEDS could be a promising approach for poorly soluble drugs like astilbin [58].

8.6 CONCLUSION

SMEDDS is principally amalgam of oil, surfactant, and co-surfactant. The latest studies have revealed its capability to progress the solubility and bioavailability of the oral nutraceutical delivery. The restrictions of the liquid SMEDDS formulation can be effortlessly overcome by solidifying into a solid form. There are methods for the alteration of liquid SMEDDS into a solid form. These methods are currently receiving additional apprehension to discover their efficacy for economical manufacturing.

There are limitations that should be accounted, predominantly in the manufacturing and progression of the SMEDDS for oral nutraceutical delivery. The CQAs should be cautiously allotted to inhibit batch disasters or unaccepted conditions. All the critical attributes should be appropriately structured and well-ordered directive to construct the superiority of the formulation. A sound understanding of the system may be desired to regulate and exceeds the unsuccessful records.

Lastly, it is essential that SMEDDS with proper solidification should be executed for the progress of suitable pharmaceutical dosage form for the patient. Also, this expertise covers the way for oral delivery of nutraceuticals to move to remarkably suitable pharmaceutical dosage form.

KEYWORDS

- **cardiovascular disease**
- **insoluble dietary fiber**
- **lipid formulation classification system**
- **liquid-crystalline**
- **new chemical entities**
- **soluble dietary fiber**

REFERENCES

1. Dangre, P. V., & Chalikwar, S. S., (2019). Self-emulsifying drug delivery system (SEDDS): Formulation development and quality attributes. In: Vakhrushev, V., Kodolov, V., Haghi, A., & Ameta, C., (eds.), *Carbon Nanoparticles and Nanotubes* (1st edn., pp. 241–258). AAP, CRC Press, (Taylor & Francis group).

2. Gursoy, R. N., & Benita, S., (2004). Self-emulsifying drug delivery systems (SEDDS) for improved oral delivery of lipophilic drugs. *Biomed. Pharmacother., 58*, 173–182.

3. Tang, B., Cheng, G., Gu, J. C., & Xu, C. H., (2008). Development of solid self-emulsifying drug delivery systems: Preparation techniques and dosage forms. *Drug Discov., 13*(13, 14), 606–612.

4. Pouton, C. W., (2006). Formulation of poorly water-soluble drugs for oral administration: Physiochemical and physiological issues and the lipid formulation classification system. *Eur. J. Pharm. Sci., 29*(3, 4), 278–287.

5. Andersen, O., Zweidorff, O. K., Hjelde, T., & Rødland, E. A., (1995). Problems when swallowing tablets: A questionnaire study from general practice. *Journal of the Norwegian Large Association: Journal of Practical Medicine, Nyraekke, 115*(8), 947–949.

6. Slowson, M., & Slowson, S., (1985). *What to do When Patients Cannot Swallow Their Medications* (Vol. 51, pp. 90–96). Pharm, Times.

7. Lindgren, S., & Janzon, L., (1993). Dysphagia: Prevalence of swallowing complaints and clinical finding. *Med. Clin. North Am., 77*, 3–5.

8. Chang, R. K., Xiaodi, G., Burnside, B. A., & Couch, R. A., (2000). Fast-dissolving tablets. *Pharma Tech., 24*(6), 52–58.

9. Das, L., Bhaumik, E., & Raychaudhuri, U., (2012). Role of nutraceuticals in human health. *J. Food Sci. Tech., 49*(2), 173–183.

10. Nasri, H., Baradaran, A., Shirzad, H., & Kopaei, M. R., (2014). New concept in nutraceuticals as alternative for pharmaceuticals. *Int. J. Prev. Med., 5*(12), 1487–1499.

11. Gul, K., Singh, A. K., & Jabeen, R., (2015). Nutraceuticals and functional foods: The foods for the future world. *Cri. Rev. Food Sci. Nutr., 56*(16), 2617–2627.

12. Tsirigotis-Maniecka, M., Lamch, Ł., Chojnacka, I., Gancarz, R., & Wilk, K. A., (2017). Microencapsulation of hesperidin in polyelectrolyte complex micro beads: Physico-chemical evaluation and release behavior. *J. of Food Engg., 214*, 104–116.

13. Assini, J. M., Mulvihill, E. E., & Huff, M. W., (2013). Citrus flavonoids and lipid metabolism. *Current Opinion in Lipidology, 24*(1), 34–40.

14. Rafieian-Kopaei, M., (2014). Identification of medicinal plants affecting on headaches and migraines in Lorestan province, West of Iran. *Asian Pac. J. Trop. Med., 7*, 376–379.

15. Ghorbani, A., Rafieian-Kopaei, M., & Nasri, H., (2013). Lipoprotein (a): More than a bystander in the etiology of hypertension? A study on essential hypertensive patients not yet on treatment. *J. Neuropathol., 2*, 67–70.

16. Behradmanesh, S., & Nasri, P., (2012). Serum cholesterol and LDL-C in association with level of diastolic blood pressure in type 2 diabetic patients. *J. Renal. Inj. Prev., 1*, 23–26.

17. Nasri, H., (2012). Comment on: Serum cholesterol and LDL-C in association with level of diastolic blood pressure in type 2 diabetic patients. *J. Renal. Inj. Prev., 1*, 13, 14.

18. Asgary, S., Keshvari, M., Sahebkar, A., Hashemi, M., & Rafieian-Kopaei, M., (2013). Clinical investigation of the acute effects of pomegranate juice on blood pressure and endothelial function in hypertensive individuals. *ARYA Atheroscler., 9*, 326–331.

19. Nasri, H., Sahinfard, N., Rafieian, M., Rafieian, S., Shirzad, M., & Rafieian-kopaei, M., (2013). Effects of Allium sativum on liver enzymes and atherosclerotic risk factors. *J Herb Med Pharmacol., 2*, 23–28.

20. Rafieian-Kopaei, M., (2012). Medicinal plants and the human needs. *J Herb Med Pharmacol., 1*, 1–2.

21. Hu, F. B., & Willett, W. C., (2002). Optimal diets for prevention of coronary heart disease. *JAMA, 288*, 2569–2578.

22. Behradmanesh, S., & Nasri, H., (2013). Association of serum calcium with level of blood pressure in type 2 diabetic patients. *J. Nephropathol., 2*, 254–257.
23. Hajivandi, A., & Amiri, M., (2014). World kidney day 2014: Kidney disease and elderly. *J. Parathyr Dis., 2*, 3–4.
24. Shahbazian, H., (2013). World diabetes day. *J. Renal. Inj. Prev., 2*, 123, 124.
25. Asgary, S., Sahebkar, A., Afshani, M., Keshvari, M., Haghjooyjavanmard, S. H., & Rafieian-Kopaei, M., (2013). Clinical evaluation of blood pressure lowering, endothelial function improving, hypolipidemic and anti-inflammatory effects of pomegranate juice in hypertensive subjects. *Phytother. Res.*
26. Willis, M. S., & Wians, F. H., (2003). The role of nutrition in preventing prostate cancer: A review of the proposed mechanism of action of various dietary substances. *Clin Chim. Acta, 330*, 57–83.
27. Khoo, S. M., Humberstone, A. J., Porter, C. J., Edwards, G. A., & Charman, W. N., (1998). Formulation design and bioavailability assessment of lipidic self-emulsifying formulations of halofantrine. *Int. J. of Pharm, 167*, 155–164.
28. Mandić, J., Zvonar, Pobirk, A., Vrečer, F., & Gašperlin, M., (2017). Overview of solidification techniques for self-emulsifying drug delivery systems from an industrial perspective. *Int. J. of P'ceutics., 533*(2), 335–345.
29. Barkat, A. K., Satar, B., Haroon, K., Tariq, M., & Akhtar, R., (2012). Basics of self micro emulsifying drug delivery system. *J. of Pharm. and Alt. Med., 1*, 2222–5668.
30. Dangre, P. V., Gilhotra, R. M., & Dhole, S. N., (2016). Formulation and development of solid- self micro-emulsifying drug delivery systems (S-SMEDDS) containing chlortha-lidone for improvement of dissolution. *J. Pharm. Inv., 46*(7), 633–644.
31. Kawakami, K., Yoshikawa, T., Moroto, Y., Kanakao, E., Takahuani, K., Nishihara, Y., & Masuda, K., (2002). Microemulsion formulation for enhanced absorption of poorly soluble drugs. I. Prescription design. *J. of Contr. Rel., 81*, 75–82.
32. Zeisel, S. H., (1999). *Regulation of "Nutraceuticals" Science, 285*, 1853–1855.
33. Shah, N. H., Carvajal, M. T., Patel, C. I., Infeld, M. H., & Malick, A. W., (1994). Self-emulsifying drug delivery systems (SEDDS) with polyglycolyzed glycerides for improving *in vitro* dissolution and oral absorption of lipophilic drugs. *Int. J. Pharm., 106*, 15–23.
34. Jain, D., & Shalom, D. B., (2014). Alginate drug delivery systems: Application in context of pharmaceutical and biomedical research. *Drug Dev. Ind. Pharm., 40*(12), 1576–1584.
35. Zhang, Y., Bai, Y., Chen, H., Yuan, P., & Zhang, L., (2017). Preparation of colon specific sustained- release capsule with curcumin loaded SMEDDS alginate beads. *RSC Adv., 7*(36), 22280–22285.
36. Sookkasem, A., Chatpum, S., Yuenyongsawad, S., & Wiwattanpatapee, R., (2015). alginate beads for colon specific delivery of the beads of curcumin. *J. Drug Deliv. Sci. Tech., 29*, 159–166.
37. Sriraksa, S., Sermkaewn, N., & Setthacheewakul, S., (2012). Floating alginate beads as carriers for self emulsifying systems. *Adv Materials Res., 506*, 517–520.
38. Yuan, D., Jacqier, C., & O'Riordan, E. D., (2017). Entrapment of proteins and peptides in chitosan-polyphosphoric acid hydrogel beads: A new approach to achieve both high entrapment efficacy and controlled *in-vitro* release. *Food Chem., 239*, 1200–1209.
39. Roy, S., (2012). Quality by design: A holistic concept of building quality in pharmaceu-ticals. *Int. J. Pharm. Biomed. Res., 3*(2), 100–108.

40. Dangre, P., Gilhotra, R., & Dhole, S., (2016). Formulation and statistical optimization of self micro-emulsifying drug delivery systems of eprosartanmesylate for improvement of oral bioavailability. *Drug Deliv. Trans. Res., 6*(5), 610–621.

41. Kumar, V. P., & Gupta, N. V., (2015). A review on quality by design approach (QbD) for pharmaceuticals. *Int. J. Drug Dev. & Res., 7*(1), 0975–9344.

42. Beg, S., Sandhu, P. S., Batra, R. S., Khurana, R. K., & Singh, B., (2015). QbD-based systematic development of novel optimized solid self-nano emulsifying drug delivery systems (SNEDDS) of lovastatin with enhanced biopharmaceutical performance. *Drug Deliv., 22*(6), 765–784.

43. Reiss, H., (1975). Entropy-induced dispersion of bulk liquids. *J. Colloids Interface Sci., 53*, 61–70.

44. Ramasahayam, B., Eedara, B. B., Kandadi, P., Jukanti, R., & Bandari, S., (2015). Development of isradipine loaded self-nano emulsifying powders for improved oral delivery: *In vitro* and *in vivo* evaluation. *Drug Dev. Ind. Pharm., 41*(5), 753–763.

45. Dangre, P., Dudhkohar, S., & Chalikwar, S., (2019). Development of alginate- neusilin US2 (Magnesium alumino-metasilicate) micro-composite hydrogel beads for oral sustained release of cilnidipine: A statistical optimization. *Polymer-Plastics Tech and Materials,* 1–15.

46. ICH harmonized tripartite guideline, (2005). *Quality Risk Management* Q9, *4.*

47. Shah, A. V., Desai, H. H., Thool, P., Dalrymple, D., & Serajuddin, A. T., (2018). Development of self-micro emulsifying drug delivery system for oral delivery of poorly water-soluble neutraceuticals. *Drug Dev. and Industrial Pharm., 44*(6), 895–901.

48. Zhang, P., Liu, Y., Feng, N., & Xu, J., (2008). Preparation and evaluation of self-micro emulsifying drug delivery system of oridonin. *Int. J. of Pharm., 355*(1, 2), 269–276.

49. Guo, R., Guo, X., Hu, X., Abbasi, A. M., Zhou, L., Li, T., Fu, X., & Liu, R. H., (2017). Fabrication and optimization of self-micro emulsions to improve the oral bioavailability of total flavones of *Hippophaë rhamnoides* L. *J. of Food Sci., 82*(12), 2901–2909.

50. Khan, A. W., Kotta, S., Ansari, S. H., Sharma, R. K., & Ali, J., (2015). Self-nano emulsifying drug delivery system (SNEDDS) of the poorly water-soluble grapefruit flavonoid Naringenin: Design, characterization, *in vitro* and *in vivo* evaluation. *Drug Deliv., 22*(4), 552–561.

51. Zhao, L., Zhang, L., Meng, L., Wang, J., & Zhai, G. (2013). Design and evaluation of a self-micro emulsifying drug delivery system for apigenin. *Drug Dev. and Industrial Pharm., 39*(5), 662–669.

52. Zhu, Y., Xu, W., Zhang, J., Liao, Y., Firempong, C. K., Adu- Frimpong, M., Deng, W., et al., (2019). Self-micro emulsifying drug delivery system for improved oral delivery of limonene: Preparation, characterization, *in vitro* and *in vivo* evaluation. *AAPS Pharm. Sci. Tech., 20*(4), 153.

53. Seljak, K. B., Berginc, K., Trontel, J., Zvonar, A., Kristl, A., & Gašperlin, M. A., (2014). self-micro emulsifying drug delivery system to overcome intestinal resveratrol toxicity and pre systemic metabolism. *J. of Pharm Sci., 103*(11), 3491–3500.

54. Mekjaruskul, C., Yang, Y. T., Leed, M. G., Sadgrove, M. P., Jay, M., & Sripanidkulchai, B., (2013). Novel formulation strategies for enhancing oral delivery of methoxy flavones in *Kaempferia parviflora* by SMEDDS or complexation with 2-hydroxypropyl-β-cyclodextrin. *Int. J. of Pharm., 445*(1, 2), 1–1.

55. Wei, Y., Ye, X., Shang, X., Peng, X., Bao, Q., Liu, M., Guo, M., & Li, F., (2012). Enhanced oral bioavailability of silybin by a supersaturatable self-emulsifying drug

delivery system (S-SEDDS). *Colloids and Surfaces A: Physicochemical and Engineering Aspects, 396*, 22–28.

56. Zhang, Y., Wang, R., Wu, J., & Shen, Q., (2012). Characterization and evaluation of self-micro emulsifying sustained-release pellet formulation of Puerarin for oral delivery. *Int. J. of Pharm., 427*(2), 337–344.

57. Xu, Y., Wang, Q., Feng, Y., Firempong, C. K., Zhu, Y., Omari-Siaw, E., Zheng, Y., Pu, Z., Xu, X., & Yu, J., (2016). Enhanced oral bioavailability of [6]-gingerol-SMEDDS: Preparation, *in vitro* and *in vivo* evaluation. *J. of Functional Foods., 27*, 703–710.

58. Mezghrani, O. K., Ke, X., Bourkaib, N., & Xu, B. H., (2011). Optimized self-micro emulsifying drug delivery systems (SMEDDS) for enhanced oral bioavailability of astilbin. *Die Pharmazie: An Int. J. of Pharm. Sci., 66*(10), 754–760.

CHAPTER 9

Microemulsions for Improvement in Bioavailability of Potential Nutraceuticals

VAISHALI KILOR, NIDHI SAPKAL, SHOBHA UBGADE, and
ABHAY ITTADWAR

*Gurunanak College of Pharmacy, Rashtrasant Tukadoji Maharaj Nagpur
University, Nagpur, Maharashtra, India*

ABSTRACT

The present chapter focuses on the microemulsion (ME)-based delivery of nutraceutical/bioactive products (curcuminoids, polyphenols, steroids, flavonoids, polypeptides, alkaloids, and fat-soluble vitamins) for plausibly enhancing the bioavailability. Various factors, essential components, and recent literature reports are discussed comprehensively.

9.1 INTRODUCTION TO NUTRACEUTICALS

Changes in basic food habits and adoption of new lifestyle by people such as consumption of junk food, stressful work culture and lack of physical activity the major population across developing countries are suffering from the number of diseases like cancer, heart-related disorders, arthritis, diabetes, and many more. Most of these diseases are chronic and treated by using synthetic drugs, which may cause irreversible adverse effects, and also, the treatment is quite expensive. Health-conscious population is interested in exploring the possibility of prevention and delaying the progression of the disease by using natural compounds in a suitable form. Any alternative treatment which is economical and devoid of harmful side effects is in demand. As there is scientific evidence that many health disorders can be prevented or treated by using nutraceuticals, an alternative treatment option has come to an existence which is very well accepted by the consumers. As nutraceuticals are obtained from natural sources, demand is growing day by day. New clinical applications of nutraceuticals are increasingly being reported [1–3].

Nutraceuticals are the upcoming class of natural products that makes the thin line between food and drug [4]. As per Braithwaite et al. nutraceuticals are used for prophylaxis and prescribed and recommended as complementary and alternative medicine to treat many chronic diseases [5]. As nutraceuticals are obtained from plants, herbs, marine sources, etc., possess less toxicity and side effects as compared to synthetic drugs. WHO also encourages the use of traditional medicines obtained from natural origin as it is comparatively a safer treatment option. Pharmaceutical companies are busy in exploring the possibility of supplying potential nutrients to the consumers in the dosage forms like tablets, capsules, oral films, drinks, etc., which contain purified and concentrated nutraceuticals/bioactive compounds [6].

9.2   WHAT ARE NUTRACEUTICALS?

The term "nutraceutical" was framed from the word "pharmaceutical," where nutritional compounds are consumed for health and medical benefits. Nutraceuticals include those bioactive compounds which possess enormous potential to treat, control or prevent various diseases because of its beneficial nutritional value if they are used in a proper form and appropriate dosage. Sources of nutraceuticals are compounds isolated from plants, dietary supplements (DS), herbs, etc., which are used to have nutritional value and are also used as medicine.

Nutraceuticals may range from:

1.   **Isolated Nutrients (from Plants):** Phytochemicals or phytonutrients are bioactive molecules derived from plants. For example, carotenoids from carrots, flavonoids from citrus fruits and grapes, iso-flavonoids from soybean, etc.

2.   **Dietary Supplements (DS):** These are the doses of nutritional supplements to be administered at high doses than normal human exposure to the nutrients present in food. It may be a concentrated version of nutrient compound formulated as tablets, capsules for the prophylactic purpose. For example, vitamins, minerals, fiber, amino acids, herbs or other plants, or enzymes in the form of pills, capsules, powders, gel tabs, extracts, or liquids [7].

3.   **Isolated Nutrients from Herbs:** Curcumin which is derived from herb *Curcuma longa*, commonly called turmeric, is a polyphenol

derivative. It is a well-known antioxidant and also has anti-carci-nogenic and anti-inflammatory properties [8]. Garlic, i.e., *Allium sativum* contains sulfur compounds, reported to be used for boosting immunity and also possess anticancer as well as help to reduce platelet stickiness [9]. Broccoli, belongs to the cruciferous vegetable family, is a rich source of antioxidant sulforaphane, vitamins, minerals, fibers, etc. Therefore, it is reported to reduce the risk of cancer by protecting the body from damaging free radicals [10].

4. **Fortified Food:** These types of nutraceuticals include breeding at the agriculture level or accumulation of well-matched nutrients to the main ingredients like flour fortified with iron, calcium, and folic acid, and milk fortified with cholecalciferol commonly used for vitamin D deficiency, minerals added to cereals, and orange juice fortified with calcium [11].

5. **Processed Food:** Such as cereals, soups, beverages that contain dietary fibers, vitamins, proteins, etc.

6. **Dairy Foods:** CUT whole milk, yogurt, cheese contains an array of bioactive compounds like probiotics, fatty acids, whey proteins, probiotics, and bioactive peptides, which are claimed to improve systemic immunity, act as antioxidants as well as promote gastroin-testinal (GI) health. For example, bio-yogurts containing *Lactoba-cillus acidophilus* and *Bifidobacteria* [12].

7. **Marine Biomaterials:** The compounds like bio-peptides, collagen, gelatine, chito-oligosaccharides derivatives (COS), sulfated polysac-charides (SPs), phlorotannins, sterols, carotenoids, and lectins are obtained and isolated from various marine sources and are isolated by bio-processing [13]. Fish oil, a very important nutraceutical is beneficial to lower the risk of cardiovascular disorders [14].

8. **Genetically Engineered Designer Food:** Genetically engineered foods are produced by introducing changes in the DNA (deoxyribo-nucleic acid) of organisms using the methods of genetic engineering. For example, genetically modified golden rice contains high nutrient value [15].

9.3 CHALLENGES IN NUTRACEUTICAL DELIVERY

Scientists have proven the therapeutic potential of nutraceuticals in the recent researches, which have attracted the attention of physicians as well as consumers towards the use of nutraceuticals as an alternative therapy for the well-being as well as prevention and treatment of various diseases. Therefore researchers are working on the development of suitable delivery options, where the safety, efficacy, and stability of nutraceuticals can be retained during processing, storage, and handling in addition to the improved bioavailability. Nutraceuticals are required to provide to the patients/consumers in a convenient dosage form depending on the route of administration like tablets, capsules, suspensions, powders, oral thin films, etc., for oral administration. The extent of bioavailability of nutraceuticals from such dosage forms is a matter of concern for a formulator as therapeutic efficacy is directly dependent upon the bioavailability of the compound. Stability of many nutraceuticals like vitamins decreases in the presence of oxygen, alkaline pH, and high temperature. Nutraceutical compounds like curcuminoids, phytosterols (PS), flavonoids, catechin, etc., are highly susceptible to degradation at pH of the stomach and also suffer from low membrane permeability (Table 9.1). Therefore, very less amount of these bioactive compounds is utilizable after consumption.

Oily and sticky extracts of nutrients obtained from plants are difficult to incorporate in a dosage form since they pose solubility and miscibility challenge during formulation development. Curcuminoids, flavonoids, and vitamin D_3 are therapeutically effective in very large doses which are difficult to incorporate in suitable dosage form to deliver by convenient delivery routes. Vitamins C and E may destabilize during handling and delivery. Vitamins (A, D, E, and K) which are fat-soluble vitamins may not release from the delivery system due to excessive lipophilicity. Consumed food-containing proteins undergo hydrolysis due to the presence of digestive enzymes to form smaller peptides which possess nutritive properties. Absorption of these peptides is limited due to their hydrophilicity and high molecular weight and therefore possesses low oral bioavailability [16]. Polyphenol, resveratrol shows good solubility in ethanol, however, it has low aqueous solubility and is easily photo-isomerized and metabolized by glucuronidation [17]. Therefore, to attune *in vivo* pharmacokinetic parameters of potential nutraceuticals, their physicochemical properties like solubility, partition coefficient, high molecular weight, etc., need to be addressed by adopting novel delivery technologies during formulation design. Thus, it is necessary to deliver nutraceuticals using suitable carriers in order to improve solubilization as well as to enhance transmembrane transport to improve bioavailability.

9.4   FACTORS AFFECTING BIOAVAILABILITY OF NUTRACEUTICALS

Bioavailability of a nutritional compound is the amount of a compound that the body can utilize to show desired nutritional or therapeutic efficacy [26, 27].

TABLE 9.1 Nutraceuticals with Potential Health Benefits and Challenges in Formulation Development

Name/Class	Example	Health Benefits	Challenge	References
Polyphenol	Curcumin	Antioxidant, anti-carcinogenic, anti-inflammatory	Extremely low serum levels, low C_{max}, low Volume of distribution, rapid metabolism, and short $t_{1/2}$	[18]
Benzoquinone derivative/ enzyme	Coenzyme Q10	Antioxidant, antioxidant, for the treatment of cardiovascular disorder, migraine headache, neurodegenerative disease such as Parkinsonism	High lipophilicity and molecular weight, poor solubility, and dissolution. Substrate for P-gp efflux therefore limited permeability	[19]
Carotenoids	β-carotene	Antioxidant, vitamin A precursor, anti-carcinogenic	Poor aqueous solubility, chemically unstable, possess low bioavailability	[20]
	Lycopene (a non-provitamin A carotenoid)	Anti-carcinogenic specially for prostate cancer	Poor aqueous solubility and low bioavailability	[21]
	Lutein	Lower risk of cataract and age-related macular degeneration	Low water solubility and low bioavailability	[22]
Polypeptide	Salmon calcitonin	Regulation of calcium homeostasis, a potent inhibitor of osteoclastic bone resorption	Low membrane permeability and unstable nature in gastrointestinal tract	[23]
Sterols	Phytosterols	Reduce cholesterol levels in the blood	Poor aqueous solubility	[24]
Flavanoid	Myricetin	Antioxidant, antiproliferative, neuroprotective, and hepatoprotective activities	Poor aqueous solubility, low bioavailability	[25]

The phenomenon of bioavailability involves several processes such as the release of the compound from a delivery system, absorption, distribution, metabolism, and elimination. In order to introduce nutraceuticals in a proper form to assure stability, bioavailability as well as a good taste of the final product, various factors need attention.

9.4.1 STRUCTURE OF NUTRACEUTICAL COMPOUND

The presence of various functional groups in the compound affects the rate of absorption. For example, the sugar moiety present in the structure of flavonoids has been affected the rate of absorption of flavonoids in humans [28]. β-glucoside chain present in flavonoids is prone to metabolite by enzymes β-glucosidase and lactase phlorizin hydrolase present in the small intestine. Isomeric configuration of the compound can also affect their absorption. *Cis*-isomer of lycopene, a bioactive carotenoid has greater membrane permeability which leads to improved bioavailability [29].

9.4.2 LIBERATION OF NUTRIENT FROM FOOD MATRICES/ NUTRACEUTICAL DELIVERY SYSTEM (BIOACCESSIBILITY)

Bio-accessibility is defined as an amount of the active compound that is released from the food matrix/delivery system into the GIT. Bioaccessibility, intestinal transport, and extent of metabolism are the major processes which determine the bioavailability of the compound [30]. Bioaccessibility is affected by the release of nutraceutical from the delivery system, solubilization of the compounds in GI fluids as well as interaction with the other compounds and enzymes present in the GIT [31]. Hydrophilic nutraceuticals are dissolved in the GI fluid easily as compared to the lipophilic nutraceuticals that need help from micelle systems available in the GI fluid. Because of the lipophilic/ hydrophobic core, these mixed micelles may solubilize water-insoluble compounds.

9.4.3 ABSORPTION/TRANSPORT

Followed by solubilization, a major portion of nutraceuticals is absorbed by the small intestine via various routes across the epithelium, specifically through the enterocytes (absorption epithelial cells) that are present in the lumen of the jejunum and finally enters the systemic circulation. Mostly solubilized nutraceuticals diffuse through the epithelial layers as a function of thermal movement and a concentration gradient across the epithelium. Hydrophilic compounds are transported across the epithelium by paracellular diffusion through the intraepithelial gaps which are few angstroms (Å) wide and lipophilic/hydrophobic compounds tend to diffuse through the phospholipid membrane and the cytosol of the epithelial cells by transcellular diffusion since those are solubilized by micelles present in GI fluid. Some molecules are transported by carrier-mediated transport where specific receptor proteins act as carriers to cross the epithelium. For example, vitamin transporters, organic anion transporters are involved in the uptake of components and enhance their transport across GI epithelium. P-gp efflux pumps present in the epithelial cell membrane acts as a barrier for some nutraceuticals such as P-glycoproteins (P-gp) and breast cancer-resistant proteins (BCRP), which negatively affect the bioavailability of nutraceuticals/drugs [32].

9.4.4   TRANSFORMATION/METABOLISM

Nutraceuticals are chemically degraded or metabolized within the GIT and get transformed into an inactive form which directly affects the bioavailability of nutraceuticals (Figure 9.1). As the bioactive compound enters the enterocyte it may subject to metabolism by CYP450 enzymes which result in modification of structure by chemical reactions such as oxidation or reduction which is different from the structure of original compound capable of showing the desirable effect [33]. Some compounds may undergo first-pass metabolism in the liver followed by absorption depending upon the extent of polarity and presence of functional groups. Highly lipophilic compounds enter directly into the systemic circulation via lymphatic transport, bypassing the first-pass metabolism. Therefore, knowledge and understanding of biological processes involved in the uptake and bioavailability of nutraceuticals is of utmost importance while designing effective delivery systems for nutraceuticals.

9.5   IMPROVING BIOAVAILABILITY OF NUTRACEUTICALS

Nutraceuticals have immense potential to prevent, control, and treat many diseases. Most of the nutraceuticals are lipophilic, unstable at the pH of GIT, and suffer from low efficacy and low absorption rate, therefore consumption of large quantities of nutraceuticals is required to ensure the desirable health benefits. Although nutraceuticals are superior to synthetic drugs, it is challenging and impractical to load very high therapeutic doses in suitable dosage forms. Therefore, the use of nutraceuticals as an alternative to conventional drug therapy is a challenge which can be overcome by exploring suitable carriers for their delivery which can protect them from the harsh environment in the GIT and improve their bioavailability.

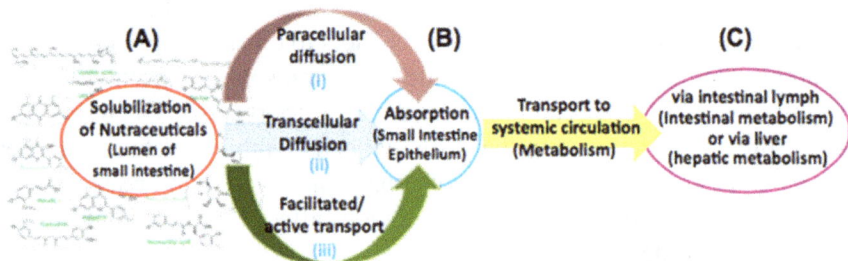

FIGURE 9.1   Important stages involved in the bioavailability of nutraceuticals.

Source: Reprinted with permisison from Ref. [34]. © 2017 Elsevier.

Literature reports various nanotechnology-based approaches explored for achieving increased bioavailability of nutraceuticals such as nanoparticles, polymeric micelles, nanoemulsions, nanodispersions. But all these delivery systems suffer from limitations such as time-consuming and complex methods of preparation, thermodynamic instability, reproducibility, etc. Therefore, requires efforts for preparation and special attention for stabilization of these delivery systems, whereas MEs are thermodynamically stable systems and the method of preparation is very simple. Oil-soluble as well as water-soluble components can be packaged in nanometer (nm)-size structures to increase their half-life and biological potency. MEs can be delivered by a variety of routes like oral, topical, transdermal, parenteral, nasal, rectal, etc. Therefore, ME can be called as the most promising vehicle for the delivery of nutraceuticals [35].

9.6   MICROEMULSIONS (MES)

Microemulsions (MEs) are isotropic, thermodynamically stable, transparent colloidal systems with droplet size ranging between 10 and 100 nm are consti-tuted of surfactant, co-surfactant, an oil phase, and an aqueous phase. Prepa-ration of ME is industrially feasible since thermodynamic stability, simple method of preparation, and low energy requirements are the key scale-up criteria of such systems. As a potentially excellent vehicle candidate for bioactive molecules, MEs can increase the solubility of bioactive materials, and can also improve absorption through human gut membranes because MEs exert extremely low surface tension. The bioactive compound could directly contact the GI epithelium cell, consequently, bioavailability could significantly be improved [36]. ME is a homogeneous system containing polar and non-polar microdomains available for solubilizing oil as well as water-soluble material (Table 9.2).

It is possible to load higher amounts of nutraceuticals in ME to achieve greater penetration through the biological membranes since the components like lipids/oils, surfactants play a very important role in improving bioavailability as well as minimizing variability in pharmacokinetics. The increased thermodynamic activity of the compound is achieved in the vehicles like MEs, resulting in an improved rate of absorption [37].

Structurally, MEs are categorized as oil-in-water (O/W), water-in-oil (W/O), and bi-continuous MEs (Figure 9.2) [38].

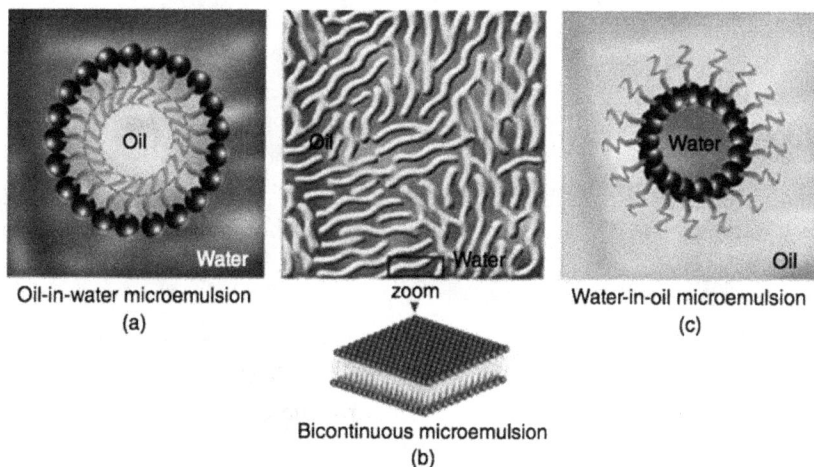

Oil-in-water microemulsion
(a)

zoom

Water-in-oil microemulsion
(c)

Bicontinuous microemulsion
(b)

FIGURE 9.2 Schematic representation of ME microstructures: (a) O/W ME; (b) bicontinuous; and (c) W/O ME.

Source: Reprinted with permisison from Ref. [39]. © 2012 Elsevier.

Hydrophobic nutraceuticals are preferably incorporated into the dispersed phase of o/w ME and tail region of the surfactant whereas hydrophilic material is solubilized by the dispersed aqueous phase of w/o ME. In terms of stability, o/w systems are superior over w/o systems since the droplet structure of o/w systems is retained upon dilution within the body. This dilution can result in either phase separation or phase inversion. However, w/o MEs are very promising for the delivery of labile nutraceuticals since many of the nutraceuticals are hydrophilic. Encapsulation of these hydrophilic materials in the aqueous droplets of w/o ME offers them protection from enzymatic degradation [40]. Thus, MEs with desirable characteristics can be generated by modifying number of parameters as well as selecting suitable components, and the resulting systems can be used for the delivery of nutraceuticals.

TABLE 9.2 Commonly Used Components of ME

Components	Category	Examples
Oil	Medium-chain triglycerides (MCTs)	Glyceryl tricaprylate: Captex 355, Miglyol 810
	Low chain triglycerides	Corn oil, soybean oil, olive oil, etc.
	Mono/diglyceride	Glyceryl caprylate, glyceryl monooleate, etc.
	Fatty acids	Oleic acid
	Propylene glycol ester	Capmul PG-8, propylene glycol monolaurate
Surfactant	HLB> 10	Tween-20, Tween-80, polyoxyl 35 castor oil, PEG-8 caprylic glyceride
	HLB < 10	Span-40, Span-80, phosphatidylcholine, polyoxyl 40 hydrogenated castor oil
Co- surfactant	Propylene glycol, polyethylene glycol, ethanol, isopropyl alcohol, isopropyl myristate, propanol, isopropanol, etc.	

9.7 COMPONENTS OF MES

Oil, surfactant, co-surfactant/co-solvent, and water are important components of microemulsion. It is desirable to use GRAS (Generally Regarded as Safe) listed components or ingredients for the development of safer and effective ME systems of nutraceuticals.

9.7.1 SURFACTANTS

The nature of surfactant used for the construction of ME systems, whether ionic or non-ionic determines the stabilizing interactions of the surfactant with the polar phase (Table 9.3). Dipole, as well as hydrogen bond interactions with the aqueous layer and hydrophilic groups of non-ionic surfactants, are involved in the stabilization of surfactant, whereas the electrical double layer stabilizes anionic surfactant which is affected by the salt concentration in the system.

TABLE 9.3 Surfactants Used in Food Preparations

General Class	Example
Lactylated esters	Pure phospholipid (e.g., phosphatidylcholine) and mixed phospholipids hydroxylated phospholipids/lecithin
Lactylated esters	Lactylic esters of fatty acids, lactylated fatty acid esters of glycerol and propylene glycol
Glycerol fatty acid esters	Polyglycerol fatty acid esters
	Polyglycerol polyricinoleate
	Propylene glycol fatty acid esters (Propane-1, 2-diol esters of fatty acids)
Partial glycerides and derivatives	Mono- and di-glycerides, monosodium phosphate derivatives of mono- and diglycerides Acetic acid esters of mono- and diglycerides
Sucrose esters	Mono-, di-, and tri-esters of sucrose with fatty acids
Sorbitan fatty acid esters	Sorbitan monostearate, Sorbitan tristearate, Sorbitan monolaurate, Sorbitan monooleate
Polyoxyethylene sorbitan fatty acid esters	Polyoxyethylene [20]
Other	Ox bile extract, propylene glycol, sodium lauryl sulfate

9.7.2 CO-SURFACTANT

A co-surfactant is an amphiphilic molecule that substantially accumulates with the surfactant at the interfacial layer. A blend of co-surfactant with high and low HLB is used in order to adjust the HLB of the system. Co-surfactants increases loading capacity of ME since it helps in increasing solubility of the compound and stability of the dispersed phase. Ethanol, as well as non-ionic surfactants, can function as co-surfactants by molecularly dispersing surfactant and improving solubilization of nutraceuticals within hydrophobic pockets created by co-surfactants in the continuous phase, i.e., water [41].

9.7.3 OIL PHASE

The oily phase is considered to be the most vital component in the formulation of the ME not only because of its ability to solubilize the desired quantity of the lipophilic drugs but it can also enhance the transport of lipophilic compounds through the intestinal lymphatic system leading to enhanced absorption. Selection of appropriate oil phase is very important since the chosen oil must possess a good solubilizing potential for the selected substance as well as the chosen oil must result in enhanced ME forming region. The solubilizing capacity of chosen oil depends upon the length of the hydrocarbon chain. Short hydrocarbon chains in oils are desirable for the formation of ME than that of the oils with long hydrocarbon chain [42]. Orange oil, lemon oil [43] as well as dietary lipids like olive oil, sunflower oil, corn oil, soybean oil, palm oil, and animal fats has been incorporated in MEs of nutraceuticals as the oils and carrier lipids.

9.7.4 AQUEOUS PHASE

The aqueous phase is a very important component of ME since it is responsible for reducing the overall viscosity of the formulation as well as to solubilize hydrophilic components. Usually, aqueous phase may possess dissolved excipients in it like isotonic agents, buffers, preservatives, etc., which may affect the stability of ME. For example, effect on the thickness of the electrical double layer or salting out of dissolved surfactant. Therefore, it is required to maintain a neutral pH of the ME system [44].

9.8 MICROEMULSION AS A VEHICLE FOR BIOAVAILABILITY ENHANCEMENT OF NUTRACEUTICALS

In order to improve solubility, bioavailability, and stability of bioactive molecules for better obtaining nutritional and therapeutic efficacy, ME is proven to be a very promising vehicle by various researchers and formulators. These delivery vehicles containing bioactive agents entrapped in nano-sized oil/water droplets enable improved delivery of antioxidants, essential oils, vitamins, flavonoids, PS as compared to formulation developed conventionally [45].

Microemulsion formulation technique can be applied for the delivery of oil-soluble or water-soluble bioactive compounds as those are entrapped within a nanosized protective matrix composed of oil, surfactant/co-surfactant, and water. The droplet size of ME, the solubility of nutraceutical compound in the dispersed phase, type of oil phase used and pH of the system determines the extent of bioavailability improvement of the nutraceutical compound in question [46].

Curcumin, obtained from turmeric is a polyphenolic compound which possesses noteworthy anti-cancer and anti-inflammatory, as well as antioxidant properties, suffer from poor bioavailability, which affects its bioactivity. Hu et al. developed ME system for the enhancement of solubility and bioavailability of curcumin which was composed of Capryol 90 as oil, Cremophor RH40 as a surfactant, and Transcutol P aqueous solution as co-surfactant. The solubility of curcumin significantly increased in the form of ME (up to 32.5 mg/mL) as compared to its aqueous solubility (<0.1 mg/mL). *In vivo* pharmacokinetic studies of curcumin ME performed in rats showed improvement in C_{max} and AUC (area under the curve) as compared to curcumin suspension (Figure 9.3). It can be concluded from the results of pharmacokinetic studies that lipid-based components used in the formulation have contributed significantly for enhancement of the oral bioavailability of. It may be due to the stimulation of lymphatic transport and increased membrane permeability as well as avoidance of first-pass metabolism and inhibition of P-gp efflux pump activity [48].

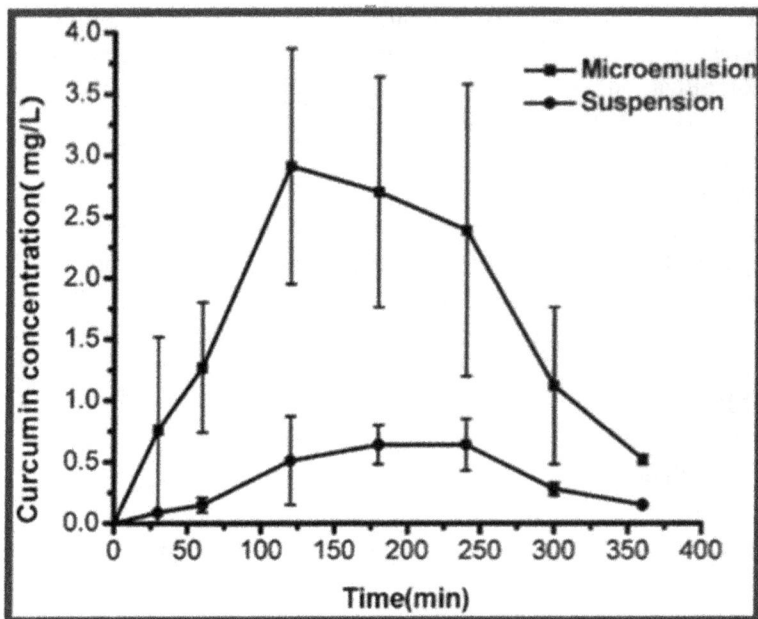

FIGURE 9.3 Blood concentration-time profile of curcumin after oral administration of suspension and ME to rats.
Source: With permission from: Liandong et al. [47]. © 2012 American Chemical Society.

Berberine, a type of isoquinoline alkaloid, an active constituent is an active constituent of the Chinese herb *Rhizoma coptidis* is poorly absorbed on oral administration. Berberine has a broad antifungal spectrum and also possesses antitumor, anti-diabetic, and anti-ischemic activity. ME formulations of berberine were developed by Sh et al. which consisted of oleic acid (15%), Tween-80 (17%), PEG400 (17%), and water (51%). Noticeable enhancement in pharmacokinetic parameters was observed after oral administration of berberine ME to male Sprague-Dawley rats when compared with berberine tablet suspension [49].

Phytosterols are chemical mixtures of sterols, stanols, phytosteroids produced only in plants. PS are structurally similar to cholesterol; therefore, it possesses cholesterol-lowering effects. As PS shows poor oil as well as aqueous solubility, it is required to be consumed in large doses to achieve low levels of body cholesterol. Therefore, food, as well as the pharmaceutical industry, is working on the development of effective delivery systems to achieve a decrease in cholesterol levels using smaller doses of PS with improved bioavailability. Rozner et al. prepared MEs of PS to improve its bioavailability, where Tween 60 was used as an emulsifier, (R-(+)-limonene) as oil phase, and propylene glycol and ethanol as co-surfactants. The solubilization capacity of phytosterol was increased 6-fold following incorporation in R-(+)-limonene [50].

Tang et al. carried out studies to understand the mechanism by which MEs enhance the oral bioavailability of puerarin, an isoflavone glycoside reported to be used to treat hypertension, coronary heart disease, and diabetic retinopathy. O/W ME of puerarin was prepared using cremophore RH 40 and propylene glycol as a surfactant, and co-surfactant in (2:1) ratio and W/O ME was prepared using lecithin and ethanol in (1:1 w/w ratio), while ethyl oleate was used as an oil phase. As compared to the O/W ME, the W/O ME showed better permeability through the intestinal membrane, as evident from the results of lymphatic transport analysis (Figure 9.4). Thus, it was concluded that the components ME and their content significantly contributed to the oral bioavailability enhancement of puerarin [51].

A high molecular weight polypeptide, Salmon calcitonin (sCT), molecular weight 3,500-Da, found in salmon is very effective than its human analog in treating osteoporosis, hypercalcemia, and Paget's disease. Though, a potent inhibitor of osteoclastic resorption its therapeutic use is limited by its low permeability and instability at GIT pH. To protect it from degradation as well as to improve its membrane permeability W/O ME formulation was developed by Fan et al. by choosing appropriate components like medium-chain triglyceride, Tween 80, and Span 80/soybean phosphatidylcholine, propylene glycol and phosphate saline for improving the absorption of intraduodenally administered sCT. The enhanced hypocalcemic effect was observed followed by intra-duodenal administration of W/O sCT ME in rats (Figure 9.5). Encapsulation in ME droplets provided protection to sCT molecule from proteolysis and acid degradation as well as nanometer-size droplets (6 nm to 134 nm) provided a large surface area for rapid absorption of sCT from the intestine [23].

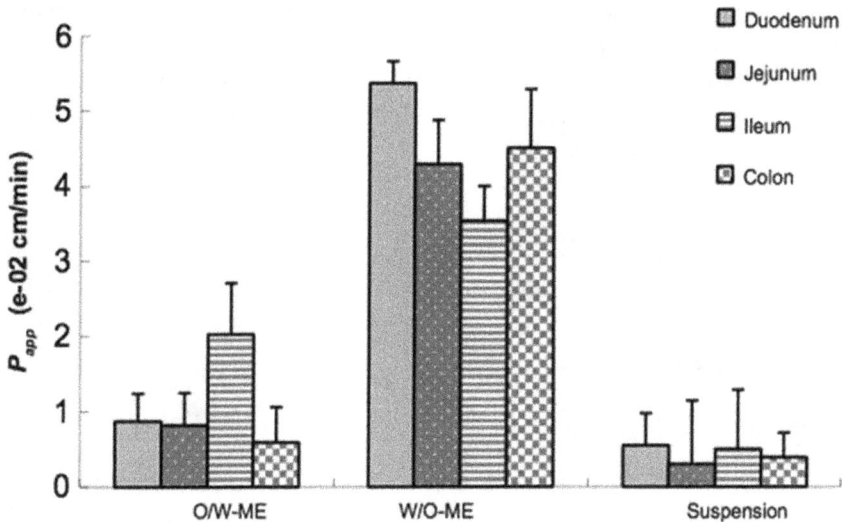

FIGURE 9.4 The apparent permeability coefficients (Papp) of MEs obtained for *in-situ* perfusion in the single-pass intestinal perfusion model for four different intestinal segments (mean ± SD (n=6).

Source: With permission from: Tang et al. [51].

Most commonly occurring flavonoid, ampelopsin contains anti-bacterial, anti-cancer, antioxidant, hepatoprotective, and anti-hypertensive activities. Use of ampelopsis as a nutraceutical is limited due to its poor aqueous solubility. The bioavailability of ampelopsin was improved by developing a nano-carrier system, microemulsion, for oral delivery, where medium-chain triglyceride, Capmul MCM was used as a lipid phase, Cremophor EL as a surfactant, and Transcutol as co-surfactant. ME formulation showed higher *in-vitro* release, as compared to plain ampelopsis suspension and the suspension of the commercially available tablet. These results demonstrate the potential use of ME for improving the bioavailability of poorly water-soluble compounds, such as ampelopsin [54].

Propolis, a resinous material collected by honey bees from leaf buds and cracks in the bark of the poplar genus and other tree species, possess a wide range of therapeutic properties, such as hepatoprotective, anti-tumor, anti-oxidative, anti-microbial, anti-inflammatory, and immune-enhancing properties [55]. Flavonoids are the important contributors for therapeutic properties, and therefore, Propolis possess low oxidation stability and poor aqueous solubility [56]. To address these limitations, propolis flavonoid (PF) was encapsulated in oil in water (o/w) ME carrier system. The prepared ME was evaluated for immune-enhancing activity by using CTX-induced immunosuppressive chickens. The study revealed that PF ME at high and medium doses improved lymphatic proliferation and concentrations of IgG and IgM. Thus, as a result of improved bioavailability, immune-enhancing activity of PF showed significant increase [57].

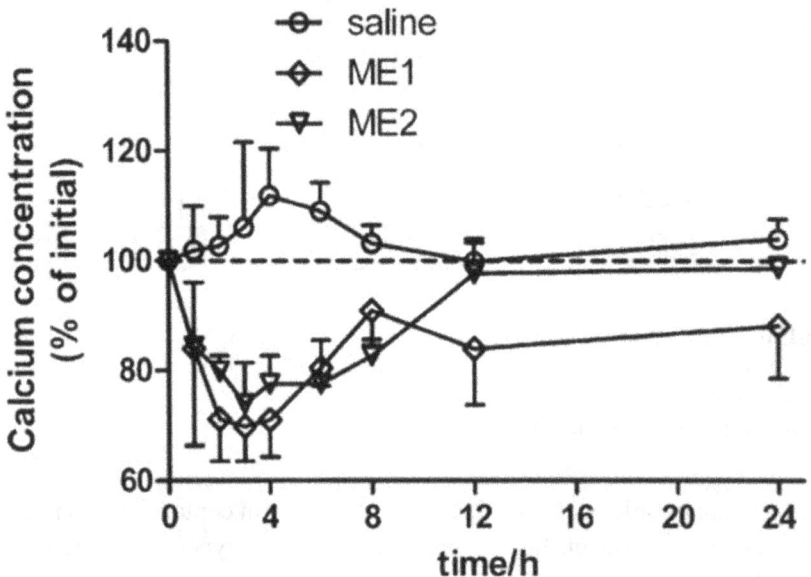

FIGURE 9.5   Serum calcium level profiles after intra-duodenal administration of sCT-loaded MEs to rats at a single dose of 275 mcg/kg (n = 5). ME1: MCT/tween 80-SPC/PG/PBS; ME2: MCT/tween 80-SPC/PG/PBS with 1% Carbopol 980 (CP).

Source: Reprinted with permisison from Fan et al. [23]. © 2011 Elsevier.

Pepper fruit, a popularly used spice contains a pungent alkaloid, Piperine (PIP) which is known to have activity against CNS disorders. Recently, many papers suggested the beneficial physiological actions of PIP on the central nervous system. This potentially useful alkaloid possesses high log P value (2.25), poor aqueous solubility, very high lipophilicity, and it is prone for first-pass metabolism [58], which limits its therapeutic application.

When lipid components like Caproyl 90, surfactant (Tween 80/Cremophore RH40), and co-surfactant Transcutol HP were used to develop ME system of PIP, improved bioavailability was observed as evident from *in vivo* studies. Negative zeta potential and nano size of the ME droplets (150 nm) contributed to show improved activity in the treatment of Alzheimer's disease (AD) over free PIP [59].

Myricetin (MYR), a polyphenolic compound derived from various natural sources like vegetables, tea, nuts, fruits, etc., possess antioxidant and antiproliferative activity. Polyphenolic compounds are poorly water-soluble and therefore requires special efforts to solubilize for utilizing it as a nutraceutical. Thus, oral ME formulation of MYR was developed by Guo et al. to improve antiproliferative activity of MYR against human cancer cell HepG2. Significant enhancement in the activity was observed when MYR-ME was administered orally in Sprague-Dawley rats as compared to MYR-CMC-Na suspension (Table 9.4) [25]. This might be due to the presence of formulation components like Cremophore RH-40 and Tween-80, which are known to inhibit P-gp efflux pumps present on the GI enterocyte membrane, improving permeability and subsequent bioavailability of MYR [51].

TABLE 9.4 Pharmacokinetic Parameters of MYR-Suspension (25 mg/kg) and MYR-ME (25 mg/kg) After Oral Administration of Rats (Mean ± SD, n = 6)

Parameters	Formulations	
	MYR-Suspension	**MYR-ME**
C_{max} (µg/mL)	0.48 ± 0.08	8.11 ± 0.69
T_{max} (h)	4.16 ± 0.28	2.25 ± 0.21
$t_{1/2}$ (h)	3.53 ± 0.30	5.20 ± 0.58
AUC (µg.h/mL)	3.73 ± 0.31	53.83 ± 3.38
Relative bioavailability (%)	100	1443.16

Source: With permission from: Guo et al. [25]. © 2016 American Chemical Society.

Quercetin, a flavonoid compound, is considered as one of the most powerful natural antioxidants [60]. *In vitro* and *in vivo* experiments demonstrate that quercetin can protect keratinocytes from exogenous oxidizing agents, scavenge free radicals, prevent endogenous antioxidant depletion, and inhibit lipid peroxidation upon exposure to UV irradiation. The therapeutic effect of quercetin is limited due to the poor water solubility, low permeation into the skin, and instability under light, pH, and temperature. Therefore, Lv et al. developed a nano vehicle, ME for topical application by using essential oils like peppermint oil, rosemary oil, clove oil as oil phase and Cremophore EL and 1,2-propanediol as surfactant and co-surfactant, respectively to improve pH stability, photostability, solubility, and skin permeation of Quercetin [61]. The presence of essential oils in ME enhanced the skin permeation rate to many folds as compared to the aqueous solution of quercetin.

Lin et al. developed a ME system of curcumin by using soybean oil and soybean lecithin to investigate the cytotoxicity of curcumin on the HepG2 cell line. It was observed from the cytotoxicity studies that the curcumin ME with smaller particle size (30 nm) resulted in the lowest cell viability as shown in Figure 9.6. The cellular uptake of the curcumin ME was investigated using fluorescence microscopy. The increased delivery of curcumin to the target sites might have taken place by fusion of ME droplets with cellular membranes [62].

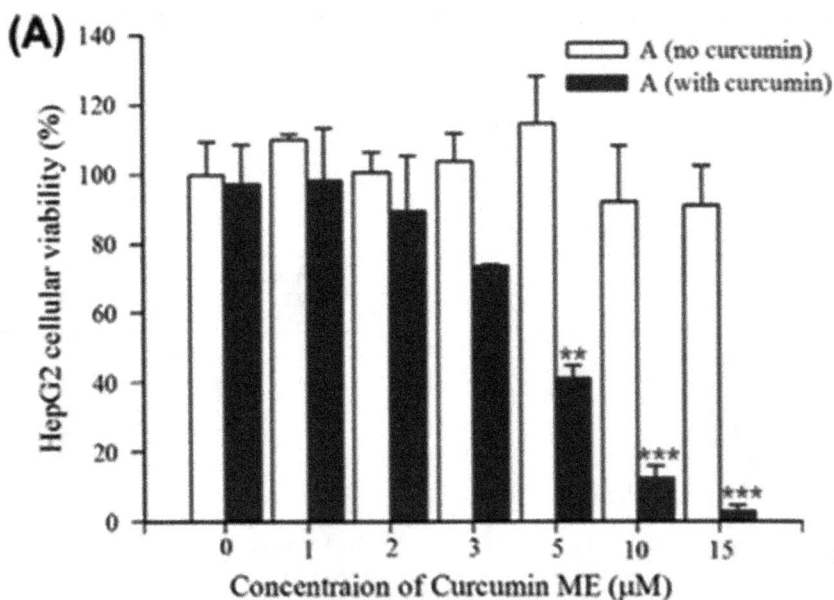

FIGURE 9.6 The cell viability of HepG2 cells treated with various concentrations of curcumin MEs. Comparison of the effect of curcumin-free and curcumin loaded ME on the viability of HepG2 cell lines (**P<0.00, ***P<0.0001) statistically analyzed by students' t-test. *Source:* With permission from Lin et al. [62]. © 2016 Elsevier.

Carotenoids are the colored fat-soluble pigments, an important class of active phytochemicals found in a variety of fruits and vegetables. Carotenoids possess strong cancer-fighting properties [63], as well as activity against heart disease [64] and colorectal adenomas [65]. Carotenoids are converted by the body to vitamin A which is essential for good vision, body growth, and development. Roohinejad et al. developed O/W MEs of β-carotene using Capmul MCM oil with medium-chain monoglycerides for the evaluation of the cytotoxic activity of β-carotene using Caco-2 cells. It was evident from the study results that ME containing higher loading of β-carotene showed a significant reduction in the cell viability, confirming improved bioavailability and permeation of β-carotene ME [20].

MEs can also act as a delivery vehicle for sensitive lipophilic nutraceuticals which can be solubilized in the oil phase of emulsions for potential protection from degrading enzymes, pH, heat, light, etc. For example, carotenoids are prone to degrade under the influence of heat, light, and/or oxygen during handling and storage. Literature reports slowing down of the rate of reduction of β-carotene when it is solubilized in the oil phase of emulsions containing lecithin as an emulsifier, as lecithin possess effective antioxidant property and prevents the penetration of peroxyl radicals [52, 66].

Chen and coworkers reported that when β-carotene encapsulated in ME composed of peppermint oil/Tween 20/sunflower lecithin, its degradation under UV radiation and thermal treatment was greatly suppressed as compared to the solution control. The transparent β-carotene ME having droplet size less than 10 nm remained stable for 65 days under ambient storage conditions. Thus, it is observed that the homogeneous ME system can ensure delivery of poorly soluble, sensitive nutraceuticals in the form of elegant consumer products [52].

9.9 CONCLUSION

Nutraceutical is a very fast-growing area of attention for research and product development as consumers are inclined to use nutraceuticals for a healthy life as well as for prophylactic purpose due to their presumed safety and promising nutritional and therapeutic outcomes. The development of nutraceuticals is equally important for pharmaceuticals as well as food industries as it has a broad scope. The limitations in the delivery of nutraceuticals can be successfully overcome by designing ME systems. MEs improve the bioavailability of nutraceuticals by enhancing their solubilization in GI fluids, protecting the microemulsified nutrients from oxidation and enzymatic degradation as well as enhancing membrane permeability and lymphatic transport. Lack of nutraceutical/drug precipitation upon aqueous dilution of ME plays a very important role in the improvement of bioavailability of nutraceuticals. Thermodynamic stability, ease and spontaneity of formation, and spontaneous formation, as well as bioavailability improvement of lipophilic nutraceutical compounds make them a potential delivery vehicle. Successful application of ME to maximize the bioavailability of nutraceuticals requires keen control on the selection of components, bioavailability class of nutraceutical, compatibility as well as knowledge of biological function and metabolism of nutraceutical in the body. By controlling droplet size, composition, and surface properties, MEs can also be developed for targeted delivery of nutraceuticals.

KEYWORDS

- **bioavailability**
- **insoluble dietary fiber**
- **lipid formulation classification system**
- **liquid-crystalline**
- **microemulsions**
- **nano vehicles**
- **new chemical entities**
- **nutraceuticals**

REFERENCES

1. Sangiovanni, E., Piazza, S., Vrhovsek, U., et al., (2018). A bio-guided approach for the development of a chestnut-based proanthocyanidin-enriched nutraceutical with potential anti-gastritis properties. *Pharmacological Research, 134*, 145–155.
2. Radke, M., Picaud, J., Loui, A., et al., (2016). Starter formula enriched in prebiotics and probiotics ensures normal growth of infants and promotes gut health: A randomized clinical trial. *Pediatric Research, 81*(4), 622–631.
3. Fabian, C., Kimler, B., & Hursting, S., (2015). Omega-3 fatty acids for breast cancer prevention and survivorship. *Breast Cancer Research, 17*(1).
4. Adelaja, A. O., & Schilling, B. J., (1999). Nutraceutical: Blurring the line between food and drugs in the twenty-first century. *Mag. Food Farm Resour., 14*, 35–40.
5. Braithwaite, M. C., Tyagi, C., Tomar, L. K., Kumar, P., Choonara, Y. E., & Pillay, V., (2014). Nutraceutical-based therapeutics and formulation strategies augmenting their efficiency to complement modern medicine: An overview. *J. Funct. Foods., 6*, 82–99.

6. Lockwood, B., (2007). *Nutraceuticals* (2nd edn., p. 1). Pharmaceutical Press, London, UK.

7. Caprio, M., Infante, M., Calanchini, M., Mammi, C., & Fabbri, A., (2016). Vitamin D: Not just the bone. Evidence for beneficial pleiotropic extraskeletal effects, eating and weight disorders-studies on anorexia. *Bulimia and Obesity, 22*(1), 27–41.

8. Moghadamtousi, S., Kadir, H., Hassandarvish, P., Tajik, H., Abubakar, A., & Zandi, K., (2014). A review on antibacterial, antiviral, and antifungal activity of curcumin. *BioMed Research International, 12*.

9. Schäfer, C., & Kaschula, (2014). The immunomodulation and anti-inflammatory effects of garlic organosulfur compounds in cancer chemoprevention. *Anti-Cancer Agents in Medicinal Chemistry, 14*(2), 233–240.

10. Li, Y., Zang, T., Korkaya, H., et al., (2010). Sulforaphane, a dietary component of broccoli/broccoli sprouts, inhibits breast cancer stem cells. *Clin Cancer Res., 16*(9), 2580–2590.

11. Casey, C., Slawson, D., & Neal, L., (2010). Vitamin D supplementation in infants, children, and adolescents. *American Family Physician, 81*(6), 745–748.

12. Genís, S., Sánchez-Chardi, À., Bach, Fàbregas, F. & Arís, A., (2017). A combination of lactic acid bacteria regulates Escherichia coli infection and inflammation of the bovine endometrium. *Journal of Dairy Science, 100*(1), 479–492.

13. Zhang, C., Li, X., & Kim, S. K., (2012). Application of marine biomaterials for nutraceuticals and functional foods. *Food Sci. Biotechnol., 21*, 625–631.

14. Chaisa, G., Busnelli, M., Stefano, M. S., & Parolini, C., (2016). Nutraceuticals and bioactive components from fish for dyslipidemia and cardiovascular risk reduction. *Mar. Drugs, 14*(6)., 113.

15. Tang, G., et al., (2009). Golden rice is an effective source of vitamin A. *Am. J. Clin. Nutr., 89*, 1776–1783.

16. Renukuntla, J., Vadlapudi, A. D., Patel, A., Boddu, S. H., & Mitra, A. K., (2013). Approaches for enhancing oral bioavailability of peptides and proteins. *Int. J. Pharm., 447*, 75–93.

17. Patel, K. R., Scott, E., Brown, V. A., Gescher, A. J., Steward, W. P., & Brown, K., (2011). Clinical trails of resveratrol. *Annals of the New York Academy of Sciences, 1215*, 161–169.

18. Chauhan, D., (2002). Chemotherapeutic potential of curcumin for colorectal cancer. *Curr. Pharm. Des., 8*(19), 1695–1706.

19. Balakrishnan, P., Lee, B. J., Oh, D. H., Kim, J. O., Lee, Y. I., et al., (2009). Enhanced oral bioavailability of coenzyme Q10 by self-emulsifying drug delivery systems. *Int. J. Pharm., 374*, 66–72.

20. Roohinejad, S., Oey, I., Wen, J., Lee, S., Everett, D., & Burritt, D, (2015). Formulation of oil-in-water b-carotene MEs: Effect of oil type and fatty acid chain length. *Food Chemistry, 174*(2015). 270–278.

21. Garti, N., Amar-Yuli, I., Serpanth, A., & Hoffman, R., (2004). Transitions and loci of solubilization of nutraceuticals in U-type nonionic MEs studied by self-diffusion NMR. *Phys. Chem. Chem. Phys., 6*, 2968–2976.

22. Amar, I., Aserin, A., & Garti, N., (2003). Solubilization patterns of lutein and lutein esters in food-grade non-ionic MEs. *J. Agric. Food Chem., 51*(16), 4775–4781.

23. Fan, Y., Li, X., Zhou, Y., et al., (2011). Improved intestinal delivery of salmon calcitonin by water-in-oil MEs. *Int. J. Pharm., 416*(1), 323–330.

24. Rozner, S., & Garti, N., (2006). *Colloids and Surfaces A: Physicochem. Eng. Aspects, 282, 283*, 435–456.

25. Ruixue, G., Xiong, F., Jian, C., Lin, Z., & Gu, C., (2016). Preparation and characterization of mes of myricetin for improving its antiproliferative, antioxidative activity and oral bioavailability. *J. Agric. Food Chem., 64*(32), 6286–6294.

26. Benito, P., & Miller, D., (1998). Iron absorption and bioavailability: An updated review. *Nutr Res., 18*, 581–603.

27. Fernàndez-Garcìa, E., Carvajal-Lérida, I., & Pérez-Gàlvez, A., (2009). *In vitro* bioaccessibility assessment as a prediction tool of nutritional efficiency. *Nutr Res., 29*, 751–760.

28. Hollman, P. C., Bijsman, M. N., Van, G. Y., Cnossen, E. P., De Vries, J. H., & Katan, M. B., (1999). The sugar moiety is a major determinant of the absorption of dietary flavonoid glycosides in man. *Free Radic Res., 31*, 569–573.

29. Richelle, M., Lambelet, P., Rytz, A., Tavazzi, I., Mermoud, A. F., Juhel, C., Borel, P., & Bortlik, K., (2012). The proportion of lycopene isomers in human plasma is modulated by lycopene isomer profile in the meal but not by lycopene preparation. *Br. J. Nutr., 107*, 1482–1488.

30. Versantvoort, M., & Rompelberg, M., (2004). Development and applicability of an *in vitro* digestion model in assessing the bioaccessibility of contaminants from food. *Bilthoven. Inspectorate of Health Inspection*, 9–10.

31. McClements, D. J., Li, F., & Xiao, H., (2015). The nutraceutical bioavailability classification scheme: Classifying nutraceuticals according to factors limiting their oral bioavailability. *Annual. Rev. of Food Sci. and Tech., 6*, 299–327.

32. Kerns, E. H., & Di, L., (2008). *Transporters. Drug-like Properties: Concepts, Structure Design and Methods, from ADME to Toxicity Optimization* (1st edn., pp. 103–122). London: Elsevier.

33. Williamson, G., & Manach, C., (2005). Bioavailability and bioefficacy of polyphenols in humans. II. Review of 93 intervention studies. *Am. J. Clin. Nutr., 81*(1 Suppl.), 243S–255S.

34. Kumar, B., & Smita, K., (2017). Chapter 3 - scope of nanotechnology in nutraceuticals. In: Alexandra, E. O., & Alexandru, M. G., (eds.), *Nanotechnology Applications in Food Flavor, Stability, Nutrition and Safety* (pp. 43–63). Academic Press, Elsevier Inc.

35. Spernath, A., & Aserin, A., (2006). *Adv. in Coll. and Inter. Sci., 128–130*, 47–64.

36. Lawrence, M. J., & Rees, G. D., (2000). ME-based media as novel drug delivery systems. *Adv Drug Deliv. Rev., 45*(1), 89–121.

37. Muzaffar, F., Singh, U., & Chauhan, L., (2013). Review on ME as futuristic drug delivery. *Int. J. of Pharm. and Pharm. Sci., 5*(3), 39–53.

38. Lu, Y., Qi, J., & Wu, W., (2012). Absorption, disposition and pharmacokinetics of nanoemulsions. *Curr. Drug Metab. 13*(4), 396–417.

39. Garti, N., & Aserin, A., (2012). Chapter 9, Micelles and MEs as food ingredient and nutraceutical delivery systems. In: Garti, N., & McClements, D. J., (eds.), *Encapsulation Technologies and Delivery Systems for Food Ingredients and Nutraceuticals* (pp. 211–251). Woodhead Publishing Limited.

40. Rao, J., & McClements, D., (2011). Food-grade MEs, nanoemulsions and emulsions: Fabrication from sucrose monopalmitate and lemon oil. *Food Hydrocolloids, 25*, 1413–1423.

41. Strickley, R., (2004). Solubilizing excipients in oral and injectable formulations. *Pharmaceutical Research, 21*(2), 201–230.

42. Jha, S., Dey, S., & Karki, R., (2011). MEs- potential carrier for improved drug delivery. *Internationale Pharmaceutica Sciencia, 1*(2), 25–31.

43. McClements, D. J., Decker, E. A., & Weiss, J., (2007). Emulsion-based delivery systems for lipophilic bioactive components. *J. Food Sci., 72*(8), R109–124.

44. Graf, A., Ablinger, E., Peters, S., Zimmerb, A., Hooka, S., & Rades, T., (2008). ME containing lecithin and sugar based surfactants: Nanoparticles templates for delivery of protein and peptides. *Int. J. Pharm., 350*, 351–360.

45. Kumar, K., et al., (2011). MEs as carrier for novel drug delivery: A review. *Int. Journal of Pharm. Sci. Rev. and Res., 10*.2, 37–45.

46. Sood, A., & Panchagnula, R., (2001). Peroral route: An opportunity for protein and peptide drug delivery. *Chem. Rev., 101*, 3275–3303.

47. Liandong, H., Yanhong, J., Feng, N., Zheng, J., Xun, Y., & Kuiliang, J., (2012). Preparation and enhancement of oral bioavailability of curcumin using MEs vehicle. *J. Agric. Food Chem., 60*, 7137–7141.

48. Narang, A., Delmarre, D., & Gao, D., (2007). Stable drug encapsulation in micelles and MEs. *Int. J. Pharm., 345*(1, 2), 9–25.

49. Sh, Y., Gui, L., Wu, D., Peng, Y., et al. (2008). Preparation and evaluation of a ME for oral delivery of berberine. *Pharmazie, 63*, 516–519.

50. Rozner, S., Abraham, A., & Nissim, G., (2008). Competitive solubilization of cholesterol and phytosterols in nonionic MEs studied by pulse gradient spin-echo NMR. *Journal of Colloid and Interface Science, 321*, 418–425.

51. Tang, T., Hu, X., Liao, D., et al., (2013). Mechanisms of ME enhancing the oral bioavailability of puerarin: Comparison between oil-in-water and water-in-oil MEs using the single-pass intestinal perfusion method and a chylomicron flow blocking approach. *Int. J. Nanomedicine, 8*, 4415–4426.

52. Helgason, T., Awad, T. S., Kristbergsson, K., Decker, E. A., McClements, D. J., & Weiss, J., (2009). Impact of surfactant properties on oxidative stability of b-carotene encapsulated within solid lipid nanoparticles. *Jour of Agri and Food Chemistry, 57*(17), 8033–8040.

53. John, F., & Singh, H., (2006). MEs: A potential delivery system for bioactives in food. *Critical Reviews in Food Science and Nutrition, 46*(3), 221–237.

54. Solanki, S., Sarkar, B., & Dhanwani, R., (2012). ME drug delivery system: For bioavailability enhancement of ampelopsin. *ISRN Pharmaceutics.* doi: 10.5402/2012/108164.

55. Popova, M., Silici, S., Kaftanoglu, O., & Bankova, V., (2005). Antibacterial activity of Turkish propolis and its qualitative and quantitative chemical composition. *Phytomedicine, 12*, 221–228.

56. Banskota, A., Tezuka, Y., & Kadota, S., (2001). Recent progress in pharmacological research of propolis. *Phytother. Res., 15*, 561–571.

57. Fan, Y., Ma, L., Zhang, W., Xu, Y., Suolangzhaxi, Zhi, X, Cui, E., & Song, X., (2014). *International Journal of Biological Macromolecules, 63*, 126–132.

58. Wu, Z. J., Xia, X. J., & Huang, X. S., (2012). Determination of equilibrium solubility and apparent oil/water partition coefficient of piperine. *J. Jinan Uni. Natl. Sci. Med., 5*(33), 473–476.

59. Etman, S., Yosra, S., Elnaggar, D., Abdelmonsif, A., & Ossama, Y., (2018). Brain targeted ME for enhanced piperine delivery in Alzheimer's disease therapy: *In vitro* appraisal, *in vivo* activity and nanotoxicity. *AAPS PharmSciTech.* doi: 10.1208/s12249-018-1180-3.

60. Carocho, M., & Ferreira, I. C., (2013). A review on antioxidants, prooxidants and related controversy: Natural and synthetic compounds, screening and analysis methodologies and future perspectives. *Food Chem. Toxicol., 51*, 15–25. doi: 10.1016/j.fct.2012.09.021.

61. Lv, X., Liu, H., Ma, H., Tian, Y., et al., (2017). Preparation of essential oil-based MEs for improving the solubility, pH stability, photostability, and skin permeation of quercetin. *AAPS PharmSciTech.* DOI: 10.1208/s12249-017-0798-x.

62. Lin, C., Lin, H., Chi, M., Shen, M., Chen, H., Yang, W., & Lee, M., (2014). Preparation of curcumin MEs with food-grade soybean oil/lecithin and their cytotoxicity on the HepG2 cell line. *Food Chemistry, 154*, 282–290.

63. Albanes, D., Heinonen, O. P., Taylor, P. R., Virtamo, J., Edwards, B. K., Rautalahti, M., et al., (1996). a-Tocopherol and b-Carotene supplements and lung cancer incidence in the alpha-tocopherol, beta-carotene cancer prevention study: Effects of base-line characteristics and study compliance. *Journal of the National Cancer Institute, 88*(21), 1560–1570.

64. Omenn, G. S., Williams, J. H., Barnhart, S., Hammar, S., Goodman, G. E., Thornquist, M. D., et al., (1996). Effects of a combination of beta carotene and vitamin A on lung cancer and cardiovascular disease. *The New England Journal of Medicine, 334*(18), 1150–1155.

65. Jung, S., Wu, K., Giovannucci, E., Spiegelman, D., Willett, W. C., & Smith-Warner, S. A., (2013). Carotenoid intake and risk of colorectal adenomas in a cohort of male health professionals. *Cancer Causes and Control, 24*(4), 705–717.

66. Pan, Y., Tikekar, R. V., & Nitin, N., (2013). Effect of antioxidant properties of lecithin emulsifier on oxidative stability of encapsulated bioactive compounds. *Int. J. Pharm, 450*(1, 2), 129–137.

PART V
Advanced Innovative Nutraceutical Delivery Systems

CHAPTER 10

Challenges in Oral Delivery of Nutraceuticals: From Formulation Scale-Up to Clinical Assessment

KAUSHALENDRA CHATURVEDI,[1] HARSH SHAH,[1] and BHAVIN GAJERA[2]

[1]Lachman Institute for Pharmaceutical Analysis Laboratory at Long Island University, New York, USA

[2]Formulation Scientist, Impel NeuroPharma, Washington, USA

ABSTRACT

Nutraceuticals have grown in popularity over the past decade, and demand in the consumer sector is expected to skyrocket in the future years. They provide consumers with value-added benefits and a variety of nutritional choices. The extraction of phytochemicals with the required purity and yield is a constant problem for nutraceutical products. The use of sophisticated technology in the extraction and production of nutraceuticals is addressing these issues. Low bioavailability issues associated with nutraceutical oral administration have been effectively addressed using novel formulation methods. However, to effectively scale up production of nutraceuticals without compromising the quality of the final product, investment in new manufacturing methods and sophisticated analytical procedures is required. Due to the absence of reliable biomarkers and a lack of knowledge of nutraceutical interactions with food and medications, clinical research of nutraceuticals presents a greater difficulty. The regulatory authorities have recognized the need to improve current nutraceutical standards and offer nutraceutical-specific advice so that clinical studies may be conducted efficiently and with clear findings. Furthermore, a scientific knowledge of nutraceuticals is required, as is the evaluation of their therapeutic and pharmacological effects on people.

10.1   INTRODUCTION

The origin of the word nutraceutical is from the Latin word "nutrire" and the English word "Pharmaceuticals." The word nutrire means nourish and pharmaceuticals is the compound manufactured for medicinal purposes [1, 2]. Therefore, nutraceutical word essentially describes the potential benefits of the substance towards the medicinal purposes, which are sourced from nature. According to Wikipedia, nutraceutical word can be defined as the food containing health-giving additives and having therapeutic benefits. Nutraceutical term was first coined in 1989 by Stephen De Felice, Founder and Chairman of the Foundation for Innovation in Medicine (FIM). This chapter defines nutraceutical as the food, or parts of food, that provide medical or health benefits, including the prevention and treatment of disease [3, 4]. The dietary supplements (DS) are defined and regulated by the Dietary Supplement Health and Education Act (DSHEA) of 1994. According to the act dietary supplement is a product that is intended to supplement the diet which contains different ingredients including amino acids, botanicals, herbs, minerals, and vitamins. These supplements are designed to be ingested as a pill, capsule, tablet, or liquid; and is labeled as being a dietary supplement. There is no specific definition of nutraceutical according to the US law; however it is understood as a product derived from a human food source and dispensed for extra health benefits beyond the fundamental nutritional value found in foods [5, 6]. All these products are sold as an over-the-counter product, and no prescription is required. Different definitions of nutraceutical can be found in literature, but nutraceutical word can be simply defined as the therapeutically active substance sourced from the food or part of food which is compounded with a different ingredient to form a final dosage form which is used for the treating diseases and the prophylactic purposes. It should be noted that the pharmaceuticals in which substance is incorporated for the therapeutic purpose can be chemically synthesized or sourced from nature [7, 8], but these compounds are not from the regular diet, and they cannot be used as a supplement which makes the distinctive difference between the pharmaceuticals and nutraceuticals products.

10.2   NUTRACEUTICAL DELIVERY SYSTEM

Nutraceuticals are classified based on either their intended use or if they have been modified before making it available to consumers, e.g., traditional, non-traditional, fortified, and recombinant. In the literature different medicinal applications of nutraceuticals have been reported, including but not limited to digestion, cold, fever, diabetes, blood pressure, and heart diseases [9–14]. However, this research work was conducted using active nutraceutical ingredient which could be difficult to formulate into the finished product which can be delivered to the consumer. Extraction of phytochemicals which are an active ingredient in providing intended pharmacological activity is a difficult task [15–17]. The total amount of this active chemical present in the raw material is in microgram scale which makes it a costly process apart from the cost chemicals are very sensitive to heat, moisture, and light [18–21]. For example, ascorbic acid, catechin, anthocyanins are very sensitive to the presence of oxygen, light, and high temperature [22–24]. However, in recent few years industry is moving towards the use of sophisticated instrumentation to extract these chemicals from the sources [3, 25–27]. After extraction, it is imperative to design and formulate a dosage form which can help to deliver active compounds to the patient. Different dosage forms are currently available in the market based on the material characteristics and the intended use. Formulation and development of these active components are complicated and not cost-effective process. The market values for these products are very low compared to pharmaceuticals, and most often these nutraceuticals are not covered by the insurance plan. Which makes it very difficult for the industry to design a formulation which can help to deliver the active ingredient patient with low product cost. Like pharmaceuticals, nutraceuticals can be delivered via different dosage forms, including tablet, capsule, syrup, cream, gels, and ointments.

Dosage form selection for nutraceuticals is significant because of their chemical and physical nature. There are a few most critical aspects which could lead to either failure or success in the formulation of nutraceuticals. The total amount of active ingredient present in raw materials of nutraceuticals is in micro ranges, which means before going for the formulation development, it is vital to consider the dosing aspects. If the active ingredient is available in micrograms and the drug dose is in milligrams, then the total formulation blend for a unit dose will be grams such as multivitamin, glucosamine [28] and flavonoid tablets [29] which is not preferred by the patient. However, for medium dose compounds solid orals could be the preferred choice for the delivery. However, the tableting operation seems straightforward compared to novel delivery systems, but it has its limitations associated with the physical and mechanical characteristics of powder. Second, the solubility of the ingredients, if the actives are not water-soluble then delivering a tablet or capsules, will not work. Therefore, it is essential to come up with the alternative formulation approaches including solution, suspension, or syrups. Novel formulations such as nanosuspension or nanoemulsions can be an excellent approach to deliver these drugs. However, the cost associated with the unit operations may not align with the company's interests. Third, the chemical stability of these compounds is one of the major concerns. Some literatures are available indicating the chemical sensitivity of nutraceuticals. Most often, these chemical compounds are either moisture or heat sensitive and making it a difficult task for a formulator to develop a formulation in which material is not exposed to an unstable condition which could negatively affect the stability of the compound. Formulation operation is a complex process that involves multiple unit operations, including blending, granulation, tableting, coating, or stirring this unit operation imparts a certain amount of stress on to the material. If the content is sensitive to a specific process, then it is critical to choose an alternate approach, e.g., vitamins are very sensitive to thermal condition then, in this case, wet granulation or melt granulation may not be the best approach [30]. Broad application, safety, and rapid growth in demand for nutraceuticals impelled researchers to develop novel delivery systems which could efficiently deliver the actives to the patients [31–33]. These advances resulted into development of nanoemulsions, liposomes, phytosome, and transferosomes. The formulations can be categorized into three major categories based on the route of delivery.

10.2.1 ORAL DELIVERY

In pharmaceuticals or nutraceuticals, oral delivery is the most acceptable and preferred route administration. Patient compliance, non-invasive nature, and cost-effective manufacturing process make the oral solids as a preferred choice [34–36]. For oral delivery gastrointestinal tract (GIT) plays a significant role. Like pharmaceuticals in the literature, it has been reported that the content in the GI tract may or may not influence the absorption of the nutraceutical. Fat-soluble vitamins showed an increase in absorption in the fed state over the fasted state [37, 38]. For example, carotenoids absorption is increased with the presence of avocado or avocado oil in contrast to this in the literature, it is reported that in some women, the presence of fibers decreases the absorption of carotenoids [39, 40]. A recent study supports the finding that the absorption of B-carotene from GI tract is significantly affected when meal involves the use of sunflower oil or beef fat. This suggests that the oral delivery of nutraceuticals has its challenges which are not very different from the pharmaceuticals. Lycopene, vitamins, melatonin, creatine, green tea extract, glucosamine, and chondroitin are few of many available nutraceutical ingredients which are marketed as oral dosage forms [41–45].

10.2.1.1 FORMULATION AND SCALABILITY ISSUES FOR THE ORAL DELIVERY OF NUTRACEUTICALS

It is very well established that for oral delivery tablet, and capsules are the preferred dosage forms. However, manufacturing a tablet or capsule may not be an easy task for nutraceuticals. For a quality product in tablets, it is essential to have good friability, hardness, and organoleptic properties. Similarly, for capsules, it is crucial that formulation blend should have excellent flow properties. Powder flow property and compressibility is also very important for tablet formulation as well, if the flow property of the mixture is not good, that may lead to weight variation, so the content uniformity issues [46, 47]. In pharmaceuticals tackling the problems associated with the flow can be resolved either by granulation or by using excipients [48–50]. These solutions can be used in nutraceuticals, but the use may be minimal. It is because the most often nutraceutical product has more than three actives with some excipient leaving formulator with no space to make any changes in the formulation to resolve the powder flowability or compressibility issues. Therefore, roller compactor operation could be the best choice for the scale-up. In roller compactor operation no heat is involved, or the granulating media is engaged in making intermediate or the final product. Granulation resolves the issue related to content uniformity and the flow issues, but it may not help with other tableting defects such as sticking, picking, and capping. Tablet is sticking, and picking is one of the significant concerns in tableting operation, especially when the process is set up for hours (Figure 10.1) [51, 52]. The reason for sticking is the presence of very high moisture content in nutraceutical products which under high compression pressure leads to tablet sticking. In the literature, it has been reported that the different electroplated punches can help to resolve the problem of tablet sticking (Figure 10.2).

GI tract has a different pH range starting from 1.2 to 7.4, which changes based on the content present in the GI tract. The wide range of GI pH has could potentially impact the stability of the nutraceuticals in the body. Also, metabolic enzyme plays a crucial role in metabolizing the foreign compound which could affect the bioavailability so the therapeutic activity. For example, catechin is highly susceptible to degradation at alkaline pH. Tablet coating could be the best solution to eliminate the issues related to the pH sensitivity as well as for taste masking [53]. Therefore, before formulating an oral dosage form for nutraceutical, it is imperative to understand the physical, chemical, and mechanical properties of the active substances. Despite so many potential issues related to bioavailability, dose potency and stability consumer has shown a consistent preference for nutraceuticals. It is essential to consider a tailor-made approach to design a delivery system for a specific compound depending on the physical, chemical, and mechanical characteristics of formulation blend. In recent years a number of reports have been published regarding the use of novel oral delivery systems for the nutraceuticals, which improves different formulation factors including solubility, bioavailability, and stability.

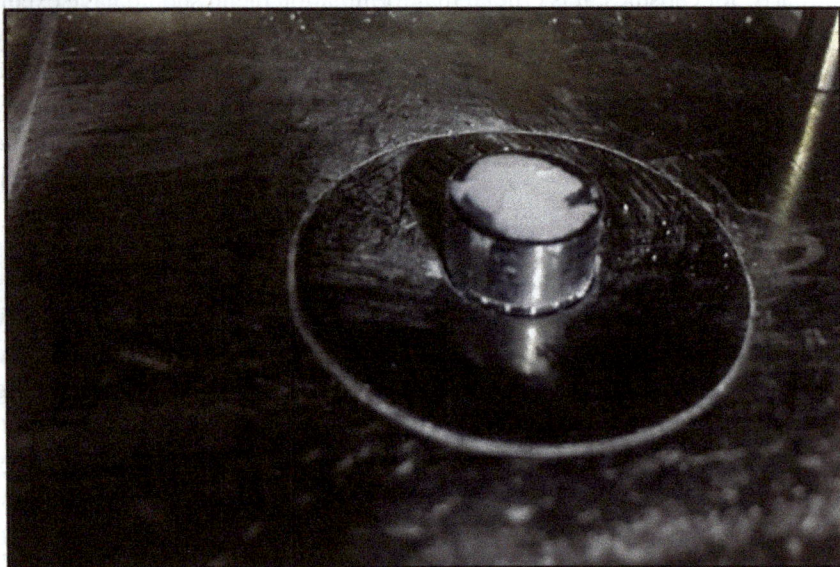

FIGURE 10.1   Tablet sticking issue.

10.2.2   *DERMAL DELIVERY*

Dermal route of delivery is one of the preferred delivery systems when the patient is suffering from local infection, inflammation, or for cosmetic purposes [54]. Although the oral delivery of nutraceuticals reported producing higher plasma concentration of bioactives compared to the dermal delivery. However, the first-pass effect, and GI environmental condition is two primary causes for nutraceuticals low therapeutic activity and bioavailability. Therefore, the dermal route of administration is one of the best alternate delivery systems for the bioactives which are very sensitive to first pass and GI effect. Nutraceutical products dermal delivery is very demanding in the cosmetic section. Consumers are getting aware of the potential harms related to the cosmetics which are made from chemically synthesized compounds. Therefore, consumers are leaning towards the natural products which are 100% organic. For example, antiaging cream made from Co-enzyme Q10 (CoQ10) and vitamin C reported showing a significant clinical result by reducing wrinkle depth in old aged skin [55]. Currently, in a market different range of cosmetics products are available which are made from the nutraceuticals like curcumin, vitamin C, gluconolactone, N-acetylcysteine, and genistein. Therefore, the primary reason for more patients searching for treatments using nutraceuticals is in association with its safety but not the potential activity compared to pharmaceuticals. Many nutraceuticals are best suited to deliver dermally instead of orally because of its access to treat the target area such as curcumin. Curcumin reported having an excellent anti-inflammatory activity which is used for the treatment of psoriasis [56]. However, the oral delivery of curcumin may not be the best idea to treat psoriasis infected area; therefore, dermal delivery is the best one. Similarly, some other products, such as hot patches, which are used for the local effect of reducing pain that contains capsaicin as an active ingredient.

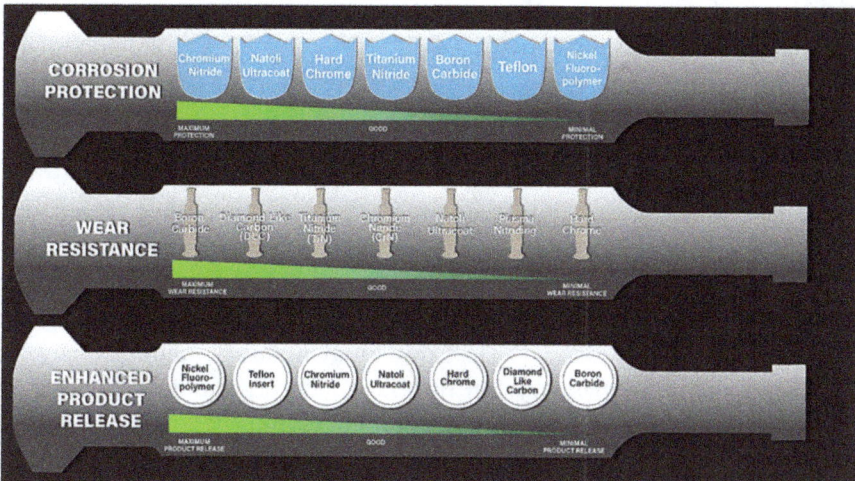

FIGURE 10.2 Different types of tooling provided by the Natoli engineering to resolve technical issues related to tableting operation.

Source: Reprinted with permission from: Natoli Engineering Website; https://natoli.com/which-coating-can-help-solve-your-tableting-issues/.

10.2.2.1   *FORMULATION AND SCALABILITY PROBLEMS IN DEVELOPING TOPICAL FORMULATIONS*

Literature supports the advances of designing the topical delivery of nutraceuticals. However, there are multiple factors which need to be considered before the formulation scale-up. Manufacturing steps of topical formulations involve complicated measures such as melting, mixing, and homogenization. During the scale-up, these unit operation time may range from minutes to hours. All these steps involve high energy which ultimately generates a high amount of stress which may negatively affect the quality of the product. Especially in cosmetic purpose nutraceutical product viscosity and texture of the product is very important. To make smooth textured formulation, the formulation approaches are to melt the bioactive into the carrier or micronization of the solid particles in micron size ranges. In the literature, it is reported that the many nutraceutical bioactives are susceptible to degradation when they are exposed to light or higher temperature. Therefore, before deciding the carrier for the formulation, it will be essential to check the melting temperature of the carrier and the bioactive. If the melting temperature of the carrier is higher than the bioactives, then that may not be the best choice because of the instability issue of actives at the approximate processing temperature. Similarly, micronization of solid particle involves milling of the particle at very high pressure, which could lead to degradation of the actives.

10.2.3   *OPHTHALMIC DELIVERY*

CoQ10, vitamin E, and lutein are few of many bioactives which can be delivered into the ocular activity because of their antioxidant, anti-inflammatory, and anti-cataract properties [57]. However, the product therapeutic performance is dependent on the residence time and the permeability of the drug [58]. Low bioavailability and efficacy of nutraceuticals is the primary limiting factor during the development of ophthalmic formulation. Different approaches like nanoemulsions and nanosuspension are researched in this area to modify the solubility as well as the residence time, which could provide the desired properties in the formulation [59]. However, at large scale manufacturing, similar problems explained in oral, and delivery could affect the product quality as well as the production rate.

10.3 GROWING DEMAND AND ITS IMPACT ON DRUG DEVELOPMENT AND CLINICAL DEVELOPMENT OF NUTRACEUTICALS

Over the years, the nutraceutical market has been developed due to the side effects associated with the pharmaceuticals, treatment cost, and sophisticated techniques for determination of qualitative and quantitative parameters. Because of these advances in the field multi-million-dollar industry is turned into a multi-billion-dollar sector. The sector growth is seen at the global level and based on the literature data, global marketing of nutraceutical was USD 128.4 billion in 2008 [60]. Approximately more than 70% of the American population take some form of dietary supplement every day, which caused that the supplement industry is currently over $28 billion in US only. Based on the study published in December 2017 by Grand View Research, Inc., the global market for nutraceuticals will reach USD 578.23 billion by 2025 [61]. The significant rise in the nutraceutical market capital indicates the growing awareness regarding the use of healthy foods as a supplement. In the market survey, it is reported that the nutraceuticals demand in the market will rapidly increase in the coming next eight years as the consumer considers these supplements are safer to use than the synthetic pharmaceuticals.

10.4 NEED FOR CHANGE IN MANUFACTURING APPROACH AND REGULATORY GUIDELINES

In ancient civilization including but not limited to Egyptian, Roman, and Indus valley the use of DS for treatment of different diseases have been reported. However, the modernization of medical science seems to be forgotten the essence of nutraceuticals for many decades. There could be a different reason, and most often but not limited to active components effectiveness, ease of use, and regulatory issues. Regarding efficacy, the nutraceutical substances are mostly non-potent in nature and treatment with these substances to treat disease may range from days to months. The second most important reason could be the lack of reported studies indicating the use of this substance for their purpose. In the literature, the pharmacological or therapeutic activity of nutraceuticals have been reported, but again most of those studies are conducted in an academic research environment. US Food and Drug Administration (FDA) guidelines regulate DS utterly different than the pharmaceuticals. For the pharmaceuticals, USFDA has strict guidelines related to the drug's effectiveness and safety before it can be brought to the market, however, for the nutraceuticals, manufacturers does not need to provide any effectiveness or safety data. In summary, there is no strict guideline pertaining to products safety also no clinical trials are required. However, it is clearly stated that the manufacturer should not specify any specific claim regarding curing or treating the disease on the product label. The explanation for not having a clinical trial is that nutraceuticals are generally recognized as safe (GRAS) based on their historical use. However, after October 15, 1994, it is a necessary requirement for the manufacturer to notify the FDA and provide reasonable evidence that the product is safe for human consumption.

The use of nutraceuticals was left behind and most of the time, not preferred by the healthcare professionals because of the aforementioned essential factors related to product effectiveness and lack of documented studies. As previously mentioned, regulations for pharmaceuticals are stringent and regulated worldwide before its launch in the market. Monitored, controlled, and documented clinical trial reports establish the effectiveness and safety of pharmaceutical products, and which ultimately provides the documented evidence for the healthcare professionals. This provides the confidence in doctors to prefer pharmaceuticals over a nutraceutical to treat a patient. Despite the lack of health care professional advice to switch to nutraceuticals, there is a steady growth in the use of nutraceuticals. According to the published report, approximately half of the adult population in the United States takes DS either for medical or fitness purposes and only about a quarter of this population takes supplements based on the advice of health care professionals. This indicates that the patients or the consumer's decisions to take nutraceuticals for their intended use are made by themselves, unlike in pharmaceuticals. DS are generally safe but not totally without risk and being in the sector of health care, it is the responsibility of industry and regulatory bodies to come with a guideline defining safety, efficacy, and quality of these nutraceutical products (Figure 10.3).

10.5   SELECTION OF THE DOSAGE FORM BASED ON CHALLENGES DURING THE PRODUCT DEVELOPMENT AND COMMERCIAL MANUFACTURING OF THE NUTRACEUTICAL INGREDIENTS

Among all the available dosage forms on the market, solid oral formulations continue to remain one of the most preferred forms [62]. Tablets and capsules form a large part of the oral solid dosage form for administration to the patients due to ease dispensing unit doses and Physico-chemical stability of the nutraceutical contents used for the desired effect [63]. Powders and granules are also used in certain situation when the major component suffers from issues related to compressibility or deprived flow properties [64]. Tablets are generally manufactured by reducing powders and granules into a compact product. The advantage that tablet offers over any other dosage form is its versatility, robustness, and accuracy, and from the commercial view-point, larger batch size production can be achieved rapidly [65]. However, from the quality perspective, the nutraceutical solid dosage forms are now expected to transition to stringent regulatory standards which are identical to those being currently used for the pharmaceutical industry [66].

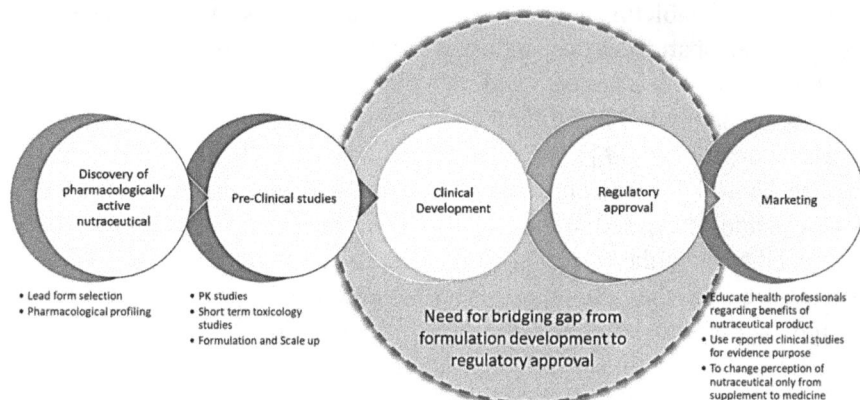

FIGURE 10.3 Life cycle for nutraceutical product development from discovery to commercialization.

As an example, multivitamin tablets may contain between about 25–50 active ingredients as well as 6–10 inactive ingredients which also include coating polymers, whereas, pharmaceutical drug products will contain a maximum of three active ingredients and 5–6 inactive ingredients [67, 68]. It becomes even more challenging due to the presence of numerous active ingredients within a nutraceutical formulation [69]. The challenges range from particle sizing, flowability, compressibility, moisture degradation, chemical interaction, and content uniformity [61, 69]. From a quality perspective, it becomes even more difficult to adopt a quality control (QC) testing method as the product must undergo lengthy or multiple analytical procedures to verify the content of each active ingredient present in the formulation [70, 71].

Each active ingredient may have a unique physical property in terms of particle size, hygroscopicity or flowability, and every individual physical property could affect the blending unit operation during the product development or commercial manufacturing of the nutraceutical product [72, 73]. The differences in the physical properties of each ingredient will ultimately affect the integrity of the tablets resulting in capping, sticking, picking or weaker strength tablets during the compression process. Affected tablets may yield variabilities in the content uniformity [74].

From the tooling perspective, the production of tablet involves punches and dies in a tablet press used to compress ingredients either in powder or granular form at high compaction pressures [75]. It is same tableting process which was invented in 1843 and evolved with further improvements [76]. The improved tableting technology available today is the only used technique in the pharmaceutical industry for making tablets [76]. Because of the reliability, cost-efficient, and robustness, tablet formulation accounts for approximately 80% of total market share among all other dosage forms available on the market [77].

The natural ingredients used in the nutraceutical products are poorly compressible, unrefined, abrasive, corrosive, and hard [78]. These properties together have the potential to damage the tablet tooling (i.e., punches, and dies) during the tableting process as these materials are required to be compressed at high compaction pressures and for longer periods of time to ensure high output and lower the manufacturing cost [79, 80]. Therefore, along with the formulation development process the tablet tooling needs to be designed depending upon the physical properties of the ingredients [80]. The tablet tooling design may include a selection of metallurgically strong alloy and a tooling design which can withstand possible harsh conditions from compacting nutraceuticals [81, 82].

The nutraceutical products are comprised of multiple active ingredients, which forms a major portion in the drug product as compared to its portion of inactive ingredients. Similarly, the high-dose pharmaceutical product can be compared to the nutraceutical products, except, pharmaceutical product would have only one ingredient in high dose product, where nutraceutical product may have up to 50 different active ingredients. The lesser amounts of excipients limit the possibility of tablets achieving desirable physical attributes, i.e., disintegration time, hardness, and friability. To develop a product with minimal quantity of excipients pose a serious challenge for the formulators in term of achieving desired product results, not only during product development but also during scale-up and commercial manufacturing.

The challenges that the formulator faces during the product development of nutraceutical products includes:

- Delivering appropriate quantity of each active ingredient in the desired dosage form;
- Studying material characteristics of active as well as inactive ingredients used in the formulation;
- Develop a formulation with minimal excipients;
- Design process, tooling, and optimize the process variables.

As an example, in the case of tablets or capsules, improper powder flow will lead to inter lot and intra lot variability in content uniformity of the active ingredients claimed to present. Compressibility problems if not identified as small scale can translate to productivity problems in the tableting process during scale-up or commercial manufacturing. Similarly, if the material is characterized to be rigid and cause abrasion, the tableting process needs to be designed such that high-quality punches and dies (with or without specific antiwear, antistick, and anticorrosion coatings) are used. While choosing suitable tooling, tablet shape, form, and compaction force needs to be considered to ensure the long life of the tooling during tablet manufacturing.

If all the mentioned criteria are addressed carefully, then it can save tedious and time-consuming efforts of resolving issues by trial-and-error during the final stage of product development.

In an effort to achieve the identification and marketing of the brand; the shape, inscription (in tablets) and printing (in capsules) serves as brand identifier and marketing tool. These pose a challenge to the manufacturer because the sticking and picking issues may intensify due to imprints and score on the tablets [83]. Furthermore, in the nutraceutical tablets, the active ingredients inherently have neutral colors such as brown or gray with mottled or textured appearance visually poses difficulty in reading the inscriptions or the symbols [84].

The nutraceutical ingredients are inherently tough and has potential to cause damage to the tablet tooling. Types of tooling damage includes pitted or worned off surfaces, which may further cause to form deformed tablets due to "capping" and "lamination" issues [85]. Despite the availability of different types of steel, only a few material choices are available to manufacture tablet tooling with the complex design and necessary functional requirements. Commonly available materials choices for nutraceutical tooling include high carbon, high chrome, and cold work tool steels [86]. Furthermore, tungsten carbide and chromium coatings have also been used to prevent the wear and deformation of the dies due to its extremely high wear resistance to withhold high compaction pressures. Wearing effects and deformation of the tooling is not limited to hydrogen embrittlement, microcracking, and environmental issues.

Oral solid formulation continues to remain the preferred dosage form among all other dosage forms, oral liquid dosage forms in certain cases might prove useful, especially when pediatric or geriatric population are targeted who may not be able to consume tablets or capsules due to dysphagia [87]. However, the problems associated with development of liquid dosage form includes:

- Freely soluble active ingredients are required;
- Stability of active ingredients in liquid form;
- Ensure dosing accuracy of the active ingredients;
- Increased interaction among active ingredients.

Liquid emulsions may offer an alternative route of administration which require careful selection of vehicles during product development in earlier stage [88, 89]. The oils and oil-soluble active ingredients can be used to formulate oil-in-water (O/W) emulsion. The preparation of liquid emulsions involves homogenization of oil with an aqueous solution yielding kinetically stable O/W emulsions. The active ingredients can be dissolved in either water or oil prior to formulating liquid emulsion. Water-soluble vitamins are often encapsulated in oil/water/oil (O/W/O) emulsions. Fechner et al. [90] reported the entrapment of vitamin B12 in the inner phase of an O/W/O emulsion, which was stabilized by caseinate-dextran conjugates [90]. The stabilization of the emulsion helped in restricting the release of the vitamin in gastric conditions. Microemulsions (MEs) can also be used to design thermodynamically stable nutraceutical formulations for water-soluble active ingredients. In the case of oil-soluble ingredients like vitamin A, vitamin D, vitamin E, vitamin K, and β-carotene, spray-dried emulsions can be formulated as drug delivery systems [89]. Currently, emulsion-based techniques and spray drying process are the most preferred strategies to achieve microencapsulation and deliver functional fatty acids as nutritional supplements [89, 91]. In order to stabilize the microcapsules in MEs, alginate-chitosan (CHT) can be used. Alginate-CHT has demonstrated its importance in improving the mechanical strength of microcapsules against *in vitro* digestion [92].

Novel liquid dosage forms like liposomes, niosomes, nanoemulsions, nanosuspension, and others have recently gained more interest in developing targeted drug delivery systems [93–98]. The applicability of liposomes as novel oral delivery systems has now been attempted to extend to dietary and nutritional supplements [99–101] in order to improve the bio-efficacy of nutraceutical ingredients. Liposomes gains the advantage of improved absorption and bioavailability rates in comparison to the conventional delivery systems (i.e., tablets and capsules). The benefits of liposomes not only include protection of nutritional ingredients against its degradation in gastric system but also aid in bypassing recognition by the immune system, that is, cells of the reticulo-endothelial system (RES) [102, 103]. Capsaicin and quercetin are poorly soluble nutraceutical ingredients with many health benefits including anti-obesity, cardioprotection, and anti-cancer. Lu et al. developed lipid-based nanoemulsion system for capsaicin and formulated nanoparticles of quercetin. Novel formulation system helped to improve the dissolution and the bioaccessibility of each drug, respectively [104].

Although the dissolution and bioaccessibility improved significantly using novel liquid delivery systems, the stability and production cost for novel processes may raise concerns during the commercialization of the nutraceutical products (Table 10.1).

10.6 PATIENT COMPLIANCE ASSOCIATED WITH COLOR, ODOR, AND TASTE

The nutraceutical tablets available on the market suffers from the patient compliance issues [105]. The compliance issues include color, odor, and taste of the nutraceutical product [106]. The color of active ingredients that are used in the nutraceutical products are inherently dull in color, and in most cases, the tablet color will mottled brown or gray [106]. In addition to this, the texture may be rough instead of smooth surface due to inherent elastic and plastic nature of the active ingredients [106]. Also, due to color differences of the active ingredients, patches may be observed on the surface of the tablet. To improve patient compliance issues arising from the color and appearance of the tablet, the film coating, which is widely used in the pharmaceutical industry, should be used. If texture or rough surface are responsible for patient compliance problems, sugar coating will be the ideal choice.

Sometimes, the active ingredients being used in the nutraceutical products have an unpleasant odor and unpleasant/bitter taste, which may lead to serious patient compliance issues, irrespective of its beneficial therapeutic effects [107]. In such cases, different flavors available on the market can be used. Commonly used flavors include vanilla, peppermint, strawberry, and others.

The active ingredients which are very abrasive and hard makes it impossible to form a compact for tableting process, hard gelatin capsules may be

TABLE 10.1 Innovations in Nutraceutical Formulations

Product	Category	Active Ingredients	Formulation	Manufacturer
Simplybiotix® Gutsy	Probiotic powder	Vitamin D, Bifidobacterium lactis Bl-04, *Lactobacillus rhamnosus* GG	Stick/powder	Healthy Directions
Equelle®	Women's health (post-menopausal)	Equol	Tablet	Otsuka
Protinex Bytes®	Nutritional supplement	Proteins, vitamins, fibers, nutrients	Cookie	Danone India
Neocate®	Digestive health	Amino acids, vitamins	Powder	Nutricia
Slim-VX1®	Weight loss	Fibers, gingerol, polyphenols	Capsules	Europharma
Natrol® Cognium	Brain health supplement	Cera Q® powder (60% silk protein hydrolysate)	Tablet	Natrol
Pure Protein Super Food®	Dietary supplement	Protein, vitamin	Powder	Nature's Bounty
New Probiotic Mix®	Dietary supplement	Bifidobacterium, *Lactobacillus*, *Streptococcus* strains	Powder	Biopolis
Hemp seed oil	Heart health	Omega 3 fatty acids, Omega 6 fatty acids	Oil	Hempco
Natural marine algae®	Heart and brain health	Omega 3 fatty acids (Eicosapentaenoic acid, docosahexaenoic acid)	Soft gel capsule	Veramaris
Reginator®	Muscle health	Amino acids	Powder, capsule, tablet	Zanda
Aptamil®	Baby formula milk	Galacto- and fructo-oligosaccharides (GOS/FOS), and contains reduced lactose, whey protein	Powder	Danone

the choice of the formulation process [108]. However, hard gelatin capsules require a specified storage condition such that 10–15% moisture is retained within the capsule shell [109]. If the relative humidity (RH) in the storage area drops to 20%, the moisture from the capsule shell begins to dry out, leading to the formation of deformed capsules or cracks on capsule shells [110]. Moreover, it is important to characterize the hygroscopicity of each active as well as inactive ingredients used in the formulation, if the ingredients are hygroscopic in nature, it may begin to sorb moisture from the capsule shell ultimately affecting the stability of the product [110].

If the materials are characterized properly, the capsule not only offers an advantage to the abrasive ingredients but also help in overcoming the patient compliance issues associated with color, odor, and taste.

Nonetheless, while considering hard gelatin capsules as a final dosage form, it is important to keep in mind the added cost associated with it. All the hard gelatin capsules require controlled room temperature conditions and a RH between 40% and 60%, and in certain case, it is 45%–55% during the storage and transportation. Also, if the active ingredients have higher bulk density, then weight variation issues may be observed during the capsule filling process [111].

10.7 SUMMARY OF ADDRESSING FORMULATION DEVELOPMENT CHALLENGES

The formulation development of nutraceutical products using modern machineries help us achieve the high-volume market requirement rapidly. However, the development process involves complexities and problems associated with the ingredients and unit process operations. With utmost caution and thorough knowledge of process and materials, robust nutraceutical product can be developed successfully [112]. Though the higher concentrations of active ingredients in nutraceutical products pose challenges to the physical attributes of the formulation, it can be overcome by making uniform particle size of all the active ingredients being used in the formulation, thoroughly characterized active ingredients, careful selection of dosage form based on material characteristics and appropriate consideration of unit process operation used for manufacturing of nutraceutical product.

Quality by design (QbD) approach can also be applied to produce quality rich and robust nutraceutical dosage form with desirable properties [113]. Irrespective of the dosage form selected, the equipment design plays a very important role in ensuring the quality of the nutraceutical product. It is equally important to achieve a good product design as it helps in avoiding the problems responsible for product failures right from the beginning of the product development, yielding end product free from any type of problems, produce quality rich products and efficient process.

If all the discussed factors are carefully considered during product design and process design, it becomes possible to attain a stable, efficacious, and safe nutraceutical product.

10.8 POSSIBLE PROBLEMS ASSOCIATED WITH NUTRACEUTICAL PRODUCTS AND IMPORTANCE OF ASSESSING THE NUTRACEUTICAL INGREDIENTS AT CLINICAL LEVEL

The amounts of each ingredient in the nutraceutical products are usually decided based upon the optimal health effects in the group that represents the larger population. However, these amounts may fail to correlate with the requirement of the subpopulations that include children, pregnant women, geriatric patients, patients with a specific medical condition, and patients already consuming other medication.

As an example, the nutraceutical products containing multiple vitamin ingredients have been a debatable to identify the safe-intake range for deficiency or toxicity among adults. Vitamin B1 and C are considered few among of the list of substances that are "generally recognized as safe" (GRAS) [114, 115]. The United States Food and Drug Administration's (USFDA) recommendation for vitamin C intake per day is between 60 and 90 milligrams for adults on a normal 2,000 calorie diet per day [116]. However, if vitamin C is consumed more than the daily intake may be considered potentially dangerous [117].

Specifically, pregnant women consuming any multivitamin product on the market containing vitamin A should consult a physician because vitamin A in excess may develop birth defects [118]. Therefore, during pregnancies, there are strict limits on the content of retinol, one of the major chemical constituents in vitamin A which are specifically addressed by prenatal formulas.

It has been published earlier that use of β-carotene, vitamin E and vitamin A in long run can increase the risk of lung cancer among excessive cigarettes smokers, former smoker and people consuming alcohol often [119]. Many nutraceutical supplement products in the United States contain active ingredients higher than the recommended daily intake among healthy people.

In certain situations, the patients suffering from extreme vitamin or mineral deficiencies, the over-the-counter nutraceutical product may be a no-starter, and patients should consult physicians for specialized formulations containing higher potencies of specific components that the patient is deprived of.

Nutraceutical products available on the market, if consumed in large quantities, poses a risk of toxicity of some components, especially iron. Tablets containing iron may prove to be fatal among children as compared to the overdose toxicity from multivitamins [119].

The Harvard School of Public Health has cleared indicated in 2008 that "multivitamins should not replace healthy eating or make up for unhealthy eating" [120].

Similarly, melatonin is often used as an effective sleeping aid. It is again controversial if melatonin can cause overdose toxicity by itself [121]. However, it is known to have drug-drug interactions with pharmaceutical ingredients used as anti-coagulants, anti-hypertensive, anti-diabetic, steroids, immune suppressors and anti-convulsant. Drug-drug interactions due to melatonin usually lowers the therapeutic effect of a particular drug [122–124].

Another problem associated with melatonin is its regulation. Melatonin is considered as a dietary supplement, and therefore it does not require to undergo US-FDA's approval process like NDA or ANDA before making the products available to the market. Later also, the products are not regulated strictly by the USFDA for its quality and uniformity in terms of possible variable introduced due to product components, product design or process design. Therefore, there is always a possibility that the actual content in the product may or may not be the same as that of the label claim. The literature report indicated that the melatonin content assayed from 31 melatonin supplements procures from different pharmacy stores and grocery stores showed 70% of the analyzed product were either sub-potent or super potent. Though the excessive consumption of melatonin has not found any reports on dying, but over dose of melatonin has resulted in severe side effects that include depression, headaches, stomach cramps, hypothermia, and irritability. Again, the melatonin supplements' use in pediatric patients and pregnant women is questionable [125].

Considering all these above given challenges of optimal dose concern for nutraceutical products, there has been a strong advocacy to decide whether clinical assessment should be required for the claimed health benefits to treat a particular disease. In our opinion, the decision that a specific ingredient listed to be used as a nutraceutical supplement should undergo clinical assessment should be based on the number of reported adverse events. As an example, if the reported adverse events are more than 100, it is a clear indicator of serious quality concerns and so that nutraceutical supplement must undergo clinical assessment.

Nutraceutical products are being more relied upon due to lesser-known side effects by the patients, therefore, the product development should also be carried out with utmost care in order to control the purity, clinical safety, and clinical efficacy of the end-product.

10.9 CHALLENGES RELATED TO THE CLINICAL ASSESSMENT OF NUTRACEUTICALS

The nutraceuticals are regulated by the Dietary Supplement, Health, and Education Act (DSHEA) of 1994. According to DSHEA, a dietary supplement is defined as "a product (other than tobacco) intended to supplement the diet that bears or contains one or more of the following dietary ingredients: vitamins, minerals, amino acids, herbs, or other botanicals; a concentrate, metabolite, constituent, extract or combination of the ingredients listed above" [126]. Additionally, it should be intended for ingestion in pill, capsule, tablet, powder, or liquid form; and it must be labeled as a 'dietary supplement.' Also, it must not be represented for use as a conventional food or as a sole item of the diet. As per the guidelines put forward by DSHEA, the dietary supplement can claim the use of nutraceuticals for management of diseases related to nutrient deficiency. However, the companies are expected to put a disclaimer stating the product has not been evaluated by the USFDA and that they are not intended to diagnose, treat, cure, or prevent any disease. FDA regulations related to cGMP manufacturing are also applicable to nutraceutical manufacturing, ensuring the quality, purity, safety, and reproducibility of the nutraceutical products.

To ensure the quality of nutraceuticals and the safety of consumers, efforts are being made by the FDA to take actions against unsafe dietary products during its shelf life. Under DSHEA, the dietary supplement manufacturer is responsible for ensuring that a dietary supplement is safe before it is marketed and that the product label information is truthful and not misleading. In the last few decades, several preclinical and clinical studies have been performed with nutraceutical products to verify the claims made by the companies and possibly inspect the use of these products for other indications. A couple of case studies related to leading diseases have been listed and discussed below wherein certain drawbacks and challenges associated with nutraceutical clinical studies have been outlined:

1. **Osteoarthritis:** This involves wearing down of protective cartilages on the end of the bones affecting the movement of body parts. It

is one of the common diseases striking and disabling the elderly. Osteoarthritis has been reported in animals as well. Vandeweerd et al. carried out a systematic review of the efficacy of nutraceuticals to alleviate clinical signs of osteoarthritis. They took into account several treatments of osteoarthritis commonly used for treatment in horses, dogs, and cats. They reported low strength of evidence in most of the nutraceuticals [127]. Also, a common drawback with most of the studies was limited numbers of rigorous randomized controlled trials. They concluded poor evidence of efficacy of nutraceuticals except diets supplemented with omega-3 fatty acids in dogs. A separate study (randomized, double-blind, placebo-controlled in 622 patients) was carried out by Kahan et al. to determine the long-term effects of chondroitins 4 and 6 sulfates (CS) on knee osteoarthritis. The patients assigned with chondroitins showed statistically significant improvement in pain compared to the placebo group at the end of two years. Although authors have reported a positive effect of CS on patients, the study has a limitation since a prescription drug was used during the study. Thus, the results cannot be generalized to other CS products [128]. Robust clinical study design is warranted to evaluate the effect of over the counter (OTC) CS products produced by different manufacturers. This shall potentially provide us the confidence of the efficacy of CS products irrespective of the source and manufacturer of the drug product.

2. **Alzheimer's Disease (AD):** This is a progressive neurogenerative disorder which leads to cognitive and memory impairment. Several nutraceuticals such as carotenoids, curcumin, quercetin, selenium, catechin, ginkgobiloba, alpha-lipoic acid, and fish oils have been routinely marketed to slow the progression of AD or reverse the disease process [129–131]. The brain tissue of AD patients has been shown to possess higher levels of oxidized protein. Natural antioxidants such as vitamin C and E were clinically tested by Kontush et al. in a population of 20 AD patients to evaluate the efficacy of these antioxidants in preventing or delaying the development of AD [132]. The study revealed positive effects of vitamin supplements and provided a biochemical rationale for the beneficial results. However, a target population of 20 patients may not provide robust and reliable results. The work performed by Luchsinger et al. included a larger study population (980 patients) and a mean period of observation of four years. They reported "neither dietary, supplemental, nor

total intake of carotenes and vitamin C and E was associated with a decreased risk of AD in this study" [133]. The longitudinal study and large study population in work performed by Luchsinger et al. instill confidence and reliance on the results.

3. **Diabetes Mellitus:** This is a group of metabolic diseases characterized by chronic hyperglycemia resulting from defects in insulin secretion, insulin action, or both. Diabetes mellitus is rising to an alarming epidemic level amongst the worldwide population. In 2015, an estimated 9.4% of the U.S. population was suffering from diabetes mellitus. Patients with diabetes often seek natural therapies as an alternative to pharmaceutical products [134]. Several natural supplements such as fenugreek, American ginseng, and cinnamon are widely used in the treatment of Diabetes Mellitus. *Panax quinque-folius* (American ginseng) is attributed to have anti-diabetic effects and was found to decrease postprandial glycemia significantly in a small placebo-controlled randomized study of 10 patients with type 2 diabetes as well as in a randomized study with a crossover design of 12 healthy subjects. Moreover, Vuksanet al. found that a 3-g dose of American ginseng lowered blood glucose levels in normoglycemic subjects if taken 40 minutes before a meal but did not affect blood glucose if taken with a meal; decreased levels of blood glucose were observed in patients with type 2 diabetes regardless of timing relative to a meal. In a meta-review by Vogler et al. of 16 PRCTs, however, a definitive benefit of ginseng root extract in patients with diabetes could not be established [135].

In 2013, a meta-analysis carried out for evaluation of cinnamon for diabetes management included 543 patients in 10 different randomized clinical trials. The total number of patients ranged from 7 to 30. The average from a bunch of small studies does not necessarily increase the statistical power of the studies. In fact, it might exacerbate the statistical issues. One of the aspects of this analysis is that it was claimed that cinnamon reduces blood glucose by 24.59 mg/dL of blood [136]. This value is significantly less than a reduction of 58 mg/dL shown by one of the more common oral diabetic medications, metformin.

Furthermore, the authors did not include the actual blood glucose level. A reduction of 24 mg/dL, may not necessarily be clinically significant and patients may still bear significant risks from complications of diabetes over both the long and short-term [137]. The study showed no reduction in hemoglobin A1C levels, a vital blood marker, which provides information about the long-term changes in a patient's blood glucose. Another meta-review concluded that Cinnamon does not appear to improve A1C or lipid parameters in patients with type 1 or type 2 diabetes. Conventional medications for diabetes, like insulin or metformin, have been shown to reduce mortality from diabetes. Cinnamon for diabetes has never been evaluated to reduce diabetes-related mortality, a key endpoint for all diabetes treatments. Also, another consideration to be made is that certain kinds of cinnamon contain coumarin, a compound that could be toxic at higher levels. While Cinnamon may have potential in managing blood glucose level type, the evidence is inconclusive, and long-term trials aiming to establish the efficacy and safety of cinnamon is needed.

4. **Cancer:** This is a leading cause of death worldwide, accounting for an estimated 9.6 million deaths in 2018. Cancer is a collective term for a large group of diseases characterized by the growth of abnormal cells beyond their usual boundaries that can then invade adjoining parts of the body and/or spread to other organs. Nutraceuticals and DS have gained popularity in recent years for aiding cancer treatment with the potential to reduce the growth rate of cancer cells. Various Phytochemicals mainly act as antioxidants and are evaluated for various mechanisms by which cancer can be inhibited such as carcinogenesis by curcumin (turmeric), Multivitamins, capsaicin (red chili), resveratrol (red grapes, peanuts, and berries), Beta-carotenes (carrots), eugenol, and isoeugenol (cloves).

    A meta-analysis of 14 RCTs for bladder cancer found that beta carotene supplementation significantly increased the risk of developing bladder cancer. An analysis of the NIH-AARP Diet and Health Study cohort that included 490,593 individuals also found no effect of multivitamin use on the incidence of upper gastrointestinal (GI) tract cancers compared with nonusers. Chang et al. published a meta-analysis of 49 intervention trials including 287,304 individuals found no link between cancer incidence and supplementation with selenium, zinc, magnesium, beta carotene, the omega-3 fatty acid, eicosapentaenoic acid (EPA), or vitamins D, C, or K [5].

The clinical assessment of nutraceuticals has inherently several challenges which need to be identified and addressed, to carry out a more robust clinical study. The drawbacks associated with the clinical study of nutraceuticals are outlined and briefly discussed below:

1. **Different Sources of Nutraceuticals:** The nutraceuticals available at different parts of the world may vary therapeutically due to the varied source of plant/animal or difference in grade or quality of nutraceuticals. There is a need to characterize nutritional products and understand their mechanism of action before carrying out any preclinical or clinical study. Several studies carried out in the past using poorly characterized herbal supplements products led to inconclusive and inconstant results [138]. Dwyer et al. have recommended "health outcomes such as changes invalidated surrogate markers for performance, functions, morbidity, and mortality from diseases or conditions are required rather than changes in biochemical measures in blood with unvalidated surrogate markers" to generate systematic evidence of bioactivity during a clinical study of nutraceuticals products.

2. **Low Bioavailability:** The most of the nutritional health products are taken orally in the form of capsules, tablets, or liquid dosage forms. There have been cases reported wherein nutritional supplements have failed to disintegrate completely. Incomplete disintegration and dissolution of DS have a negative impact on the studies of nutritional efficacy. Some of the nutraceuticals such as curcumin and coenzyme Q10 are poorly soluble in GI fluids resulting into low absorption and bioavailability. Such nutraceuticals can have a significant food effect which can skew the clinical results. Curcumin metabolizes rapidly, and it has been reported to have low serum levels, limited tissue distribution and short half-life, which worsens the overall bioavailability. Efforts must be made during clinical study to address the low-solubility and permeability issues related to nutraceuticals. Formulation approaches that overcome the solubility challenges should be adopted during the clinical trials to reduce the variability in results.

3. **Financial Challenges:** The nutraceuticals are not as potent as pharmaceuticals, and the clinical results can be easily affected by heterogeneity of subjects. Thus, a more extensive study population would be required to design a more viable study which essentially requires a larger budget. There are times when a sponsor may have to opt for a pilot study to gain better insights into clinical end results which further increases the overall cost of the project. The clinical study for nutraceuticals may require a prolonged period of monitoring of the study population which at times can be cumbersome and financially challenging.

4. **Recruitment of Participants:** Nutraceutical trials are often harder to recruit compared to pharmaceutical counterparts. Additionally, they have relatively higher drop-out rates since the participants are expected to maintain a healthy lifestyle and record-related information during the entire study period.

5. **Inclusion and Exclusion Criteria:** The inclusion and exclusion criteria set the boundaries for the systematic review. The clinical results for a nutraceutical drug product can be easily skewed by the lifestyle choices of the participants enrolled in the study. Thus, it is critical to design a study considering lifestyle variables that can be factored into the final statistical analysis. Selection of strict participant inclusion and exclusion criteria is vital here as an effect of the nutraceutical in the selected subject needs to be evidenced in the trial [139].

6. **Interactions with Prescription Medications and Food:** The interactions of nutraceuticals with other medications and food may have two key clinical effects: a) increased bioavailability of the nutraceutical due to food effect which increases the risk of adverse events, b) decreased bioavailability due to excessive metabolism or chemical interaction with food or prescription medications. The elderly patients are particularly at risk for such interactions since more than 30% of all the prescription drugs are taken by this population [140]. For example, herbal nutraceuticals can interact with prescription drugs resulting in inhibition or induction of CYP enzymes or transporters such as P-gp. As described by Anadon et al. P-gp, a transmembrane ATP-binding cassette transporter, can affect drug absorption in the intestinal tract, distribution to the brain, and elimination by the liver and kidney (Table 10.2) [141].

7. **Endpoint of the Clinical Study:** The decisions regarding the clinical endpoints of the nutraceutical products compared to pharmaceuticals products are more complicated. The impractical clinical endpoints may ultimately lead to negative clinical results or may result in inconclusive and incoherent results. At times pharmacokinetic endpoints are not a viable option with nutraceuticals. In such scenarios, logistic concerns arise whereby changes in participant's lifestyle can alter biomarker values, ultimately affecting the clinical results. The claim made by the sponsor regarding the nutritional product may also dictate the endpoint of the clinical study design.

8. **Regulatory Burden:** There is not any effective regulatory system regarding medical or health claims for nutraceuticals, even though these products have entered medicine and the consumer marketplace [156].

They lie in a gray area between medicinal food products and pharmaceuticals. The lack of appropriate regulatory guidelines leads to delays in the approval of regulatory documents, possibly complexing and delaying the entire study. This delay in clinical study leads to added clinical costs. The lack of regulatory guidance for nutraceuticals can also confuse consumers and promote misuse of nutraceuticals. As explained by Santini et al., "A clear and shared regulation system allowing the identification and classification of these products at an international level that clearly indicates requirements for quality, efficacy, mechanism of action and safety could benefit potential consumers as well as the industry" [156].

TABLE 10.2 List of Possible Interactions between Nutraceuticals and Therapeutic Medications

Medications	Nutraceuticals	References
Phenytoin, valproic acid, warfarin, aspirin, ticlopidine, clopidrogel, dipyridamole	Ginko Biloba	[142, 143]
atorvastatin	Vitamin D	[144, 145]
Warfarin	Vitamin K, ginseng, coenzyme Q10	[143, 146, 147]
Decongestants	Ephedra	[143]
Antidepressants	St. John's wort	[143, 148]
Atorvastatin, acetaminophen	Black cohosh	[149]
Phenothiazine	Primrose	[150]
Benzodiazepines	Melatonin	[151, 152]
Antipsychotic drugs	Goldenseal	[153]
Aspirin, clopidogrel, propanolol	Garlic	[154, 155]

10.10 PROSPECTS FOR CLINICAL TRIALS OF NUTRACEUTICALS

There have been several clinical studies with nutraceuticals which have led to inconsistent results. This irregularity can potentially be due to poorly designed clinical studies or lack of placebo controls and useful biomarkers. A methodological design with multicenter randomized controls and appropriate clinical endpoints has to be set up to expect a robust and definitive dataset. The study population needs to be monitored for long periods to make sure that all the drug-nutraceutical interactions and any possible side effects due to nutraceuticals are detected. In addition to designing and executing randomized controlled clinical studies, there is a need in general for regulatory authorities and healthcare professionals to judiciously collaborate and devise a strategy to maximize the therapeutic benefits of nutritional products.

In order to foster the continuous development of clinical trial methods for nutraceutical supplements, there is a need to make amendments to the conventional clinical designs. Following strategies can be adopted by nutraceuticals companies to design, manage, and execute efficient clinical trials:

1. **Flexible Study Designs:** The clinical trials with adaptive features can make the trials flexible and aid in making a range of adaptations, including any prospective dose change, increasing the size or duration of trial, or change in clinical endpoints. This offers the sponsor the advantage of making potential modifications to the clinical design without filing for a protocol amendment. The sponsor can monitor the incoming data and make necessary modifications to the protocol based on the acquired information. Unquestionably, the probable modifications to the design need to be approved by the regulatory body ahead of time. The results from flexible designs can be considered reliable if a selected number of people are provided access to the data along with maintaining the integrity of the data by blinding it. The advantages of exploratory adaptive clinical trials have identified and accepted by regulatory bodies across the world. Although there is always a risk of committing a type I error in adaptive trials, suitable precautions can be taken to design a robust clinical trial which can provide conclusive results. The adaptive designs can be advantageous for patients as well since it will guide the sponsor to continue evaluating the nutraceutical supplement or end the study.

2. **Digital Health in Clinical Trials:** Digital health technologies are recently being applied to pharmaceutical clinical trials, which has improved the quality of the data generated from clinical trials. The nutraceuticals can adopt the innovative data collection approach and ride the wave of digital health data to improve the accuracy of the trials. Digital health technologies such as wearable devices, mobile health, and patient-focused apps can aid in acquiring the raw data remotely with minimal effort. These technologies uncomplex the burdensome clinical protocols and improves the patient retention and engagement.

3. **Advances in Biomarkers:** A biomarker is defined as a characteristic that is measured as an indicator of normal biological processes, pathogenic processes, or responses to exposure or intervention, including

therapeutic interventions [157]. A better understanding of the biomarker-driven processes will assist in approaching and designing the clinical studies differently. The advancement of robust and reliable biomarkers by continuous research can promote nutraceutical product development and regulatory review.

4. **Modern Approaches in Clinical Trial Management:** Conventionally, data management focuses on providing reliable, high-quality data at the end of the clinical trial for data analysis and reporting purposes. There has been a growing consensus on adopting real-time data visualization and surveillance techniques to promote consistency across the trials. Implementing such real-time data monitoring approaches during Nutraceutical clinical trials can offer advantages of centralizing different departments and potentially reducing the human errors leading to compliance concerns.

10.11   CONCLUSION

Nutraceuticals have seen significant growth in the last decade, and its demand in the consumer market is poised to grow exponentially in the coming years. They offer value-added advantages to customers and empowers them with several nutritional options. The nutraceutical products face a continuous challenge to efficiently extract the phytochemicals of desired purity and enough yield. These challenges are being addressed by the implementation of advanced technologies in the extraction and manufacturing of the nutraceuticals. Novel formulation techniques have successfully addressed the low bioavailability concerns related to oral delivery of nutraceuticals. However, there is a need to invest in innovative manufacturing technologies and advanced analytical techniques to efficiently scale up production of nutraceuticals without affecting the quality of the end product. The clinical study of nutraceuticals poses a more significant challenge due to the unavailability of effective biomarkers and lack of understanding related to interactions of nutraceuticals with food and medicaments. The regulatory authorities have acknowledged the need to improvise the existing norms associated with nutraceuticals and provide nutraceutical specific guidance to resourcefully carry out clinical trials which can provide conclusive results. Moreover, there is a need to develop a scientific understanding of nutraceuticals and evaluate its therapeutic and pharmacological effects on humans.

KEYWORDS

- breast cancer-resistant proteins
- chito-oligosaccharides derivatives
- microemulsions
- myricetin
- P-glycoproteins
- phytosterols

REFERENCES

1. Martini, S. A., & Phillips, M., (2009). Nutrition and food commodities in the 20th century. *Journal of Agricultural and Food Chemistry, 57*(18), 8130–8135.
2. Adefegha, S. A., (2018). Functional foods and nutraceuticals as dietary intervention in chronic diseases; Novel perspectives for health promotion and disease prevention. *Journal of Dietary Supplements, 15*(6), 977–1009.
3. Das, L., Bhaumik, E., Raychaudhuri, U., & Chakraborty, R., (2012). Role of nutraceuticals in human health. *Journal of Food Science and Technology, 49*(2), 173–183.
4. Chauhan, B., Kumar, G., Kalam, N., & Ansari, S. H., (2013). Current concepts and prospects of herbal nutraceutical: A review. *Journal of Advanced Pharmaceutical Technology & Research, 4*(1), 4.
5. Winter, R., (2009). *A Consumer's Dictionary of Food Additives: Descriptions in Plain English of More Than 12,000 Ingredients Both Harmful and Desirable Found in Foods.* Crown Archetype.
6. Thompson, A. K., & Moughan, P. J., (2008). Innovation in the foods industry: Functional foods. *Innovation, 10*(1), 61–73.
7. Kitson, P. J., Marie, G., Francoia, J. P., Zalesskiy, S. S., Sigerson, R. C., Mathieson, J. S., & Cronin, L., (2018). Digitization of multistep organic synthesis in reaction ware for on-demand pharmaceuticals. *Science, 359*(6373), 314–319.
8. Tan, D., Loots, L., & Friščić, T., (2016). Towards medicinal mechanochemistry: evolution of milling from pharmaceutical solid form screening to the synthesis of active pharmaceutical ingredients (APIs). *Chemical Communications, 52*(50), 7760–7781.
9. Adejoh, I. P., Mark, A., & Agatemor, M., (2018). Anti-radical and inhibitory effect of some common Nigerian medicinal plants on alpha-glucosidase, aldose reductase and angiotensin-converting enzyme: Potential protective mechanisms against diabetic complications. *Int. J. Adv. Res. Biol. Sci., 53*, 188–201.
10. Ali, B., Al-Wabel, N. A., Shams, S., Ahamad, A., Khan, S. A., & Anwar, F., (2015). Essential oils used in aromatherapy: A systemic review. *Asian Pacific Journal of Tropical Biomedicine, 5*(8), 601–611.

11. Koulivand, P. H., Khaleghi, G. M., & Gorji, A., (2013). Lavender and the nervous system. *Evidence-Based Complementary and Alternative Medicine, 2013.*
12. Houston, M. C., (2018). The prevention and treatment of coronary heart disease and congestive heart failure with antioxidants and nutritional supplements. *Antioxidant Nutraceuticals: Preventive and Healthcare Applications.*
13. Zhang, H., & Ma, Z., (2018). Phytochemical and pharmacological properties of Capparis spinosa as a medicinal plant. *Nutrients, 10*(2), 116.
14. Tank, D. S., Gandhi, S., & Shah, M., (2010). Nutraceuticals-portmanteau of science and nature. *Int. J. Pharm. Sci. Rev. Res., 5*(3), 33–38.
15. Atanasov, A. G., Waltenberger, B., Pferschy-Wenzig, E. M., Linder, T., Wawrosch, C., Uhrin, P., Temml, V., et al., (2015). Discovery and resupply of pharmacologically active plant-derived natural products: A review. *Biotechnology Advances, 33*(8), 1582–1614.
16. Saad, B., Zaid, H., Shanak, S., & Kadan, S., (2017). Introduction to medicinal plant safety and efficacy. In: *Anti-diabetes and Anti-obesity Medicinal Plants and Phytochemicals* (pp. 21–55). Springer.
17. Sasidharan, S., Chen, Y., Saravanan, D., Sundram, K., & Latha, L. Y., (2011). Extraction, isolation and characterization of bioactive compounds from plants' extracts. *African Journal of Traditional, Complementary and Alternative Medicines, 8*(1).
18. Azmir, J., Zaidul, I., Rahman, M., Sharif, K., Mohamed, A., Sahena, F., Jahurul, M., Ghafoor, K., Norulaini, N., & Omar, A., (2013). Techniques for extraction of bioactive compounds from plant materials: A review. *Journal of Food Engineering, 117*(4), 426–436.
19. Selvamuthukumaran, M., & Shi, J., (2017). Recent advances in extraction of antioxidants from plant by-products processing industries. *Food Quality and Safety, 1*(1), 61–81.
20. Jin, P., Madieh, S., & Augsburger, L. L., (2007). The solution and solid-state stability and excipient compatibility of parthenolide in feverfew. *AAPS Pharmscitech, 8*(4), 200.
21. Jin, P., Madieh, S., & Augsburger, L. L., (2008). Selected physical and chemical properties of feverfew (Tanacetum parthenium) extracts important for formulated product quality and performance. *AAPS PharmSciTech, 9*(1), 22–30.
22. Ignat, I., Volf, I., & Popa, V. I., (2011). A critical review of methods for characterization of polyphenolic compounds in fruits and vegetables. *Food Chemistry, 126*(4), 1821–1835.
23. Wojdyło, A., Figiel, A., & Oszmiański, J., (2009). Effect of drying methods with the application of vacuum microwaves on the bioactive compounds, color, and antioxidant activity of strawberry fruits. *Journal of Agricultural and Food Chemistry, 57*(4), 1337–1343.
24. Wojdyło, A., Figiel, A., Lech, K., Nowicka, P., & Oszmiański, J., (2014). Effect of convective and vacuum-microwave drying on the bioactive compounds, color, and antioxidant capacity of sour cherries. *Food and Bioprocess Technology, 7*(3), 829–841.
25. King, J. W., (2004). Development and potential of critical fluid technology in the nutraceutical industry. *Drugs and the Pharmaceutical Sciences, 138*, 579–614.
26. Bhusnure, O., Gholve, S., Giram, P., Borsure, V., Jadhav, P., Satpute, V., & Sangshetti, J., (2015). Importance of supercritical fluid extraction techniques in pharmaceutical industry: A review. *IAJPR, 5*(12), 3785–3801.
27. Tsiaka, T., Sinanoglou, V. J., & Zoumpoulakis, P., (2017). Extracting bioactive compounds from natural sources using green high-energy approaches: Trends and opportunities in lab-and large-scale applications. In: *Ingredients Extraction by Physicochemical Methods in Food* (pp. 307–365). Elsevier.
28. Krishnan, S. K., Chidananda, B., & Ahmed, M. G., (2015). *Formulation and Evaluation of Effervescent Tablets of Glucosamine Sulphate in Combination with Ibuprofen and Vitamin-E for the Treatment of Osteoarthritis. 4*(9), 1075–1087.

29. Hadisoewignyo, L., Soegianto, L., Ervina, M., Wijaya, I., Santoso, S., Tania, N., Syawal, L. A., & Tjandrawinata, R. R., (2016). Formulation development and optimization of tablet containing combination of Salam (Syzygium polyanthum) and sambiloto (Andrographis paniculata) ethanolic extracts. *International Journal of Pharmacy and Pharmaceutical Sciences, 8*(3), 267–273.

30. Leane, M., Pitt, K., Reynolds, G., & Group, M. C. S. W., (2015). A proposal for a drug product Manufacturing Classification System (MCS) for oral solid dosage forms. *Pharmaceutical Development and Technology, 20*(1), 12–21.

31. Melocchi, A., Parietti, F., Maccagnan, S., Ortenzi, M. A., Antenucci, S., Briatico-Vangosa, F., Maroni, A., et al., (2018). Industrial development of a 3D-printed nutraceutical delivery platform in the form of a multicompartment HPC capsule. *AAPS PharmSciTech, 19*(8), 3343–3354.

32. Ghanbarzadeh, B., Babazadeh, A., & Hamishehkar, H., (2016). Nano-Phyto some as a potential food-grade delivery system. *Food Bioscience, 15*, 126–135.

33. Jafari, S. M., (2017). *Nanoencapsulation Technologies for the Food and Nutraceutical Industries.* Academic Press.

34. Thwala, L. N., Préat, V., & Csaba, N. S., (2017). Emerging delivery platforms for mucosal administration of biopharmaceuticals: A critical update on nasal, pulmonary and oral routes. *Expert Opinion on Drug Delivery, 14*(1), 23–36.

35. Chen, A., Shi, Y., Yan, Z., Hao, H., Zhang, Y., Zhong, J., & Hou, H., (2015). Dosage form developments of nanosuspension drug delivery system for oral administration route. *Current Pharmaceutical Design, 21*(29), 4355–4365.

36. Karki, S., Kim, H., Na, S. J., Shin, D., Jo, K., & Lee, J., (2016). Thin films as an emerging platform for drug delivery. *Asian Journal of Pharmaceutical Sciences, 11*(5), 559–574.

37. Harrison, E. H., & Kopec, R. E., (2018). Digestion and intestinal absorption of dietary carotenoids and vitamin A. In: *Physiology of the Gastrointestinal Tract* (6th edn., pp. 1133–1151). Elsevier.

38. Goncalves, A., Gleize, B., Roi, S., Nowicki, M., Dhaussy, A., Huertas, A., Amiot, M. J., & Reboul, E., (2013). Fatty acids affect micellar properties and modulate vitamin D uptake and basolateral efflux in Caco-2 cells. *The Journal of Nutritional Biochemistry, 24*(10), 1751–1757.

39. Cerecedo-Cruz, L., Azuara-Nieto, E., Hernández-Álvarez, A., González-González, C., & Melgar-Lalanne, G., (2018). Evaluation of the oxidative stability of chipotle chili (Capsicum annuum L.) oleoresins in avocado oil. *Grasasy Aceites, 69*(1), 240.

40. Priyadarshani, A., (2017). A review on factors influencing bioaccessibility and bioefficacy of carotenoids. *Critical Reviews in Food Science and Nutrition, 57*(8), 1710–1717.

41. Gleeson, J. P., Ryan, S. M., & Brayden, D. J., (2016). Oral delivery strategies for nutraceuticals: Delivery vehicles and absorption enhancers. *Trends in Food Science & Technology, 53*, 90–101.

42. Nunes, S., Madureira, A. R., Campos, D., Sarmento, B., Gomes, A. M., Pintado, M., & Reis, F., (2017). Solid lipid nanoparticles as oral delivery systems of phenolic compounds: Overcoming pharmacokinetic limitations for nutraceutical applications. *Critical Reviews in Food Science and Nutrition, 57*(9), 1863–1873.

43. Yao, M., McClements, D. J., & Xiao, H., (2015). Improving oral bioavailability of nutraceuticals by engineered nanoparticle-based delivery systems. *Current Opinion in Food Science, 2*, 14–19.

44. Aditya, N., Espinosa, Y. G., & Norton, I. T., (2017). Encapsulation systems for the delivery of hydrophilic nutraceuticals: Food application. *Biotechnology Advances, 35*(4), 450–457.

45. Shegokar, R., Muller, R., Ismail, M., & Gohla, S., (2018). Algal nanosuspensions for dermal and oral delivery. *Current Nanomedicine (Formerly: Recent Patents on Nanomedicine), 8*(1), 45–57.

46. Van, S. B., Grymonpré, W., Dhondt, J., Pandelaere, K., Di Pretoro, G., Remon, J., De Beer, T., et al., (2018). Impact of blend properties on die filling during tableting. *International Journal of Pharmaceutics, 549*(1, 2), 476–488.

47. Dülle, M., Özcoban, H., & Leopold, C., (2018). Analysis of the powder behavior and the residence time distribution within a production scale rotary tablet press. *European Journal of Pharmaceutical Sciences, 125*, 205–214.

48. Hancock, B. C., (2019). The wall friction properties of pharmaceutical powders, blends, and granulations. *Journal of Pharmaceutical Sciences, 108*(1), 457–463.

49. Schiano, S., Chen, L., & Wu, C. Y., (2018). The effect of dry granulation on flow behavior of pharmaceutical powders during die filling. *Powder Technology, 337*, 78–83.

50. Chaturvedi, K., Gajera, B. Y., Xu, T., Shah, H., & Dave, R. H., (2018). Influence of processing methods on physico-mechanical properties of ibuprofen/HPC-SSL formulation. *Pharmaceutical Development and Technology, 23*(10), 1108–1116.

51. Natoli, D., Levin, M., Tsygan, L., & Liu, L., (2017). Development, optimization, and scale-up of process parameters: Tablet compression. In: *Developing Solid Oral Dosage Forms* (pp. 917–951). Elsevier.

52. Swaminathan, S. (2016). *Modeling Picking on Pharmaceutical Tablets* (Doctoral Dissertation, Purdue University).

53. Ho, S., Thoo, Y. Y., Young, D. J., & Siow, L. F., (2017). Cyclodextrin encapsulated catechin: Effect of pH, relative humidity and various food models on antioxidant stability. *LWT-Food Science and Technology, 85*, 232–239.

54. Cristiano, M. C., Cilurzo, F., Carafa, M., & Paolino, D., (2018). Innovative vesicles for dermal and transdermal drug delivery. In: *Lipid Nanocarriers for Drug Targeting* (pp. 175–197). Elsevier.

55. Pérez-Sánchez, A., Barrajón-Catalán, E., Herranz-López, M., & Micol, V., (2018). Nutraceuticals for skin care: A comprehensive review of human clinical studies. *Nutrients, 10*(4), 403.

56. Khiljee, S., Rehman, N. U., Khiljee, T., Ahmad, R. S., Khan, M. Y., & Qureshi, U. A., (2016). Use of traditional herbal medicines in the treatment of eczema. *Journal of Pakistan Association of Dermatology, 21*(2), 112–117.

57. Jain, S., Yadav, V., Jain, A. K., & Yadav, A. K., (2018). Nutraceuticals: A revolutionary approach for nano-drug delivery. *Nanonutraceuticals*, 1–22.

58. Bao, Q., Shen, J., Jog, R., Zhang, C., Newman, B., Wang, Y., Choi, S., & Burgess, D. J., (2017). *In vitro* release testing method development for ophthalmic ointments. *International Journal of Pharmaceutics, 526*(1, 2), 145–156.

59. Rathod, V., (2018). *Optimization and Design of Ibuprofen-Loaded Nanostructured Lipid Carriers Using a Hybrid-Design Approach for Ocular Drug Delivery*. Long Island University, The Brooklyn Center.

60. Ruchi, S., (2017). Role of nutraceuticals in health care: A review. *International Journal of Green Pharmacy (IJGP), 11*(03).

61. Daliu, P., Santini, A., & Novellino, E., (2019). From pharmaceuticals to nutraceuticals: Bridging disease prevention and management. *Expert Review of Clinical Pharmacology, 12*(1), 1–7.

62. Liu, F., Ranmal, S., Batchelor, H. K., Orlu-Gul, M., Ernest, T. B., Thomas, I. W., Flanagan, T., & Tuleu, C., (2014). Patient-centered pharmaceutical design to improve acceptability of medicines: Similarities and differences in paediatric and geriatric populations. *Drugs, 74*(16), 1871–1889.

63. Cosgrove, J. (2009). *Tablet & Capsule Trends.* https://www.nutraceuticalsworld. com/contents/view_online-exclusives/2009-03-01/tablet-amp-capsule-trends/1560 (accessed on 31 July 2021).

64. Patra, Ch, N., et al., (2008). A Systematic Study on Flowability and Compressibility of Asparagus racemosus root Powder for Tablet Preparation. International *Journal of Pharmaceutical Sciences and Nanotechnology, 1*(2), 129–135.

65. Di Pierro, F., Putignano, P., Villanova, N., Montesi, L., Moscatiello, S., & Marchesini, G., (2013). Preliminary study about the possible glycemic clinical advantage in using a fixed combination of *Berberis aristata* and *Silybum* marianum standardized extracts versus only *Berberis aristata* in patients with type 2 diabetes. *Clinical Pharmacology: Advances and Applications, 5*, 167.

66. Parikh, D. M., (2016). *Handbook of Pharmaceutical Granulation Technology.* CRC Press.

67. Ghosh, N., & Sen, C. K., (2019). The promise of dietary supplements: Research rigor and marketing claims. In: *Nutrition and Enhanced Sports Performance* (pp. 759–766). Elsevier.

68. John, D. L., Kim, E., Kotian, K., Ong, K. Y., White, T., Gloukhova, L., Woodbridge, D. M. K., & Ross, N., (2019). Topic modeling to extract information from nutraceutical product reviews. In: *2019 16th IEEE Annual Consumer Communications and Networking Conference (CCNC)* (pp. 1–6). IEEE.

69. Fernandes, S. D., & Narayanan, A., (2019). The emergence of India as a blossoming market for nutraceutical supplements: An overview. *Trends in Food Science & Technology.*

70. Govindarajan, R., Tejas, V., & Pushpangadan, P., (2019). High-performance liquid chromatography (HPLC) as a tool for standardization of complex herbal drugs. *Journal of AOAC International.*

71. Abdallah, A., Zhang, P., Zhong, Q., & Sun, Z., (2019). Application of traditional Chinese herbal medicine by-products as dietary feed supplements and antibiotic replacements in animal production. *Current Drug Metabolism, 20*(1), 54–64.

72. Byeon, J. C., Ahn, J. B., Jang, W. S., Lee, S. E., Choi, J. S., & Park, J. S., (2019). Recent formulation approaches to oral delivery of herbal medicines. *Journal of Pharmaceutical Investigation, 49*(1), 17–26.

73. Laudon, M., & Zisapel, N., (2019). *Melatonin Mini-Tablets and Method of Manufacturing the Same.* Google Patents.

74. Singh, M. C., & Gujar, K. N., (2019). preparation and evaluation of nutraceutical product mixture of seeds of *Cucumis melo, Punica granatum, Linum usitatissimum,* for antioxidant, prebiotic and nutraceutical potential. *Pharmacognosy Journal, 11*(2).

75. Télessy, I. G., (2019). Nutraceuticals. In: *The Role of Functional Food Security in Global Health* (pp. 409–421). Elsevier.

76. Çelik, M., (1996). The past, present, and future of tableting technology. *Drug Development and Industrial Pharmacy, 22*(1), 1–10.

77. Jivraj, M., Martini, L. G., & Thomson, C. M., (2000). An overview of the different excipients useful for the direct compression of tablets. *Pharmaceutical Science & Technology Today, 3*(2), 58–63.

78. Tonon, R. V., Brabet, C., & Hubinger, M. D., (2008). Influence of process conditions on the physicochemical properties of açaí (Euterpe oleraceae Mart.) powder produced by spray drying. *Journal of Food Engineering, 88*(3), 411–418.

79. Chaudhari, S. P., Powar, P. V., & Pratapwar, M. N., (2017). Nutraceuticals: A Review. World *J. Pharm Pharm Sci. 6*(8), 681–739.

80. Lawrence, X. Y., Amidon, G., Khan, M. A., Hoag, S. W., Polli, J., Raju, G., & Woodcock, J., (2014). Understanding pharmaceutical quality by design. *The AAPS Journal, 16*(4), 771–783.

81. Blanchard, R., (2014). Scientific improvements to benefit industry: Tableting & encapsulation. *South African Pharmaceutical and Cosmetic Review, 41*(11), 44–45.

82. Dugar, R. P., (2017). *A Mechanistic Approach to Model the Realistic Dwell Time of Different Toolings Based on Compression Roller Interactions*. Long Island University, The Brooklyn Center.

83. Deakin, S., & Osborn, S., (2014). A spoonful of good design helps the medicine go down: Pharmaceutical focus. *South African Pharmaceutical and Cosmetic Review, 41*(3), 28–32.

84. Grillo, S. M., Korchok, B., Kinsey, B., Porter, S. C., Reyes, G., Burke, T. J., & Cunningham, C., (2001). *Film Coatings and Film Coating Compositions Based on Dextrin*. Google Patents.

85. Reddy, B. V., Navaneetha, K., Reddy, K. V. R., Reddy, P. P. (2014). Formulation Development and Evaluation of Emtricitabine and Tenofovir Disoproxil Fumarate Film Coated Tablets. *Journal of Pharmaceutical and Biomedical Analysis Letters. 2*(2), 148–157.

86. Reed, K., Davies, C., & Kelly, K., (2015). Tablet sticking: Using a 'compression toolbox' to assess multiple tooling coatings options. *Powder Technology, 285*, 103–109.

87. Schiele, J. T., Penner, H., Schneider, H., Quinzler, R., Reich, G., Wezler, N., Micol, W., et al., (2015). Swallowing tablets and capsules increases the risk of penetration and aspiration in patients with stroke-induced dysphagia. *Dysphagia, 30*(5), 571–582.

88. Appelqvist, I. A., Golding, M., Vreeker, R., & Zuidam, N. J., (2007). Emulsions as delivery systems in foods. *Encapsulation and Controlled Release Technologies in Food Systems*, 41–81.

89. McClements, D., Decker, E., & Weiss, J., (2007). Emulsion-based delivery systems for lipophilic bioactive components. *Journal of Food Science, 72*(8), R109–R124.

90. Fechner, A., Knoth, A., Scherze, I., & Muschiolik, G., (2007). Stability and release properties of double-emulsions stabilized by caseinate-dextran conjugates. *Food Hydrocolloids, 21*(5, 6), 943–952.

91. Sanguansri, L., & Augustin, M. A., (2010). *Microencapsulation in Functional Food Product Development* (Vol. 1, pp 1–23). Chapter.

92. Urbanska, A. M., Bhathena, J., & Prakash, S., (2007). Live encapsulated *Lactobacillus acidophilus* cells in yogurt for therapeutic oral delivery: Preparation and *in vitro* analysis of alginate-chitosan microcapsules. *Canadian Journal of Physiology and Pharmacology, 85*(9), 884–893.

93. Merisko-Liversidge, E., Liversidge, G. G., & Cooper, E. R., (2003). Nanosizing: A formulation approach for poorly-water-soluble compounds. *European Journal of Pharmaceutical Sciences, 18*(2), 113–120.

94. Rabinow, B., (2005). In pharmacokinetics of nanosuspensions. *Proceedings of the Nanotechnology for Drug Delivery Conference.*

95. Panagiotou, T., & Fisher, R. J., (2008). Form nanoparticles via controlled crystallization. *Chemical Engineering Progress, 104*(10), 33–39.

96. Panagiotou, T., & Fisher, R. J., (2011). Enhanced transport capabilities via nanotechnologies: Impacting bioefficacy, controlled release strategies, and novel chaperones. *Journal of Drug Delivery, 2011.*

97. Panagiotou, T., Mesite, S. V., & Fisher, R. J., (2009). Production of norfloxacin nanosuspensions using microfluidics reaction technology through solvent/antisolvent crystallization. *Industrial & Engineering Chemistry Research, 48*(4), 1761–1771.

98. Lasic, D. D., (1997). *Liposomes in Gene Delivery.* CRC press.

99. Panagiotou, T., & Fisher, R. (2012). Improving product quality with entrapped stable emulsions: From theory to industrial application. *Challenges, 3*(2), 84–113.

100. Gomez-Hens, A., & Fernandez-Romero, J., (2006). Analytical methods for the control of liposomal delivery systems. *TrAC Trends in Analytical Chemistry, 25*(2), 167–178.

101. Reza, M. M., Johnson, C., Hatziantoniou, S., & Demetzos, C., (2008). Nanoliposomes and their applications in food nanotechnology. *Journal of Liposome Research, 18*(4), 309–327.

102. Mozafari, M., & Mortazavi, S., (2005). *Nanoliposomes: From Fundamentals to Recent Developments.* Trafford Pub. Ltd. Oxford, UK.

103. Bender, D. A., (2003). *Nutritional Biochemistry of the Vitamins.* Cambridge university press.

104. Lu, M., (2017). *Delivery of Nutraceuticals Using Novel Processing Methods and Emulsion-Based Formulations with Enhanced Dissolution, Bioaccessibility and Bioavailability.* Rutgers University-School of Graduate Studies.

105. Dureja, H., Kaushik, D., & Kumar, V., (2003). Developments in nutraceuticals. *Indian Journal of Pharmacology, 35*(6), 363–372.

106. Heyland, D. K., (2001). In search of the magic nutraceutical: Problems with current approaches. *The Journal of Nutrition, 131*(9), 2591S–2595S.

107. D'silva, J., (2008). *Preparing for Individualized Dosage Forms of Medicaments.* Google Patents.

108. Ku, M. S., Li, W., Dulin, W., Donahue, F., Cade, D., Benameur, H., & Hutchison, K., (2010). Performance qualification of a new hypromellose capsule: Part I. Comparative evaluation of physical, mechanical and processability quality attributes of VCaps Plus®, Quali-V® and gelatin capsules. *International Journal of Pharmaceutics, 386*(1, 2), 30–41.

109. Chang, R. K., Raghavan, K. S., & Hussain, M. A., (1998). A study on gelatin capsule brittleness: Moisture transfer between the capsule shell and its content. *Journal of Pharmaceutical Sciences, 87*(5), 556–558.

110. Kathpalia, H., Sharma, K., & Doshi, G., (2014). Recent trends in hard gelatin capsule delivery system. *Journal of Advanced Pharmacy Education & Research, 4*(2).

111. Cole, E. T., Cadé, D., & Benameur, H., (2008). Challenges and opportunities in the encapsulation of liquid and semi-solid formulations into capsules for oral administration. *Advanced Drug Delivery Reviews, 60*(6), 747–756.

112. Narang, A. S., & Badawy, S. I., (2019). Emerging paradigms in pharmaceutical wet granulation. In: *Handbook of Pharmaceutical Wet Granulation* (pp. 825–840). Elsevier.

113. Benjasirimongkol, P., Piriyaprasarth, S., Moribe, K., & Sriamornsak, P., (2019). Use of risk assessment and Plackett-Burman design for developing resveratrol spray-dried emulsions: A quality-by-design approach. *AAPS PharmSciTech, 20*(1), 14.

114. Naidu, K. A. (2003). Vitamin C in human health and disease is still a mystery? An overview. *Nutrition Journal, 2*(1), 1–10.

115. Roseli, C., (2008). Vitamin and mineral fortification of bread. In: *Technology of Functional Cereal Products* (pp. 336–361). Elsevier.

116. Hathcock, J. N., (2004). *Vitamin and Mineral Safety*. Council for responsible nutrition.

117. Gershoff, S. N., (1993). Vitamin C (ascorbic acid): new roles, new requirements? *Nutrition Reviews, 51*(11), 313–326.

118. Hovdenak, N., & Haram, K., (2012). Influence of mineral and vitamin supplements on pregnancy outcome. *European Journal of Obstetrics & Gynecology and Reproductive Biology, 164*(2), 127–132.

119. Bjelakovic, G., Nikolova, D., Gluud, L. L., Simonetti, R. G., & Gluud, C., (2012). Antioxidant supplements for prevention of mortality in healthy participants and patients with various diseases. *Cochrane Database of Systematic Reviews*, (3).

120. Guenther, P. M., Reedy, J., Krebs-Smith, S. M., & Reeve, B. B., (2008). Evaluation of the healthy eating index-2005. *Journal of the American Dietetic Association, 108*(11), 1854–1864.

121. Kunz, D., & Bes, F., (2019). Melatonin therapy of RBD. In: *rapid-eye-movement Sleep Behavior Disorder* (pp. 315–331). Springer.

122. Vigo, D. E., & Cardinali, D. P., (2019). Melatonin and benzodiazepine/Z-drug abuse. In: *Psychiatry and Neuroscience Update* (pp. 427–451). Springer.

123. Farzaei, M. H., Hajialyani, M., & Naseri, R., (2019). Melatonin. In: *Nonvitamin and Nonmineral Nutritional Supplements* (pp. 99–105). Elsevier.

124. Leu, R. M., (2019). Melatonin. In: *Sleep in Children with Neurodevelopmental Disabilities* (pp. 339–350). Springer.

125. Darien, I. L. (2017). *Study Finds that Melatonin Content of Supplements Varies Widely.* https://aasm.org/study-finds-that-melatonin-content-of-supplements-varies-widely/ (accessed on 31 July 2021).

126. Food, U., & Administration, D., (1995). *Dietary Supplement Health and Education Act of 1994, 1.*

127. Vandeweerd, J. M., Coisnon, C., Clegg, P., Cambier, C., Pierson, A., Hontoir, F., Saegerman, C., et al., (2012). Systematic review of efficacy of nutraceuticals to alleviate clinical signs of osteoarthritis. *Journal of Veterinary Internal Medicine, 26*(3), 448–456.

128. Kahan, A., Uebelhart, D., De Vathaire, F., Delmas, P. D., & Reginster, J. Y., (2009). Long-term effects of chondroitins 4 and 6 sulfate on knee osteoarthritis: The study on osteoarthritis progression prevention, a two-year, randomized, double-blind, placebo-controlled trial. *Arthritis & Rheumatism: Official Journal of the American College of Rheumatology, 60*(2), 524–533.

129. Mecocci, P., Tinarelli, C., Schulz, R. J., & Polidori, M. C., (2014). Nutraceuticals in cognitive impairment and Alzheimer's disease. *Frontiers in Pharmacology, 5*, 147.

130. Lieberman, S (2012). Nutraceuticals Against Alzheimer's Disease. https://www.a4m.com/assets/pdf/bookstore/aamt_vol7_23_lieberman.pdf.

131. Kelsey, N. A., Wilkins, H. M., & Linseman, D. A., (2010). Nutraceutical antioxidants as novel neuroprotective agents. *Molecules, 15*(11), 7792–7814.

132. Kontush, A., Mann, U., Arlt, S., Ujeyl, A., Lührs, C., Müller-Thomsen, T., & Beisiegel, U., (2001). Influence of vitamin E and C supplementation on lipoprotein oxidation in patients with Alzheimer's disease. *Free Radical Biology and Medicine, 31*(3), 345–354.

133. Luchsinger, J. A., Tang, M. X., Shea, S., & Mayeux, R., (2003). Antioxidant vitamin intake and risk of Alzheimer disease. *Archives of Neurology, 60*(2), 203–208.

134. Kharroubi, A. T., & Darwish, H. M., (2015). Diabetes mellitus: The epidemic of the century. *World Journal of Diabetes, 6*(6), 850.

135. Mechanick, J. I., Brett, E. M., Chausmer, A. B., Dickey, R. A., Wallach, S., Bergman, D. A., Garber, J. R., et al., (2003). American Association of Clinical Endocrinologists medical guidelines for the clinical use of dietary supplements and nutraceuticals. *Endocrine Practice, 9*(5), 417–470.

136. Allen, R. W., Schwartzman, E., Baker, W. L., Coleman, C. I., & Phung, O. J., (2013). Cinnamon use in type 2 diabetes: An updated systematic review and meta-analysis. *The Annals of Family Medicine, 11*(5), 452–459.

137. Akilen, R., Tsiami, A., Devendra, D., & Robinson, N., (2012). Cinnamon in glycaemic control: Systematic review and meta-analysis. *Clinical Nutrition, 31*(5), 609–615.

138. Dwyer, J., Coates, P., & Smith, M., (2018). Dietary supplements: Regulatory challenges and research resources. *Nutrients, 10*(1), 41.

139. Team, S. C., (2018). *Nutraceuticals Trials: Demand, Design and Challenges.* https://www.quanticate.com/blog/nutraceutical-trials-design (accessed 10 August 2021).

140. Shils, M. E., & Shike, M., (2006). *Modern Nutrition in Health and Disease.* Lippincott Williams & Wilkins.

141. Anadón, A., Martínez-Larrañaga, M. R., Ares, I., & Martínez, M. A., (2016). Interactions between nutraceuticals/nutrients and therapeutic drugs. In: *Nutraceuticals* (pp. 855–874). Elsevier.

142. Kupiec, T., & Raj, V., (2005). Fatal seizures due to potential herb-drug interactions with Ginkgo biloba. *Journal of Analytical Toxicology, 29*(7), 755–758.

143. Biloba, G., (1999). Herbal remedies: Adverse effects and drug interactions. *Am. Fam. Physician, 59*(5), 1239–1244.

144. Schwartz, J., (2009). Effects of vitamin D supplementation in atorvastatin-treated patients: A new drug interaction with an unexpected consequence. *Clinical Pharmacology & Therapeutics, 85*(2), 198–203.

145. Robien, K., Oppeneer, S. J., Kelly, J. A., & Hamilton-Reeves, J. M., (2013). Drug-vitamin D interactions: A systematic review of the literature. *Nutrition in Clinical Practice, 28*(2), 194–208.

146. Butterweck, V., Derendorf, H., Gaus, W., Nahrstedt, A., Schulz, V., & Unger, M., (2004). Pharmacokinetic herb-drug interactions: Are preventive screenings necessary and appropriate? *Planta Medica, 70*(09), 784–791.

147. Lee, S. H., Ahn, Y. M., Ahn, S. Y., Doo, H. K., & Lee, B. C., (2008). Interaction between warfarin and Panax ginseng in ischemic stroke patients. *The Journal of Alternative and Complementary Medicine, 14*(6), 715–721.

148. Lantz, M. S., Buchalter, E., & Giambanco, V., (1999). St. John's wort and antidepressant drug interactions in the elderly. *Journal of Geriatric Psychiatry and Neurology, 12*(1), 7–10.

149. Shi, S., & Klotz, U., (2012). Drug interactions with herbal medicines. *Clinical Pharmacokinetics, 51*(2), 77–104.

150. Williamson, E. M., (2003). Drug interactions between herbal and prescription medicines. *Drug Safety, 26*(15), 1075–1092.

151. Niles, L., (1991). Melatonin interaction with the benzodiazepine-GABA receptor complex in the CNS. In: *Kynurenine and Serotonin Pathways* (pp. 267–277). Springer.

152. Cardinali, D. P., Vigo, D. E., Olivar, N., Vidal, M. F., & Brusco, L. I., (2015). Therapeutical implications of melatonin in Alzheimer's and Parkinson's diseases. In: *Tryptophan Metabolism: Implications for Biological Processes, Health and Disease* (pp. 197–238). Springer.

153. Urrutia, A., Peral, J., & Padierna, J. Á., (2015). Clinically relevant psychopharmacological interactions in the elderly. *Psychopharmacological Issues in Geriatrics, 49*.

154. Gardiner, P., Phillips, R., & Shaughnessy, A. F., (2008). Herbal and dietary supplement-drug interactions in patients with chronic illnesses. *Am. Fam. Physician, 77*(1), 73–78.

155. Asdaq, S., Inamdar, M., Asad, M., & Nanjundan, P., (2008). Interaction of propranolol with garlic in isoproterenol induced myocardial infarction in rat. *J. Pharmacol. Toxicol., 3*(6), 414–424.

156. Santini, A., Cammarata, S. M., Capone, G., Ianaro, A., Tenore, G. C., Pani, L., & Novellino, E., (2018). Nutraceuticals: Opening the debate for a regulatory framework. *British Journal of Clinical Pharmacology, 84*(4), 659–672.

157. Robb, M. A., McInnes, P. M., & Califf, R. M., (2016). Biomarkers and surrogate endpoints: Developing common terminology and definitions. *JAMA, 315*(11), 1107, 1108.

CHAPTER 11

Solid Dispersion Techniques for Improvement of Dissolution and Bioavailability of Nutraceuticals

ABHIJEET D. KULKARNI, UNNATI M. PATEL, PALLAVI S. KANDALKAR,
ANKITA A. GORHE, ANJALI S. SABALE, ASMITA K. KEDAR,
SNEHAL S. JAGTAP, and VAIBHAV A. MAHALE

Department of Pharmaceutical Quality Assurance,
SRES's Sanjivani College of Pharmaceutical Education and Research,
Kopargaon, Maharashtra, India

ABSTRACT

Bioavailability of some hydrophobic bioactive like carotenoids, polyphenols, fat solvent nutrients, phytosterols (PS), and unsaturated fats are constrained due to their restricted water dissolvability, and in some occurrence chemical stability. The week bioavailability rate of such bio-actives might be because of low bio-accessibility, poor absorption, inside the gastrointestinal tract (GIT). Hydrophobic bio-actives compounds of nutraceutical's bioavailability can be improved utilizing solid dispersion methods. These approaches are considered actual progression in beating restricted aqueous dissolvability and oral ingestion issues. This chapter features the potential systems for expanding the nutraceutical's oral bioavailability dependent on SDs methods. Also, this chapter audits the different manufacturing procedures of SDs and gathers a portion of the ongoing innovation technology. The various sorts of SDs dependent on the molecular arrangement have been featured. A portion of the applied facts to be taken care while preparing SDs, for example, determination of carrier and strategies for physicochemical portrayal, alongside knowledge into the molecular arrangement of action of medications in SDs are discussed.

11.1   INTRODUCTION

The value and part of fundamental nutrients in wellbeing, support, and in body development are well acknowledged. Food contributes not only energy but also nutrients and non-nutrient like (minerals, lipids, proteins, various vitamins, carbohydrates, enzyme inducers, prebiotics, probiotics, antioxidants, and fibers) respectively, further man body make use of said fragments of the food more accurately [1]. Indeed, as it is a very tedious process to understood thoroughly. Present series of molecules like polyphenols and classes, antioxidants, and above-stated nutrients have been the trend of research. Once those composites are separated from a food medium, they are termed as nutraceuticals,' which was defined in 1979 by DeFelice as food or its portion that deliver medicinal or health aids, counting the treatment and anticipation of disease [2].

A Greek physician, Hippocrates quoted let the food be as medicine and medicine as food," to predict the connection between nourishment for wellbeing and their particular helpful advantages. In Ayurveda, the ancient Indian science of medicine, a great deal of accentuation is given to role of sustenance in wellbeing and infection [3]. The expression "Nutraceutical" was authored as a half-breed of nourishment and Pharmaceutical in 1989 by Dr. Stephen DeFelice [4]. A nutraceutical is any material that might be viewed as nourishment or components of sustenance and medicinal offer therapeutic or health advantages, encompassing prophylaxis and cure of disease. Nutraceuticals can be additionally characterized as dietary segments that give helpful or carnal rewards past the basic healthy wants and include a wide scope of compounds, for example, bioactive peptides, phenolic compounds, carotenoids, lipids, nutrients [4], etc.

The nutraceutical field demand is tremendous, both as far as kinds of mediations and the assortment of wellbeing results. Reasonably, the zone can be viewed as situated between restorative medications and fundamental nutrition, with methodologies and products on the most distant closures of the range either stressing the 'ceutical' (for example looking like pharmaceuticals approaches) or the 'nutri' (i.e., Towards nutritional concepts) portions of the word nutraceuticals. On one side, there are products that are only or basically consumed for their practical impacts. These products frequently discover their foundations in conventional medication, for example, many herbal compounds [5], and are regularly promoted and expanded in manners that imitate parts of standard pharmaceuticals, as capsules or liquid formulations, regularly with explicit dosing regimens [5, 6].

The classification of nutraceuticals likewise shifts in various nations: the US depicts them as them as Nutritional Complements, in Canada, they're alluded to as Natural Health Products" and Japan records them as Foods for Special Health Use (FOSHU). These terms may be common or obvious; there are particular definitions and guidelines for nutritional complements and useful foods in the US, Canada, and Europe, while in Japan, both dietary enhancements and functional foods are administered under a similar arrangement of guidelines [7]. The US and Canada list the qualities that a product should be known as a nutraceutical, though Europe and Japan simply give general guidelines on the feature that product ought to must be named in that capacity. Conventional and herbal remedies are incorporated into the meaning of dietary/nutritional complements in Canada. The revelation, advancement, and marketing of food supplements, nutraceuticals, and related product areas of now the quickest developing portions of the food industry, the main issue is nutraceuticals which are significant for interpretation of their acceptance as innovative and modern forms for benefit of natural substances. Because of rapid adjunct round there, the upgrading of a few perspectives is considered as it could impact the eventual fate of the market agents of the nutraceuticals group were presented as forte enhancements. The nutritional complements in Italy (1.424 million), trailed by Russia (888 million) and Germany (967 million). For 2020 a development by 14% (0%–21% as indicated by nations) is expected. The US DS marketplace is ca three to 8 times greater and came to in 2015 the US $40–121 billion "Pharmaceuticals" might be considered as medications utilized chiefly to treat sicknesses, while "nutraceuticals" are those that are expected to avert disease [7–9].

The core fact is that nutraceuticals efficacy and safety is guaranteed by the manufacturers and perhaps long-haul use, the pharmaceuticals' general adequacy and safety are ensured by guaranteed by the approval of the health authority. It has been expressed that they work by expanding the supply of significant building blocks to the body. The supply of these fundamental building blocks should be possible by two different ways. By lowering signals of the disease as buffering mediators for relief and by directly providing benefits for the health of the individuals. Novel nutraceuticals are being developed as extra enhancements for youths, who effectively partake in games, tumbling, and for various kinds of trainings, and different customers to treat the different malady [9].

11.1.1   CLASSIFICATION OF NUTRACEUTICALS

11.1.1.1   BASED ON BIOAVAILABILITY

Depending on bioavailability, they are grouped in three major classes on their bioaccessibility, absorption, and alteration within the GI tract. Inside these three noteworthy classes, there are subclasses identified with the specific physicochemical or physiological mechanisms that influence bioavailability [10]:

- **Bioaccessibility:**
  - o Liberation;
  - o Solubilization;
  - o Interactions.
- **Absorption:**
  - o Mucus layer;
  - o Tight junction transport;
  - o Bilayer permeability;
  - o Active transporters;
  - o Efflux transporters.
- **Transformation:**
  - o Chemical degradation;
  - o Metabolism.

1. **Bioaccessibility (B*):** This type of the limiting factors is linked to the bioaccessibility of the nutraceutical within the GIT fluids. In the NuBACS (nutraceutical bioavailability classification scheme), nutraceuticals with relatively high bioaccessibility are represented as B* (+), whereas those with comparatively poor bioaccessibility are represented as B* (−). High bioaccessibility is defined as when more than 75% of the nutraceutical available for absorption in an appropriate form at the suitable absorption place like small intestine.

2. **Liberation Limit:** The nutraceutical's bioaccessibility may be insufficient depending on their characteristic to get released from food complex. Enhancing the release of these group of Nutraceuticals from food complex will be a dynamic approach for enhancing their bioavailability. Which can be accomplished through modifying factors for food processing (like cooking, shearing, or other), also, by modifying eating pattern (like mastication time), or by modifying food matrix properties (such as composition and structure).

3. **Solubility Limited:** Nutraceuticals bioaccessibility is also restricted depending on their property to get solubilized in intestinal fluids. Bioaccessibility of these types of substances may consequently be enhanced by using food complex or factors that increase their intestinal solubility.

4. **Interaction Limited:** In this type, nutraceuticals bioavailability is narrow because of its interface with another substance in GI fluids. These interfering components may arise from the ingested food matrix, or they may be naturally present inside GIT. The bioaccessibility of certain Nutraceuticals may also fewer by the existence of specific constituents inside ingested food pattern, like chelating agents or ionic polymers.

5. **Mucin Layer Transport Limited:** The epithelial tissues facing GIT are surrounded through a mucus layer that acts as a defensive coating restricting the flow of few substances. If bioactive substance size is greater than the pores size of gel-like mucus layer, it may affect their migration, apparently around 400 NM. Because of interlinkage of molecular structure that form mucus layer, the pharmacokinetics of few nonpolar molecules or electrically charged may be restricted.

6. **Bilayer Permeability Limited:** The major hurdle affecting the Nutraceuticals passive absorption by epithelium cells is their characteristic to migrate through the nonpolar phospholipid bilayer, which is a vital portion of the cell membrane. Bioactive compound with greater the hydrophobicity (higher LogP), the higher the bilayer membrane permeability. In the pharmaceutical industry, a molecule with a LogP greater than 1 (i.e., KOW > 10) is assumed to have high epithelium cell permeability. The same standards may also be a base for the grouping of nutraceuticals. If log P < 1, then the bioavailability is inadequate by bioactive compound bilayer permeability.

7. **Tight Junction Transport Limited:** The presence of Tight junctions within the epithelial cell layer will not be affected the migration of some bioactive molecules having a less bilayer membrane permeability. Tight junctions occur within the region that joins neighboring epithelial cells and consist of thin networks that permits minor molecules or particles to travel through them adequately. Slightly larger substance than tight junctions will have the ability to migrate through the epithelium tissues layer.

8. **Active Transport Limited:** Active transporter mechanisms around the epithelium tissues allows transport of some kinds of bioactive

molecules having a low bilayer membrane porousness, as this method comprises of solitary protein or a type of proteins fixed within the epithelium bilayer membrane. Hence active transporters as basis of energy are required that is proficient for conveying particular kind of molecules around cell membranes.

9. **Efflux Transporter Limited:** After absorption by intestinal epithelium cells, few Nutraceuticals are migrated revert in GI lumen through efflux transporters fixed inside epithelial cell membranes. These efflux transporters result in uptake of few Nutraceuticals inside systemic circulation. There are below two possible ways due to which bioavailability may fall down:

   i.   A nutraceutical is discharged through the epithelium tissue; and
   ii. The metabolism degree raised as nutraceutical is repeatedly absorbed and effluxed. A bioactive the bioactive substance which transported out of the epithelium tissues and back into the GI lumen by this process as efflux transporter inadequate.

10. **Transformation:** Nutraceutical inactive form conversion inside the GIT disturbs its absorptions. These molecular transformations are categorized in two subclasses based on their origin.

11. **Chemical Degradation Limited:** Few nutraceuticals go through the chemical transformations inside food or post-ingestion that alter their biological activity, e.g., oxidation, reduction, or hydrolysis reactions.

12. **Metabolism Limited:** Because of occurrence and metabolism of enzymes within the GIT, e.g., Resveratrol, quercetin, and epicatechin, lipid loving Nutraceutical's polarization increases as they get attached to hydrophilic adjacent clusters of a parent molecule. Hence, endorsing reabsorption and excretion from the kidney through urine is observed. Oxidation, hydrolysis, and reduction are usually detected in Phase I metabolism reactions, where numerous groups of enzymes like esterases, dehydrogenases, etc., are engaged in this stage. Whereas, Phase II reaeration generally linked with conjugation reactions among core bioactive substances or endogenous substances and metabolites of phase I.

13. **B*A*T* Designations:** Overall, a particular nutraceutical can be denoted by a B*A*T* label rendering to the key factors limiting its bioavailability. Such physicochemical factor is designated (+) nonlimiting and (−) limiting, respectively. For example, a hydrophilic nutraceutical whose overall bioavailability is inadequate by weaker absorption (due to poor bilayer permeability and tight junction transport) and high chemical

transformation (due to metabolism) inside GIT aspiringly grouped as B*(+) A*(–) BP, TJ T*(–) M. Nutraceuticals also grouped based on food source mechanism of action and chemical nature (Table 11.1).

11.2 CHALLENGES IN THE NUTRACEUTICAL DELIVERY

The nutraceutical companies are immense and developing. Nutraceutical products are being sold based on wellbeing claims, ordinarily with deficient or even totally without supporting epidemiological research proof. From a few enormous scale mediations considers the world over, there is clear proof that dietary supplementation to enough supported populaces do not give extra medical advantages as decreases in sickness hazard, or may really expand illness chance. Nothing precluding the incentive from claiming appropriate nourishment got from eating "great sustenance" for wellbeing support and malady counteractive action [11]. These include:

- Quality control (QC) issues identified with chemical constitute (e.g., plant determination, source, constituents, and contaminants);
- Standard protocols for formulation and testing (both synthetic and pharmacological profiles);
- Safety testing (which is typically accepted, yet not demonstrated);
- Identification of mechanism-based on biomarkers to assess advantageous/destructive impacts;
- Prospective clinical trials. Well-planned further epidemiological examinations are required while some have just been led, a one-year usage of a grape nutraceutical containing resveratrol to produce human evidence for the advantages/damages of utilizing nutraceuticals (Figure 11.1) [12].

All fundamental nutraceutical experience carriage and possible issues from, water, light, rancidity stickiness, and potential binding. Tablets are hard, by, and large unpalatable and stacked with bearers important to help make the tablet. These are accepted with numerous pharmaceuticals, yet not considered as the option of supplementation Liquids (water, oils) are feasible options, however numerous oils go rancid effectively which energizes obliteration of nutraceuticals [13]. Alike, water can build obliteration of numerous compounds. With the appropriate adjustment, these alternatives are truly practical. Organized tidbit is an ideal structure with few nutraceuticals, yet the high heating can rapidly pulverize by the substances which are affected by hat such as probiotics, flavonoids, and chemicals. Comparable

TABLE 11.1 Grouping of Nutraceuticals based on Origin, Mode of action, chemical nature.

Source	Examples
Plant	Genestein, zinc, Cellulose Gallic acid, Ascorbic acid, Allicin, Quercetin, Luteolin, Cellulose, Lutein, Pectin, Daidzein, Lycopene, Selenium, Zeaxanthin, Geraniol.
Animal	Spingolipids, Choline, Lecithin, Calcium, Coenzyme Q10, Selenium, Zinc, Creatine, Minerals.
Microbes	*Saccharomyces boulardii* (yeast), *Bifidobacterium bifidum, B.longum, B.infantis, Lactobacillus acidophilis* (LC1). *L.acidophilus* (NCFB 1748). *Streptococcus salvarius* (Subs. Thermophilus).
Classification on the basis of mode of action	
Action	**Example**
Anticancer	Capsaicin, Genestein, Daidzein, α-Tocotrienol, γ- Tocotrienol, *Lactobacillus acidophilis,* Spingolipids, Limonene, Dailly sulfide, Ajoene, α-Tocopherol, Enterollactone, Glycyrrhizin
Antioxidant activity	Indole-3-carbonol, α-Tocopherol, Indole-3-carbonol, Ellagic acid, Lycopene, Lutin, Glutathione, Hydroxytyrosol, Luteolin, Oleuropein, Catechins, Gigerol, Chlorigenic acid, Tannins.
Anti-inflammtory	Linolenic acid, Capsaicin, Quercetin, Curcumin.
Osteogenetic or Bone Protective	Calcium, Genestein, Daidzein.
Classification on the basis of chemical nature	
Class	**Example**
Carotenoids	Alpha-carotene, Beta-carotene, Lutein, Lycopene, Zeaxanthin,
Collagen Hydolysate	Collagen Hydolysate
Dietary Fibre	Insoluble fibre, Beta glucan, Soluble fibre, Whole Grains,
Fatty Acids	Omega-3 fatty acids,
Flavonoids	Anthocynidins, Catechins, Flavanones, Flavones,
Glucosinolates, Indoles, Isothiocyanates	Sulforaphane

TABLE 11.1 *(Continued)*

Source	Examples
Phenol	Caffeic acid, Ferulic acid,
Plant Sterol	Stanol ester
Prebiotics/Probiotics	Fructo-oligosaccharides (FOS), Lactobacillius
Sponins	Sponins
Phytoestrogens	Isoflavones-Daidzen, Genistein, Lignans
Sulfides/Thiols	Dailly sulfide, Allyl methyl trisulfide, Dithiolthiones.
Tannins	Proanthocyanidins

contentions may prepare about expelled treats, which face high weight and heat, high dampness with drying surroundings. Soft-moist treats are often observed as a tasteful option for supplementation, yet huge moisture and acidity may discredit suitability [14]. Whatever delivery form is utilized, the formulator must know about the ways of devastation, potential interactions, and by and large strength during the proposed timeframe of realistic usability. We realize that pet sustenance loses around 30% of half of the nutrients during handling and more elevated amounts must be strengthened to meet 12 to the 18-month timeframe of realistic usability necessities.

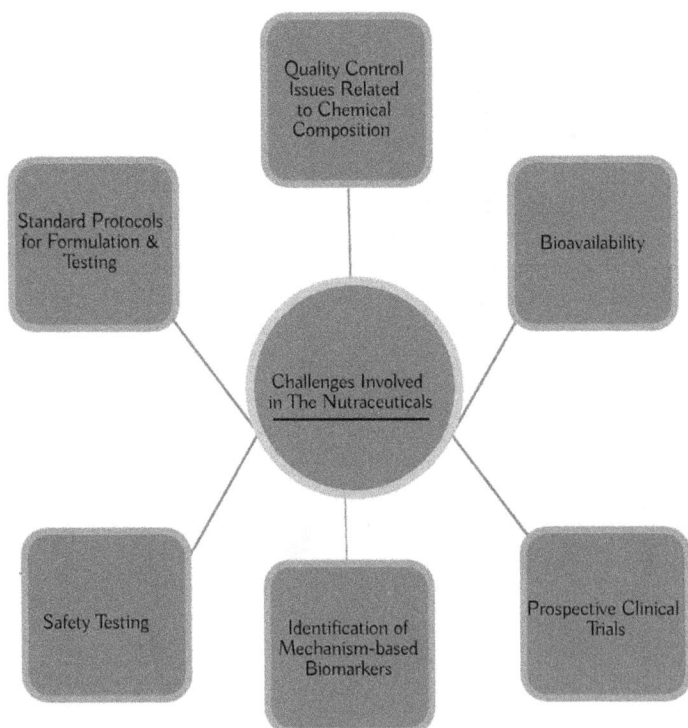

FIGURE 11.1   Challenges Involved in Nutraceutical

Different difficulties incorporate the necessity to counteract the unfortunate interaction of nutraceutical with the end and components of the food matrix, limit the degradation of the nutraceutical when it is consolidated under conditions applied for nutriment processing, stabilize out the food between the time span of usability of the completed item, and guarantee the nourishment containing the nutraceutical gives the intended health advantage after ingestion. As numerous bioactive is insecure after they are disconnected from their common food source, there may likewise be a need to embody the nutraceutical to create progressively stable fixing positions before it is utilized in the manufacture of formulated functional foods [15].

11.3 SOLID DISPERSION

To conquer such issues, SDs systems have been verified in literature for the improvement dissolution characteristic of weekly water-soluble drugs. The significant perspectives to be considered during preparation of SDs viz., properties of polymer and making procedures of strong SDs which influence dissolution profile [13]. SDs have pulled in impressive choice as a proficient method for the enhancement of dissolution profile, and henceforth, bioavailability is in the scope for hydrotropic drugs.

Around 40% novel synthetic substances found by pharma companies today are inadequately soluble or lipophilic compounds [17]. SDs of inadequately water-dissolvable medications with water-soluble carriers diminish the amount of these issues and improve dissolution. SDs are the most encouraging methodologies for improvement in the solubility. The term solid dispersion termed to a category of materials in solid form comprising of minimum 2 diverse constituents, commonly a hydrophilic medium [18].

The compound may be either in amorphous or crystalline form. Based on biopharmaceutical classification class II of drugs having poor solubility with high penetrability are the promising possibility for development of bioavailability by solid dispersion. Factors to take care while preparing the SDs are choice of carrier, molecular structure of drugs in SDs are highlighted in this chapter [19]. Choice of a great species of polymers that are self-weekly soluble or which have a tendency to swell due to aqueous medium recommends that SDs have marvelous scope in the field of controlled release dosage forms.

The compound may either in amorphous or crystalline form. The phenomena solid dispersion assigned to the type of solid materials composed of 2 ideal portions in all conditions, by hydrophilic medium and a hydrophobic medication. The grid can be either crystalline or amorphous. The medication either dispersed molecularly as indistinct clusters as crystalline materials. The drug bioavailability relies upon its dissolvability or potentially disintegration rate, hence endeavors to build disintegration of drug with constrained water solvency is frequently required. Improvement in the disintegration rate of inadequately dissolvable medications after oral administration is a standout amongst the most pivotal difficulties in present-day pharmaceutics [20].

11.3.1 SOLID DISPERSIONS (SDS) CLASSIFICATION

Based on the physical form of a carrier like crystalline or amorphous, the SDs are alienated in crystalline SDs and amorphous SDs accordingly. They may group into 4 generations depending on composition they possess [21].

11.3.1.1 FIRST GENERATION

The first-generation SDS are crystalline dispersions. Where, a drug in crystalline form dispersed inside a crystal-line carrier shaping a eutectic or monotectic blend. In the eutectic blend, the dissolving purpose of the blend is lower than the softening purpose of the medication and transporter though in the monotectic blend, the liquefying purpose of carrier and drug are consistent. Eutectic mixture is of great choice because both (drug and carrier) have tendency to be crystalize at the same time in cooling procedure, leading in a finely dispersed form of drug inside carrier, hence improving dissolution rate [22].

Crystalline carriers of first-generation SDs composed by urea also sugars like sorbitol and mannitol. These carriers, more particularly sugars, have more melting point that is not suitable for manufacturing SDs by this method. Urea possesses strong solubility in aqueous field also in numerous general organic solvents and sugars retains week solubility in maximum organic solvents; hence, sugar is not of great choice over other carriers [23].

11.3.1.2 SECOND GENERATION

Second-generation SDs comprise amorphous carriers which are generally polymers. Amorphous SDs can be ordered into amorphous solid solutions and amorphous solid suspension according to physical condition of the drug. In amorphous solid solution carrier and drug are totally miscible to frame molecularly homogenous blend amorphous solid-suspension comprises of two separate stages: amorphous solid-suspension is framed once the drug has constrained carrier solubility or has a higher melting point [21]. In these arrangements, the tiny drug particles fundamentally in amorphous form are dispersed into amorphous carriers. It has been noticed that API frequently occurs in more states than single in solid dispersions (SDs), for example, API can either break down or suspend in carrier or remain in amorphous and crystalline form simultaneously. In amorphous SDs, API is dispersed in minute size and remain in supersaturated condition amorphous carriers on account of constrained solubilization [24]. Amorphous carriers may likewise build with drugs wettability or dispersibility just as restrain the precipitation procedure of drug once amorphous SDs liquified in aqueous field. These characteristics alongside the quick dissolution profile of amorphous carriers due to low thermodynamic stability of amorphous form carriers increases the medication solvency and discharge rate [21].

11.3.1.3 THIRD GENERATION

Behind the proven concept that amorphous SDs may develop drug re-lease rate, the ensuing supersaturation condition of drug which may produce precipitation of the drug and lower down the quantity of drug *in vitro* or *in vivo*, respectively, along these lines contrarily influencing the drug bioavailability. This concept is common, particularly for sugar SDs. During the formulation procedure and while storage drug can appear in recrystallize form from amorphous. In the third-generation SDs, surface-active agents are presented as transporters or additives also displayed drastic progress in resolving the stated issues like precipitation or maybe recrystallization. These surfactants are utilized as process aids which plays a vital role to advance the biopharmaceutical efficiency of supersaturation systems. The surfactants presentation in SDs enhances not only dissolution rate but also drugs physicochemical stability. Further, surfactants having amphiphilic structure can upgrade the miscibility of medications and transporters and in this way diminish the recrystallization pace of drugs. Additionally, surfactants also recover the wettability of drugs and stop the drug precipitation because of supersaturation by engrossing to the external layer of drug particles or framing micelles to encapsulate drugs [26].

11.3.1.4 FOURTH GENERATION

The fourth-generation SDs are the controlled release dispersions having week aqueous solubility for the drugs having little biological half-life. CRSD (controlled release solid dispersion) drugs require two targets: solubility enhancers and prolonged controlled release fashion. The molecular dispersion of drugs having week aqueous solubility with carriers in CRSD, advance the drug solubility, and aqueous insoluble polymers or swellable polymers may be utilized to retard drug release in dissolution matrix. As CRSD may provide an acceptable quantity of drug for a prolonged time hence offer various benefits like minimization of adverse reactions and maximization of patient compliance by reducing dose regimen also better controlled therapeutic efficiency for weekly aqueous soluble drugs. Some of the common polymers utilized for retarding the release of weekly aqueous soluble drugs in CRSD are Eudragit, RS, RL, poly(ethylene oxide) (PEO), ethylcellulose and carboxy vinyl polymer (Carbopol). Sustention of releases of week aqueous soluble drugs is supported by these polymers. CRSD system combines and utilize these sustainable polymers or may use additional substances which has high solubility efficiency and sustaining pawer [27, 28].

11.3.2   *SOLID DISPERSION ADVANTAGES*

11.3.2.1   *REDUCED PARTICLE SIZE*

As SDs, molecular dispersions, shows the decreased particle size in the final state, where the drug is dispersed molecularly in the medium after carrier dissolution. This principle is applied by SDs for drug delivery by making a blend of a drug with week aqueous-soluble and highly soluble carriers. A high area of surface is obtained, bringing about an improved dissolution pace and, therefore, bioavailability is enhanced [29].

11.3.2.2   *IMPROVED WETTABILITY*

Surface activity carriers, for example, bile salts and cholic acid. When utilized, can essentially enhance the drug's wettability property. Indeed, uniform carriers having no surface activity, for example, urea, improved wettability of drug. By straight dissolution it impacts dissolution rate of drug which can be enhance by carriers' effects [31].

11.3.2.3   *HIGHER POROSITY*

SDs particle having higher level of porosity have been found. The porosity expands additionally relies upon the carrier properties; for example, bigger, and more porous particles are produced by linear polymers of SDs over reticular polymers and, hence, bring about a higher dissolution pace. The solid dispersion particles increased porosity additionally rushes the drug deliverance profile [21, 31].

11.3.2.4 DRUG AMORPHOUS STATE

Crystalline drugs which are poorly water-soluble, when get modified to amorphous state have higher solubility. The improvement in drug deliverance can often be accomplished utilizing drug amorphous state, owing to no energy is required for separation of crystal lattice at the time of dissolution. For low crystal energy drugs (fusion heat or low melting temperature), the amorphous composition is basically directed by the melting variation can be acquired by carrier selection, which display explicit interaction with them temperature among medication and carrier [31, 32].

11.3.3 SDS DISADVANTAGES

The SDs significant disadvantages are instability related, many systems with aging have indicated crystallinity variation and a fall in disintegration pace. Temperature and moisture have a greater extent of degradation impact on SDs over physical blends. Few SDs will not be simple in handling of due to tackiness [33].

11.3.4 DRUG RELEASE MECHANISM OF SDS

Controlled release is the core drug release mechanism of the SDs. These SDs usually dispersed in an aqueous field where carriers frequently absorb or dissolve inside aqueous field quickly due to their hydrophilic characteristics and form a thick carrier layer in some circumstances [34]. And in terms of carrier-controlled release mechanism, drug gets dissolve within layer and if thickness the layer is high enough for stopping the drug diffusion by it, later rate restricting phase led to carrier diffusion in the bulk phase. And when the drug is not able to get soluble in this thick layer, it may be released completely and interact with water, and here dissolution rate will depend on characteristics of drug substances like particle size, Polymorphism nature, and solubility. As drug may be moderately soluble or capsulated in the precipitated carrier layer, these two mechanisms frequently happen simultaneously [22]. These two mechanisms state the diverse release patterns of SDs and figure out the method for improving SDs dissolution rate. A number of the researches proved the novelty of drug dissolution profile once the proportion of carriers in SDs was increased because the drug was dispersed well and the drug crystallinity reduced. In SDs the core mechanism for release is drug-controlled release. In comparison, other research outcomes proved the reduction in dissolution profile once the proportion of carrier in SDs was high.

This may be demonstrated by the carrier-controlled mechanism where the thick carrier layer is produced and behaves as a diffusion blockade to prolong drug release. The release mechanism also gets disturbed by the proportion of drug carrier in SDs (Figure 11.2) [36].

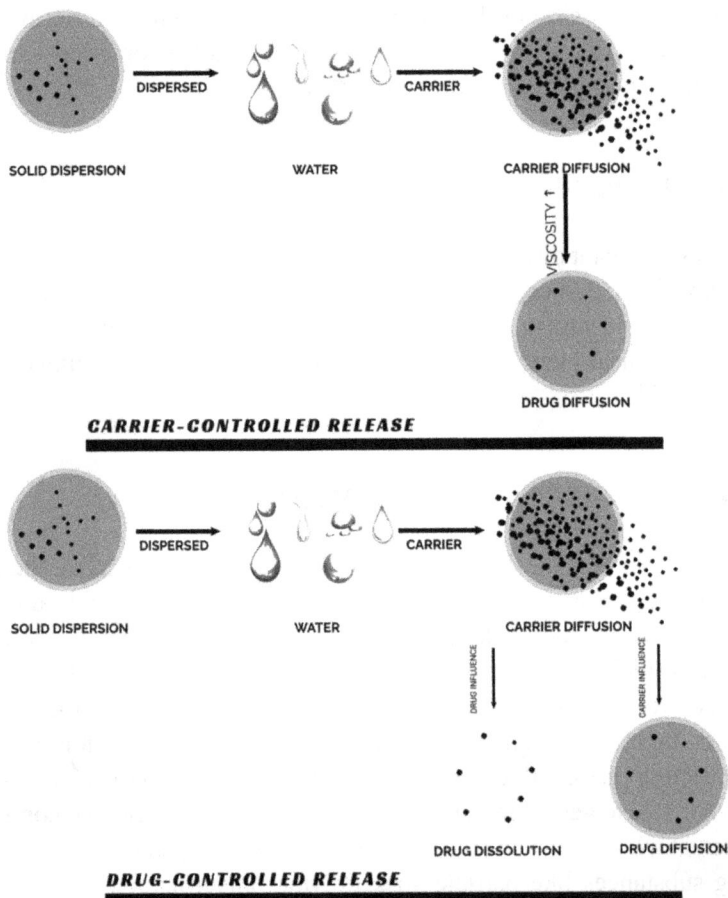

FIGURE 11.2   Mechanism action of solid dispersion

11.3.5   TYPES OF SOLID DISPERSIONS (SDS) [31]

11.3.5.1   EUTECTIC MIXTURES

A common eutectic complex comprises of two complexes which are thoroughly miscible in the liquid state but to a limited rate in the solid-state, which is processed through quick solidification of bonded melt of two compounds that revel whole liquid miscibility but insignificant solid-solid solution.

11.3.5.2   CRYSTALLINE MATRIX AND AMORPHOUS PRECIPITATION

It is similar to simple eutectic complex with variable that drug have tendency to precipitated out in a non-crystalline form.

11.3.5.3   SOLID SOLUTION

These are analogous to liquid solutions, comprising of only single-phase irrespective of the number of components. In the event of solid solutions, particle size of drug has been decreased to its absolute least viz. The molecular dimensions as well as dissolution profile are demonstrated by carrier dissolution amount. They are grouped based on their miscibility (continuous versus discontinuous solid solutions) or second, depending on the way by which solvate molecules are dispersed in solvendum (substitutional, interstitial, or amorphous).

11.3.5.4   CONTINUOUS SOLID-SOLUTIONS

In this type, components are miscible in all ratios. Hypothetically, it is understood that bonding strength among the two compounds is strong as compare to the bonding strength among the molecules of each of the individual components.

11.3.5.5   DISCONTINUOUS SOLID-SOLUTIONS

In Solid Solutions of discontinuous type, the solubility of each of the components in another component is inadequate. Based on practical approaches it had recommended by Goldberg et al. [14] that the terminology 'solid solution' would only be functional when the shared solubility of 2 components is more than 5%.

11.3.5.6   SUBSTITUTIONAL SOLID DISPERSIONS (SDS)

This term is probable only when solute molecules size varies or is below than 15% or so from that of solvent molecules. Classical solid solution has crystalline form, where solute molecules may fit into the interstices among the solvent molecules or are auxiliary for crystal lattice among the solvent molecules.

11.4   VARIOUS APPROACHES OF NUTRACEUTICAL SDS DELIVERY

For nutraceuticals by SDs, three significant major preparation approaches are present, including melting approach, solvent approach and melting solvent approach. In fact, the solvent approach and melting approach are more typical over the melting solvent approach [22].

11.4.1   MELTING METHOD

The melting or fusion strategy, includes the combination of drug physical blend with a water-soluble carrier and directly heating until it melts. The melted blend is then quickly solidified under rigorous mixing in an ice-bath. The resulting solid mass was further crushed, pulverized, and sieved. Properly this has experienced numerous up-gradation in the homogenous melt pouring onto a ferrite or a stainless-steel plate as thin layer and cooled by air stream or water on the contrary plate side. Additionally, a solute/medication supersaturation in a system can be usually acquired by melt quenching quickly from an elevated temperature. In such conditions, the s molecules of solute are captured in the matrix solvent by the prompt solidification process [22].

Scientists researched on enhancing curcumin dissolution with solid dispersion by Hydroxypropyl Methylcellulose. By the melting method SDs were set up by the melting method to upgrade curcumin dissolution pace utilizing HPMC, PEG 6000, 4000, HPMC 6, and PEO as carriers. Required amount of PEG 6000 was melted in a beaker at 190°C until a molten liquid appeared. Curcumin was added into the beaker and stirred in a desired time. HPMC later dispersed in molten mixture until a uniform mixture was obtained. These SDs then were cooled at room temperature. The obtained

SDs was preserved through covering beaker with aluminum foil and keeping in a dry place for a protection from light for further use [39].

11.4.2 SOLVENT EVAPORATION METHOD

In this approach, a solid dispersion is obtained after solvent evaporation from drug + carrier solution. The solvent approach has tackled prime issues of the melting technique relating with drug + carriers' deterioration on higher temperature owing for the solvent method, the solvent evacuation can be performed without heating, for example, freeze-drying approach. A few polymers rarely utilized as carriers in dissolving strategy due to their high softening point can be applied in the melting technique. A significant essential of this technique is the adequate solubility in solvent or co-solvent for drug + carrier. Finding an appropriate non-lethal solvent is at times troublesome owing to hydrophilic carriers with hydrophobic drugs. The solvents utilized in this approach may incorporate ethanol, methylene chloride, methanol, ethyl acetic acid derivation, water, acetone, and mixtures. A few surfactants, for example, SLS, Tween-80 can be employed to extend the solubility of drugs + carriers in solvents (Table 11.2) [20].

11.4.3 HOT MELT EXTRUSION

This approach has been known as the most widely recognized technique for preparing solid dispersion as this method possess high scalability and applicability. In this method, drug + carrier is blended, heated, liquefied, homogenized in the shape of tablets, pellets, rods, milled, and mixed with different additives for various purposes at the same time. The intense blending and force of agitation by the rotation screw during the operation leads to disaggregation of drug particles in the molten polymer, bringing about a homogeneous dispersion. By heating and intense blending, change in solid mass of intertwined particles into aqueous solvent or semisolid mass id done. The extruded system of hotmelt is made out of one to more meltable polymers, and drugs, additive substances, for example, plasticizers, and pH modifiers. The degree of melting is basically influenced by physical and rheological attributes of the polymer. The degree of melting is much quicker when polymers are amorphous and low viscous. Hot-melt extrusion of miscible parts may prompt a high pattern of development of amorphous solid dispersion, hence refining drug dissolution rate [41].

TABLE 11.2 Nutraceutical Prepared by different Technique

Formulation Strategy	Nutraceuticals	Salient Features/Benefits	Reference
Solid Dispersions	Vitamin A palmitate	Liquid crystals for timed release	Patravale and Mandawgade (2008)
	Coenzyme Q10	Solid dispersion with solubility, stability and dissolution	Nepal et al. (2010)
	Resveratrol	Solid dispersion for improved stability	Weigel et al. (2013)
Particle Coatings	Coenzyme Q10	TMC-coated liposomes containing coenzymeQ10 with improved corneal retention time and stability	Zhang & Wang (2009)
	Vitamin E	Vitamin E coated contact lenses for prolonged release of bioactive	Peng et al. (2010)
	Gastric-sensitive Nutraceuticals Hesperetin	Chitosan/ b-lactoglobulin core–shell nanoparticles for protection from gastric pH and pepsin and enhanced absorption Hesperetin loaded NLC's coated with chitosan, alginate and methoxypectin enhanced release and stability	Chen and Subirade (2005), Fathi and Varshosaz (2013)
Solvent Evaporation Technique	Quercetin	improvement in solubility, dissolution and other physicochemical properties	Vikas Verma et.al 2017
Spray Drying	Gallic acid	Apparent solubility drug increased in water	K.R. Shyam et.al 2012
	Glycyrrhizic Acid	Improved Cmax	Jingze Zhang et.al 2011
	Catechin	Increasing the stability, protecting from oxidation and incorporation	Ferreira et al. 2007
	β-carotene	Improving dispersibility, coloring strength and bioavailability	De Paz et al. 2012
	D-Limonene	Increasing the retention, stability during process	Jafari et al. 2007
Freeze drying	Capsicum oleoresin	Improving the stability and Rehydrating to study the dispersion characteristic	Nakagawa et al. 2011
	α-Tocopherol	improving stability and Protecting Improving stability and Protecting from environmental factor	Luo et al. 2011

TABLE 11.2 *(Continued)*

Formulation Strategy	Nutraceuticals	Salient Features/Benefits	Reference
	Vitamin E	increasing the stability, retention percentage and extending the shelf-life	Zhao et al. 2011
	Curcuminoids	Improving the stability	Tiyaboonchai et al. 2007
	Catechin	Protecting catechin from degradation	Dube et al. 2010
		creasing the stability, protecting rom oxidation and incorporation	Ferreira et al. 2007
	β-carotene	Improving dispersibility, coloring strength and bioavailability	De Paz et al. 2012
	D-Limonene	increasing the retention, stability during process	Jafari et al. 2007

11.4.4   *VACUUM DRYING AND ROTARY EVAPORATION*

A challenge of phase separation can emerge during the solvent evacuation process. The procedure of heating can increase the mobility of molecules bringing about separation of phase. Hence, at a moderate temperature, vacuum drying and rotational evaporation are utilized to evade that prevent and risk the drug degradation and carriers at elevated temperature. After the solvent evaporation process, with the help of vacuum desiccator, the subsequent solid dispersion might be kept for complete evacuation of residual solvent. Although the fact that these approaches are uncomplicated for performing as the procedures are very much time consuming. Hence, the separation of phase and drugs recrystallization can take place easily while drying [21].

11.4.5   *SPRAY DRYING*

For SDs manufacturing, this is an effective approach based on the fact that it allows very quick solvent dispersal leading to quick change of API-carrier solution to solid particles of API-carrier. In this approach, from the compartment, API-carrier solution or suspension is moved to the nozzle opening by means pump and atomized into fine beads having large explicit area of surface. These beads bring about fast dispersal of solvent and solid dispersion formation in few seconds. The solid dispersion size particles formed by this techniques can be modified by regulating the bead size through nozzle to meet the prerequisites for later processing/applications. The API is solid made by this approach are usually in amorphous state; hence, the solubility and dissolution profile are significantly expanded. As it is a well-known approach used to make solid dispersion in a larger scale with high recoveries (greater than 95%) due to the chance of ease of scalability, continuous manufacturing, cost-effectiveness, and good uniformity of molecular dispersion [43].

11.4.6   *FREEZE DRYING*

This is another approach for SDs drying. This approach guarantee as an appropriate procedure for the supercritical fluids (SCFs) permits the precise control for numerous drugs solubilization. When CO_2 as a solvent is utilized, drug + carrier is dissolved and sprayed in a vessel by a nozzle lesser pressure application. The fast development initiates quick nucleation of undissolved drugs + carriers, prompting solid dispersion particles formation with a preferable distribution of in an extremely short span of time. At the point when supercritical CO_2 as a anti-solvent is utilized, simultaneously with drugs + carriers' solution in organic solvent, CO_2 is transported in the nozzle. At the point when solution is sprayed, by the supercritical CO_2, the solvent is immediately extricated prompting solid dispersion particles precipitation [44].

11.4.7 FLUID-BED COATING

In this approach, the drug along with carrier in solvent are initially dissolved in the fluid-bed coater, this mixture solution sprayed by a nozzle onto the nonpareil pellet surface [45]. By drying air stream, solvent is expelled immediately after the co-precipitate settle on the prime pellets surface [46]. This approach benefit is that without further handling granules/pellets of SDs may be set for tableting or encapsulation into capsule.

11.4.8 CO-PRECIPITATION METHOD

Co-precipitation is an appropriate approach for SDs preparation of poorly water-dissolvable drugs which have low dissolvability in usually utilized organic solvents and high melting tine that cannot be handled by melting and another solvent approaches. In this approach, a drug with carrier is entirely solubilized in organic solvent prior to adding to an anti-solvent which leads to concurrent precipitation of drug with carrier. The subsequent suspension is then filtered and washed to expel leftover solvents. The micro precipitated bulk powder (MPD) is the co-precipitated material got after filtration and drying which is a drug and carrier's solid dispersion. In co-precipitation approach the polymers utilized frequently have solubility depending on pH, for example, polymethylmethacrylate, polymethyl acrylate, cellulose acetic acid derivation phthalate, polyvinyl phthalate, HPMCAS, and HPMCP while a few solvents, for example, dimethylformamide, N-methyl pyrrolidone, and dimethylacetamide, are predominantly utilized by their magnificent power of solvency, especially for elevated atomic weight polymers [22].

11.4.9 VACUUM DRYING AND ROTARY EVAPORATION

Phase separation is a challenge that can arise during the solvent removal process. The heating process can increase the molecular mobility resulting in phase separation. Therefore, vacuum drying and rotary evaporation at a moderate temperature are used to avoid that risk and prevent the degradation of drugs along with carriers at elevated temperature. Subsequent to solvent vaporization process, the SDs resulted may be kept for the entire elimination of residual solvent in vacuum desiccator. No doubt this technique is quite easy to carry out, but the method is very tedious, due to the consumption of the time drug recrystallization may takes place between the drying process and phase separation is observed [22].

11.5   REGULATORY ASPECTS OF NUTRACEUTICALS

Nutraceuticals are emerging rapidly as feasible and substitute for a variety of prophylactic treatment and therapeutic applications. That had not only huge influence on cost for health care worldwide but also in emerging nations like India. Hence strict guidance is essential in order to safe and effective usage of such agents. Considering the continuously changing scenario the currently available, there is always potential for amendment and updating. The FSSAI (2006) and the Drugs and Cosmetics Rule (1945) together ensure that many of these contentious issues are resolved [47].

11.5.1   GLOBAL REGULATORY SCENARIO FOR NUTRACEUTICALS

In U.S. guidance for manufacturing and advertising of nutraceuticals was approved in 1994 and also Dietary Supplement Health and Education Act (DSHEA) title. Guidelines by DSHEA are not quite the same as those covering traditional nutriments and medicinal products. Under DSHEA-1994, the dietary products or dietary content manufacturer is in charge for product safety assurance before marketing it and (FDA) is liable for making a move against any perilous nutritional supplement goods after it arrives in the market. In 2007, the federal (GMP) guideline (21 CFR, Part 111) was presented, and GMP enforcement was the FDA and the department of health and human services (HHS) liability. Guidelines indicate that national and multinational industries engaged in manufacturing, packaging, labeling nutraceuticals, incorporating those associated by testing, QC, and distribution of nutraceutical in the US, have the responsibility of assuring the safety of food materials prior and post introduction to the market. Companies give the confirmation of ingredients safety, utilized in their products, assessing the quality, purity, identity, strength, and composition of dietary supplements (DS), and preparing, packaging, and keeping products in consultation with FDA's recent (cGMP) guidance. They should also submit reports of serious adverse events to the FDA. In European Union, oversee food legislation with a special emphasis on food supplements is govern by the European Food and Safety Authority (EFSA). Europeans' states food supplements as nutrient's concentrated sources (e.g., proteins, vitamins, also other constituents which have the valuable nutritional outcome [42].

11.5.2 NUTRACEUTICAL'S REGULATORY ASPECTS IN INDIA

Nutraceuticals, in India, are for the most field of classifications called functional foods (braced food items and beverages) and dietary add-on (minerals, vitamins, protein supplements, and herbal products). As pharmaceuticals are under the supervision of the Drugs and Cosmetic Act of 1940, where nutraceuticals are commonly exempted from this act. Hence, Numerous other acts had come in force for governance of nutraceuticals. Like, Prevention of Food Adulteration Act was passed in 1954, Alike, the Meat Food Products Order in 1973, the Edible Oils Packaging (Regulation) Order in 1998. Fruit Product Order was approved in 1955, and Essential Commodities Act in 1955 subject to food were created [42, 47]. To drive the whole Act under solo rooftop and to unite together licensing process, alike application form and process for food industry registration, central licensing, safety, and sanitary and hygienic conditions, the Prime Minister's chamber on industry and trade delegated as single regulatory authority for food in 1998 that recommends a unified rule for agricultural and food industries. In 2002, a nonprofit national association was established with the prime objectives of this association were that every food manufacturer must provide scientific proof of safety and efficacy of their product to consumers. In 2003, the Health Ministry expert group for food law reported these products mandatory safety determination [40]. In 2005, parliament's standing committees on agriculture and other committees given in their twelfth document, which dictates a solo regulatory body and law integrated. Eventually, the Indian government executed the Food Safety and Standards Authority of India (FSSAI) in 2006. This act was formed to coordinate laws of food safety in the nation to systematically and scientifically build-up for industries engaged in food processing and to make a change in perspective from a regulatory routine to self-consistence. The act came with 2 core objectives: (i) to include a solo statute relating to food and (ii) to provide scientific advancement for industries in food processing. These products regulatory guidance all over their life cycle should be known for effectual marketing techniques, like, a quick and cost effectual forms.

The industrial regulatory prerequisites include product registration, yet in addition necessities from their development to post-marketing surveillance, such as site registration, approval process, report, and recall plan, has to be submitted. The FSSA consist of 12 parts with two schedules and 101 areas. An aggregate of 8 rules under FSSA (2006) controls the food segment and built up FSSAI, that manages the division and other united panels, including the chairperson and 22 individuals from the FSSAI. The FSSAI chairperson can be either a government official, of position not lower than of secretary, or a prominent food scientist. Seven ex-officio individuals from various services are present and they ought not be below the joint secretary post. By rotation, five individuals are appointed at every three years, from the states as well union territories. The Authority has two delegates each from food industry and consumer associations, two individuals from the association of farmers, three food technologists, and one member from a retail organization. FSSAI functions with an Advisory Committee along with numerous scientific panels to set standards for food safety. They give rules on different issues, like, ingredients specifications, pollutants, pesticide, label, biological risk, and others, for maintaining food standard. The D and C Rules of 1945 and its Schedule Y regulate the numerous facets dealing with exploration, development, and utilization of phytopharmaceuticals. It describes the information/data required for approval in India for clinical trials and/or to import/production new medications for marketing. For this reason, it is accordingly outlined to globally approved formats, suchlike criteria for ICH (International Council for Harmonization) and FDA. There are several subsections of appendices dealing with the dissimilar features included in this regulatory exercise. It also incorporates New Drug Approval Committee and a New Drug Advisory Committee. According to the Gazette Notification (GSR 702) of 2013, a phytopharmaceutical drug incorporates plants derived crude or processed standard material or portions thereof or blend of plants portions, concentrates, or formulation's fraction for internal/external utilization by animals/humans and is expected to be utilized for determination, treatment, prevention/mitigation of any ailment or disorder in animals/humans, however does exclude parenteral route administration. Recently, the unprocessed standardized material term should not be utilized has been endorsed [38].

11.5.3   REGISTRATION AND LICENSING REQUIREMENTS

A manufacturer cannot start his/her business until he/she is registered or is been licensed in a valid manner. The inspection of premises is carried out after the issue of ID number in the way which is ordered by FSSAI act by the safety official. Under this regulation, the license which is granted shall be in effect and existing, until not specified, for 15 years period. Manufacturers have to register with the state office commissioner and those makers with larger than 12 lakhs turnover to have to validly get a license from FSSAI office. Even the same goes for petty food manufacturer. In form B of schedule 2, a license grant application shall be prepared, it should be filled so that the license can be granted. And within 60 days this permit should be issued from the application ID number issue date.

11.5.4 NECESSITIES FOR INGRESS IN INDIAN NUTRACEUTICAL MARKET

Concerning advancing situation in the region of nutraceuticals in India, it is basic to streamline and amend rules from time to time. Important aspects to consider are product evaluation, product analysis, license procurement, and development of specific health claims. Formulations are commonly used; therefore, in quantity assessment, proper measurement of each ingredient should be taken care of. The active constituent with additives should be evaluated with reference to factors like regulations that have taken care of many of these complications, however there is always potential for updating and amendment, keeping in view the continually evolving scenario. The D and C Rule (1945) together with the FSSAI (2006) guarantee that many of these contentious complications are settled. Taking into account the existing overlap in the different classes of nutraceutical nomenclature, a portion of these rules should be returned to, streamlined, and refined in the intrigue of the consumer and other stakeholders in the nutraceutical market [37].

11.6 INTELLECTUAL PROPERTY GENERATED

In the nutraceutical industry, rights for intellectual property are a significant deliberation. Speculation in licensed innovation rights, suchlike, trademarks, and patents protect nutraceutical from contenders and makes organizations more significant and profitable and pleasing to investors. A new product launching by a nutraceutical organization should take into accounts about the kinds of intellectual property protection by patents, trademarks, and trade secrets [30].

11.6.1 PATENT

The patent law concedes a patentee's exclusive power by law to acquire commercial benefits out of his innovation with an intention to motivate inventors to contribute their intellectual understanding, realizing that for a particular time, nobody else would be capable of duplicating their innovation. In India, the patent is granted for 20 years from the date filling. Although, for approved patents pursuant to filed applications under the PT, the 20 years span starts from the international filing date. Patent protection is accessible for the two products and processes [25].

US has patented a patent regarding the improvement in nutraceutical bioavailability by formulation that induces micro ionization and sustain deliverance. The innovative procedure can be utilized to enhance solubility and lipophilic bioavailability and moderately water dissoluble nutraceuticals by incorporating excipients that increases solubility and SR of active compound. Appropriate pharmaceutical compositions covering aerosol delivery to a subject that incorporate curcumin lipid vehicle dispersion, wherein the lipid has a temperature transition of smaller than about 15°C. Additionally, techniques for pathological condition treatment in a subject that incorporate giving asserted pharmaceutical compositions and its administering to the subject are divulged. For instance, hyperproliferative disorder may be a pathological condition, similar to malignant growth, a pulmonary disease, or an inflammatory disease.

11.6.2 CLINICAL TRIAL

The regular credence that if a polyherbal formulation has been prepared as per the conventional system of medicine, it will undoubtedly effective and safe is untrue. If one might desire the herbal formulation to have an edge over the vying then health benefit assert is necessary. Well framed dual blind randomized clinical trials can demonstrate alike healthy assert. Traditional system has a protocol designed to achieve the client's definite requisites in the area of clinical enrollment of novel pharmaceutical product from phase 1 to phase 4 including bioequivalence, bioavailability, pharmacokinetic or pharmacodynamic study statistical assessment and data management stringently clinging to ICH and GCP (good clinical practice) rules. According to regulations, the justification for nutraceutical's benefits is required through clinical and scientific proof for their therapeutic claim for market compliance.

11.7 FUTURE PERSPECTIVES

SDs has prominent potential both for increasing the drug's bioavailability and control release formulation development. In this way, to resolve issues of bioavailability as for inadequately water-dissolvable drugs, method for SDs has quickly developed. The development of formulation with its preparation utilizing modest quantities of drugs substances in beginning times of drug advancement methods. Although SDs have numerous advantages, issues with preparation, reproducibility, formulation, scale-up and stability has restricted its utilization in commercial formulation for inadequately water-dissolvable drugs [35]. For pre-clinical, clinical, and commercial utilization, the SDs systems effective advancement has been workable from last few years owing to accessibility of self-emulsifying and surface-active carriers with low melting. The formulation preparation includes the medication in melted carriers solubilization and the filling of the hot solution into hard gelatin capsule on account of the uncomplicated manufacturing and scale-up operations, the physicochemical attributes, and thus, the SDs bioavailability are not expected to essentially vary through the scale-up. Owing to this reason, the solid dispersion system's popularity to resolve troublesome bioavailability issues of ineffectively water-dissoluble medications will quickly extend. As the formulation, can be evolved and produced utilizing dash of medication substance in initial drug development stage, the system may have a superiority over such other generally utilized bioavailability upgrading methods, suchlike, micritization, and soft gelatin encapsulation [16]. For solid dispersion, one significant point to focus on in upcoming research will be recognizing self-emulsifying and new surface-active carriers for strong scattering. Presently for oral usage, just a few such carriers are accessible. A few carriers for topical uses of drug might be capable for oral application by performing suitable toxicological testing. In development of SDs systems one constraint is insufficient drug dissolvability in carrier, so a more extensive selection of carrier, will expand the dosage accomplishment from development.

11.8 CONCLUSION

After looking at literature and current works on Nutraceuticals, one can easily conclude that its usage in numerous forms is widely increasing for the various prophylactic as well as therapeutic reasons. That led to noticeable crash on health care cost in India and globally. Though there is noteworthy guarantee of Nutraceuticals in the human health advancement and disorder avoidance, so regulatory toxicologist, nutritionists, and health expert, ought to work strategically together to design proper guideline to give a paramount health and therapeutic advantage to humankind. Hence, to uniform the standard of nutraceutical industries, enforcement of regulatory agencies is an essential part. As maximum promising nutraceuticals are very low water-soluble medications, which may introduce an absence of therapeutic impact, owing to their poor bioavailability. SDs are among the most pleasing procedures to refine drugs' week aqueous solubility. Advancement in the drug-polymer dissoluble, porosity, shapeless division, wettability of particles and amorphous fraction may enhance the solid dispersion's stability and efficiency of 3rd generation. SDs may improve drugs dissolution profile with poorly water-soluble but deliberation is needed for these systems stability. Still in a solid dispersion, carrier along with drug's physicochemical stability is a vital development issue, hence future research requires to focus and list the numerous stability issues. As stated, earlier improvement in drug-polymer solubility, amorphous, fraction, practical porosity with wettability results in drastic increase the stability and efficiency of solid dispersion, furthermore novel optimized manufacturing methods which are efficient also on the way for academic and commercial research whose validation and measurement of the method will be an integral part.

KEYWORDS

- **Dietary Supplement Health and Education Act**
- **Food and Drug Administration**
- **gastrointestinal tract**
- **generally recognized as safe**
- **nutraceuticals**
- **oil/water/oil**
- **over the counter**
- **quality control**
- **SDs technique**
- **solid dispersion**

REFERENCES

1. Prakash, V., Martinus, A. J. S., & Van, B., (2010). Nutraceuticals: Possible future ingredients and food safety aspects. *Ensuring Global Food Safety* (pp. 333–338). Academic Press.

2. Dudeja, P., & Singh, A., (2016). Let food be your medicine and medicine be your food: A step forward for celiac disease cases. *Indian Journal of Nutrition.,* 1–3.

3. Paolo, A. M., Pier, S. C., Francesco, M., Giacinto, M., Lorenzo, M., & Daniele, M. (2014). *Food for Healthy Living and Active Ageing* (Vol. 203, pp. 32–43). IOS press book. http://ebooks.iospress.nl/publication/37277 (accessed on 31 July 2021).

4. Williams, R. J., Kochupurackal, P. M., & Philip, M. B., (2015). *Neuro-Nutraceuticals: The Path to Brain Health Via Nourishment is Not So Distant* (pp. 1–6). NCS. https://doi.org/10.1016/j.neuint.2015.08.012.

5. Sharma, V., et al., (2016). The nutraceutical amino acids-nature's fortification for robust health. *Br. J Pharm [Online],* 1–20. http://www.sdiarticle2.org/prh/BJPR_14/2016/Revised-ms_BJPR_24415_v1.pdf (accessed on 31 July 2021).

6. Latham, M. C., (2014). Perspective on nutritional problems in developing countries: Nutrition security through community agriculture. *Improving Diets and Nutrition,* 1.

7. Bagchi, D., (2019). *Nutraceutical and Functional Food Regulations in the United States and Around the World* (2nd edn., pp. 257–562). Academic Press.

8. No-Seong, K., David, J. J., (2001). Functional foods. Part 1. the development of a regulatory concept. *Food Control,* 99–107.

9. Télessy, I. G., (2019). Nutraceuticals. *The Role of Functional Food Security in Global Health* (pp. 409–421). Academic Press.

10. McClements, D. J., Fang, L., & Hang, X., (2015). The nutraceutical bioavailability classification scheme: Classifying nutraceuticals according to factors limiting their oral bioavailability. *Annual Review of Food Science and Technology,* 299–327.

11. Gonzales, G. B., (2016). Flavonoid-gastrointestinal mucus interaction and its potential role in regulating flavonoid bioavailability and mucosal biophysical properties. *Food Research International.* 342–347.

12. Acosta, E., (2009). Bioavailability of nanoparticles in nutrient and nutraceutical delivery. *Current Opinion in Colloid & Interface Science,* 3–15.

13. Madaan, T., (2017). Lutein, a versatile photo-nutraceutical: An insight on pharmacology, therapeutic indications, challenges, and recent advances in drug delivery. *Pharma Nutrition,* 64–75.

14. Montes, C., Ma Jesús, V., & Ángel, R., (2019). Analytical control of nanodelivery lipid-based systems for encapsulation of nutraceuticals: Achievements and challenges. *Trends in Food Science & Technology.*

15. Mahabir, S., (2014). Methodological challenges conducting epidemiological research on nutraceuticals in health and disease. *Pharma Nutrition,* 120–125.

16. Kawabata, Y., (2011). Formulation design for poorly water-soluble drugs based on biopharmaceutics classification system: Basic approaches and practical applications. *International Journal of Pharmaceutics,* 1–10.

17. Miller, J. M., (2012). A win win solution in oral delivery of lipophilic drugs: Supersaturation via amorphous solid dispersions increases apparent solubility without sacrifice of intestinal membrane permeability. *Molecular Pharmaceutics,* 2009–2016.

18. Khadka, P., (2014). Pharmaceutical particle technologies: An approach to improve drug solubility, dissolution and bioavailability. *Asian Journal of Pharmaceutical Sciences*, 304–316.

19. Hasegawa, A., (1986). Solid dispersions of poorly water-soluble drugs with enteric coating agents. *Journal of Pharmacobio-Dynamics*. [Online] https://ci.nii.ac.jp/naid/110003638244/ (accessed June 12, 2019).

20. Baghel, S., Helen, C., & O'Reilly, N. J., (2016). Polymeric amorphous solid dispersions: A review of amorphization, crystallization, stabilization, solid-state characterization, and aqueous solubilization of biopharmaceutical classification system class II drugs. *Journal of Pharmaceutical Sciences*, 2527–2544.

21. Vasconcelos, T., Bruno, S., & Paulo, C., (2007). Solid dispersions as strategy to improve oral bioavailability of poor water-soluble drugs. *Drug Discovery Today*, 1068–1075.

22. Le-Ngoc, C. V., Chulhun, P., & Beom-Jin, L., (2013). Current trends and future perspectives of solid dispersions containing poorly water-soluble drugs. *European Journal of Pharmaceutics and Biopharmaceutics*, 799–813.

23. Van, D., & Guy, V. D. M., (2016). The role of the carrier in the formulation of pharmaceutical solid dispersions. Part I: Crystalline and semi-crystalline carriers. *Expert Opinion on Drug Delivery*, 1583–1594.

24. Rehman, S., (2019). Polysaccharide-based amorphous solid dispersions (ASDs) for improving solubility and bioavailability of drugs. *Polysaccharide Carriers for Drug Delivery*, 271.

25. Posner, R. A., (2005). Intellectual property: The law and economics approach. *Journal of Economic Perspectives*, 57–73.

26. Paudel, A., & Guy, V. D. M., (2012). Influence of solvent composition on the miscibility and physical stability of naproxen/PVP K 25 solid dispersions prepared by cosolvent spray-drying. *Pharmaceutical Research, 29*(1), 251–270.

27. Zhang, X., (2018). Pharmaceutical dispersion techniques for dissolution and bioavailability enhancement of poorly water-soluble drugs. *Pharmaceutics*, 74.

28. Hallouard, F., (2016). Solid dispersions for oral administration: An overview of the methods for their preparation. *Current Pharmaceutical Design*, 4942–4958.

29. Van, D. M. G., (2012). The use of amorphous solid dispersions: A formulation strategy to overcome poor solubility and dissolution rate. *Drug Discovery Today: Technologies*, 79–85.

30. Chaudhary, A., & Neetu, S., (2012). Intellectual property rights and patents in perspective of Ayurveda. *Ayu*. 20.

31. Singh, J., Manpreet, W., & Harikumar, S. L., (2013). Solubility enhancement by solid dispersion method: A review. *Journal of Drug Delivery and Therapeutics, 3*(5), 148–155. https://doi.org/10.22270/jddt.v3i5.632.

32. Aleksovski, A., Chris, V., & Rok, D., (2016). Hot-melt extrusion and prilling as contemporary and promising techniques in the solvent free production of solid oral dosage forms, based on solid dispersions. *Maced. Pharm. Bull., 62*, 3–24.

33. Das, S. K., (2012). Solid dispersions an approach to enhance the bioavailability of poorly water-soluble drugs. *International Journal of Pharmacology and Pharmaceutical Technology*, 37–46.

34. Karavas, E., (2007). Investigation of the release mechanism of a sparingly water-soluble drug from solid dispersions in hydrophilic carriers based on physical state of

drug, particle size distribution and drug-polymer interactions. *European Journal of Pharmaceutics and Biopharmaceutics*, 334–347.

35. Deshmane, S., (2018). Enhancement of solubility and bioavailability of ambrisentan by solid dispersion using *Daucus carota* as a drug carrier: Formulation, characterization, *in vitro*, and *in vivo* study. *Drug Development and Industrial Pharmacy*, 1001–1011.

36. Langham, Z. A., (2012). Mechanistic insights into the dissolution of spray-dried amorphous solid dispersions. *Journal of Pharmaceutical Sciences*, 2798–2810.

37. Singh, A. K., (2018). *Nutraceuticals: Meaning and Regulatory Scenario. Pharma Innovation.* 7(8), 448–451.

38. Nooreen, Z., Vineet, K. R., & Narayan, P. Y., (2018). Phytopharmaceuticals: A new class of drug in India. *Ann. Phytomed.*, 7(1), 27–37.

39. Ngoc-Gia, T. N., (2015). Dissolution enhancement of curcumin by solid dispersion with polyethylene glycol 6000 and hydroxypropyl methylcellulose. In: 5th *International Conference on Biomedical Engineering in Vietnam*. Springer, Cham.

40. Ahmad, & Faruque, M., (2011). Nutraceutical market and its regulation. *Am. J. Food Technol.*, 342–347.

41. Crowley, M. M., (2002). Stability of polyethylene oxide in matrix tablets prepared by hot-melt extrusion. *Biomaterials*, 4241–4248.

42. Yadav, Sanjay, K., Patil, S. M., & Gupta, S. K., (2013). Nutraceutical a bright scope and opportunity of Indian healthcare market. *International Journal of Research and Development in Pharmacy and Life Sciences*, 478–481.

43. Paudel, A., (2013). Manufacturing of solid dispersions of poorly water-soluble drugs by spray drying: Formulation and process considerations. *International Journal of Pharmaceutics*, 253–284.

44. Niwa, T., & Kazumi, D., (2013). Design of self-dispersible dry nanosuspension through wet milling and spray freeze-drying for poorly water-soluble drugs. *European Journal of Pharmaceutical Sciences*, 272–281.

45. Zhang, X., et al., (2009). Piroxicam/2-hydroxypropyl-β-cyclodextrin inclusion complex prepared by a new fluid-bed coating technique. *Journal of Pharmaceutical Sciences*, 665–675.

46. Lu, Y., et al., (2009). Physical characterization of meloxicam-β-cyclodextrin inclusion complex pellets prepared by a fluid-bed coating method. *Particuology*, 1–8.

47. Ray, A., Jagdish, J., & Kavita, G., (2016). Regulatory aspects of nutraceuticals: An Indian perspective. *Nutraceuticals*, 941–946. Academic Press.

CHAPTER 12

Potential Applications of Polyelectrolyte Complexes in Pharmaceutical and Nutraceutical Delivery

CHANDRAKANTSING V. PARDESHI,[1] DEBARSHI KAR MAHAPATRA,[2] VEENA S. BELGAMWAR,[3] and SANJAY J. SURANA[1]

[1]R. C. Patel Institute of Pharmaceutical Education and Research, Shirpur, Maharashtra, India, Tel.: +91-9881414752, E-mail: chandrakantpardeshi11@gmail.com (C. V. Pardeshi)

[2]Department of Pharmaceutical Chemistry, Dadasaheb Balpande College of Pharmacy, Nagpur, Maharashtra, India

[3]Department of Pharmaceutical Sciences, RTM Nagpur University, Nagpur, Maharashtra, India

ABSTRACT

The polyelectrolyte complexes (PECs) are multifaceted carriers normally formed by electrostatic interactions amid oppositely charged polyions. High biocompatibility, low toxicity, cost-effective, energy-efficient production, excellent biodegradability, and environment-friendly, makes PECs a carrier of preference for extensive multiplicity of utilizations including gene, drug, vaccine delivery, and protein-peptide. The current purpose of this book chapter is to present the discrete descriptions of PECs, mechanism(s) in the formation of PEC, structural models of the PECs, imperative interactions usually involved in the PEC formation, steps involved in the fabrication process of the PEC, critical factors that affect the PECs formation, and biomedical and nutraceutical applications of PECs.

12.1 INTRODUCTION

The electrostatic interactions, often referred to as Coulombic interactions play a dominant role in the polyelectrolyte complexes formation owing to the physical contact of the positively charged polyionic components with the negatively charged polyionic component [1–3]. A very stable and homogeneous nanodispersion having a colloidal dimension range is the typical characteristic of this delivery system [4, 5]. The absence of cross-linking components in the system successfully eliminates the adverse effects as well as toxic responses that are frequently encountered by these agents [6].

The diversified structural features offer different characteristics that favor multifarious scientific applications in cosmetics, tissue engineering, nutraceuticals, biotechnology, pharmacy, biomaterials, biomedicals, medicine, etc. [7]. The non-toxic, biocompatible, and biodegradable nature of these polyelectrolyte complexes make them pharmaceutically privilege for biomedical and therapeutic applications [8].

The book chapter exclusively and comprehensively focuses on the basic aspects of polyelectrolyte complexes, their structural aspects, fabrication techniques, factors affecting the product development, stability aspects, characterization methods, and applications in nutraceutical and pharmaceutical delivery.

12.2 MECHANISM OF PEC FORMATION

As an outcome of strong Coulomb's electrostatic forces, the PECs are developed through the interactions of oppositely charged polyelectrolytes [1–3]. PECs are considered quantitatively as non-stoichiometric (one polymer taken in a surplus quantity compared to another polymer) or stoichiometric (polymers taken in an equimolar ratio) [9].

The global agreement amid the modern-day researchers is that the formation of the PEC is an entropy-oriented occurrence. The causative strength in the creation of PECs in the aqueous solutions is the liberation of low molecular weight counterions (that were beforehand connected with the charged groups over the chains of polymer) that leads to an increase in the levels of entropy by the prevailing system [10–12]. Kabanov and Zezin [13] were the first investigators who revealed the complex formation kinetics and stop-flow measurements where they reported <5 ms time in the formation of the complex [13].

The PEC formation mechanism may be studied from the overall consequence of both counteracting processes [12] *viz.*

- Electrostatic charge recompense leads to the arranging of two oppositely charged (positive and negative) polyions to a complex molecule and this happens in connection with supportive outcomes bringing some conformational alteration complimentary for mutual charge recompense;
- A "disorganized" aggregation of polycations and polyanions with merely limited mutual charge recompense and a substantial amount of ionic position still charge-compensated by these low molecular weight counterions.

The primary PEC formation mechanism, as exemplified in Figure 12.1, it entails three chief steps *viz.*

- Primary complex formation;
- New bond formation within the intracomplexes; and
- Intercomplex aggregation.

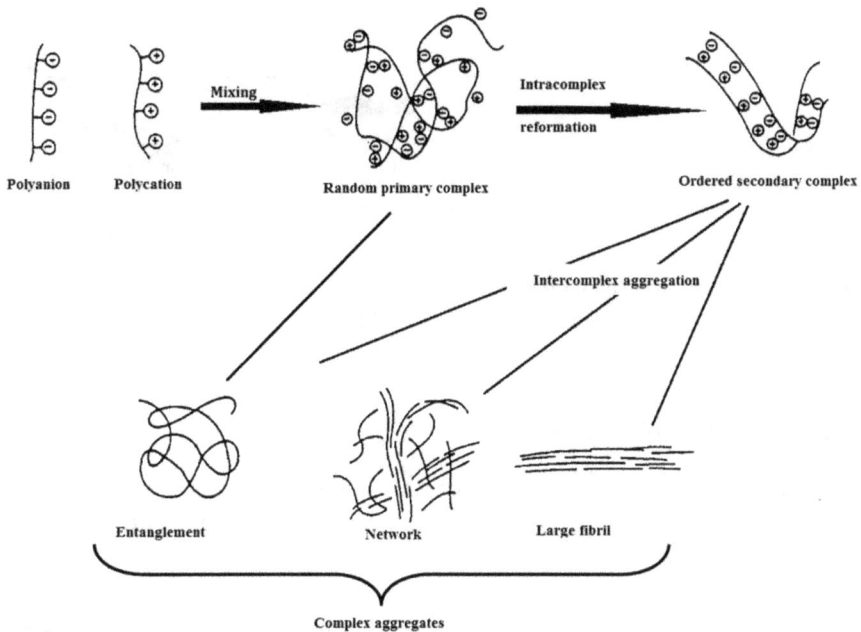

FIGURE 12.1 Depiction of the major steps in the aggregation of the PECs.

Source: Modified after Tsuchida [14].

Instantly subsequent to the combination of contrary charged polyelectrolyte solutions, the initial action continues rapidly with the organization of Coulomb's interactions, the secondary binding force. The subsequent stride advances within an hour and engrosses the development of novel bonds and/or the modification of the alteration of the polymer chains to characterize new polymer chain conformation. The final action engrosses the secondary complexes aggregation, chiefly via the hydrophobic interactive forces. The ultimate PECs aggregates are usually insoluble in regular solvents, and the polymer constituent's molar ratio in the aggregates is approximately unity [14].

On the basis of the supermolecular order of the PEC polymeric chains, two models (Figure 12.2) have been proposed; *Scrambled egg* model with disordered packing and *ladder-like* model with an ordered chain packing [11]. From every investigational validation accessible nowadays, it has been concluded that the above-mentioned models correspond to the restrictive cases, with the authenticity being active in linking these two models, but the earlier to the final than to the previous model [12].

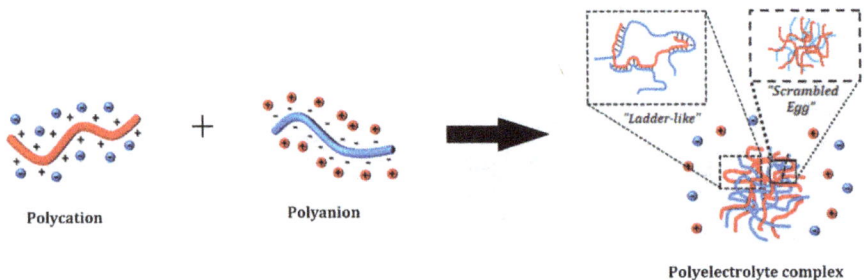

FIGURE 12.2   Mechanism(s) of the formation of PEC.
Source: Reprinted with permission from Pergushov, Muller, and Schacher [11]. © 2012 Royal Society of Chemistry.

12.3   STRUCTURAL MODELS OF PECS

The types of structures reported from polycation-polyanion interactions in the solution; *viz.* (i) water-soluble; (ii) colloidally stable; and (iii) two-phase systems [7].

At the molecular scale, these *water-soluble* aggregates are produced when the polyelectrolytes comprised of several weak ionic groups and outsized disparity in the molar mass of the components are combined in a non-stoichiometric ratio (where the ratio of anionic functional groups to the cationic functional groups is either < 1 or > 1. These structures comprise of sequentially complexed long host molecules with a shorter guest opposite charge poly-ions. The stability of water-soluble PECs is greatly affected by the charge ratio of the polyelectrolytes and the soluble salts concentration. The components coexist in the solution with colloidally stable PECs and show precipitation [7, 16].

Macroscopically heterogeneous systems and highly aggregated systems are seen when high molecular weight polyelectrolytes are employed for the formation of the complex. At the molecular scale, water-soluble aggregates are formed when polyelectrolytes of dissimilar molar masses are mixed in non-stoichiometric ratios. Although, these aggregation process may be halted at moderate to low ionic strengths under non-stoichiometric conditions in enormously diluted solutions, to form *colloidally stable* PECs [16, 17].

The *two-phase systems* are formed by mixing the high molecular weight polyelectrolytes at higher concentrations and nearer the stoichiometric ratio where a PECs-rich phase and a liquid phase exist. The salt concentrations and properties of the polyelectrolytes directly influence the rheological characteristics of the PECs-rich phase. The characteristics are comparable to the soft-solids or component having liquid-like properties, that are known as complex coacervates [17].

12.4   INTERACTIONS INVOLVED IN PEC FORMATION

The chief interactions that exist between the polyelectrolytes during the complex formation are the hydrophobic interactions, Coulomb's interactions, dipole interactions, hydrogen bonding, and Van der Waals interactions [7, 9, 12, 16]. The intermolecular interaction that strongly exist between the polyanion and polycation in the formation of the complex is often referred to as *Coulomb's interactions*. The formation of the PECs through this process is dependent on the polymeric nature. Sæther et al. [18] projected the core-shell model of the PECs on the basis of electrostatic interactions between the alginate and chitosan (CHT) (Figure 12.3).

The formation of small, non-aggregating particles has been seen when the zeta potential has higher values (either negative or positive) under the excess concentration of alginate or CHT. Owing to a surplus quantity of the major constituent, this non-aggregating behavior is perceived as a result of a steady shell around every particle. At $K\sim1$, at the intersect from the negative zeta potential value to positive zeta potential value, an enhancement in the PECs average size is seen owing to the formation of aggregates and flocks. An analogous result was monitored in close proximity to the net charge neutrality for dextran sulfate and CHT [2]. The potential to assemble big agglomerates or aggregates chiefly takes place closer to $K\sim1$. Figure 12.4 corresponds to the formation methodology and structural model of the PECs signifying the core-shell topography of the prepared PECs [18].

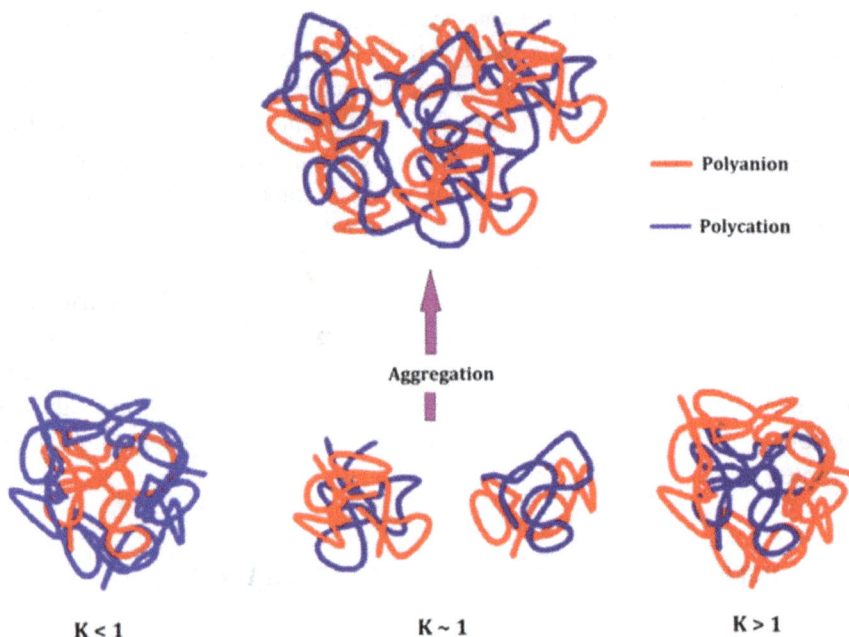

FIGURE 12.3   Representation of the core-shell model for PECs of chitosan (polycation) with alginate (polyanion) at various net charge ratios.

Source: Reproduced from: Sæther et al. [18]; with kind permission of Elsevier.

12.5   FABRICATION OF PECS

The polyelectrolyte complexes are in general prepared by three approaches which are discussed in subsections [20].

12.5.1   INITIALLY PREPARING THE POLYELECTROLYTE SOLUTION

In an appropriate dispersion medium (such as deionized (DI) water), the positively charged polyelectrolyte and the negatively charged polyelectrolyte are dispersed in a range of concentrations or stoichiometric ratios or molar concentrations to produce the required solutions. The desired ionic strength is achieved by employing the polysalt such as NaCl and penultimately, the desired value of pH is achieved through adjustment. The above content was filtered through a Millipore membrane of average pore size 0.22 μm.

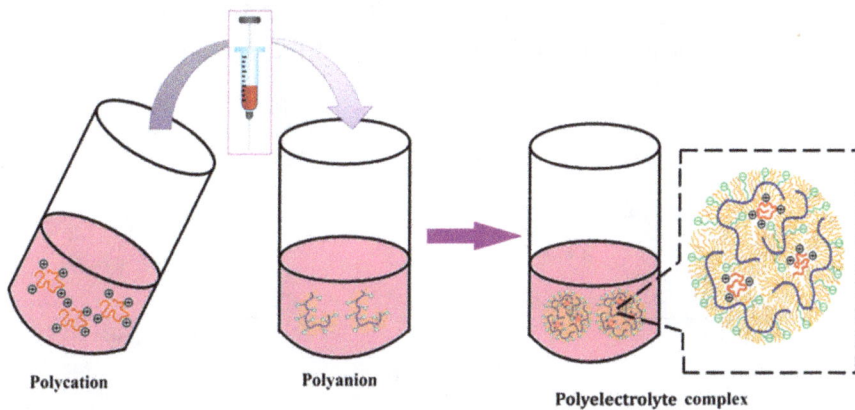

FIGURE 12.4 Formulation methods involved in the PEC formation and structural model of the PECs on the basis of polymer chains arrangement.
Source: Reprinted with permission from Lu et al. [19]. © 2016. Elsevier

12.5.2 PEC FORMATION

The solutions of polyanion and solutions of polycation act as the starting material for the polyelectrolyte complexes formation at room temperature. The fabrication of polyelectrolyte complexes involves adding the solution of a polyelectrolyte at a single-go to another solution of the polyelectrolyte of comparable ionic potency at the room temperature under a constant stirring condition. In other technique, slow dropwise addition of a particular solution of a polyelectrolyte with slow manual stirring also yields polyelectrolyte complexes.

12.5.3 PARTICLE REFINEMENT

For the complete removal or avoidance of physical adsorption of the free polymers over the previously fabricated polyelectrolyte complexes, the process of centrifugation is typically employed for the particle refinement. The acquired product was then lyophilized for improving the stability characteristics and further re-suspended in a little quantity of DI water.

12.6 FACTORS AFFECTING THE FORMATION AND STABILITY OF PEC PARTICLES

A polymer-rich phase (referred to as milky phase) gets separated from the polymer-depleted phase (referred to as clear phase) when the oppositely charged polyelectrolytes are mixed [21]. Figure 12.5 depicts a variety of factors that critically affects the formation and the overall stability of the PECs.

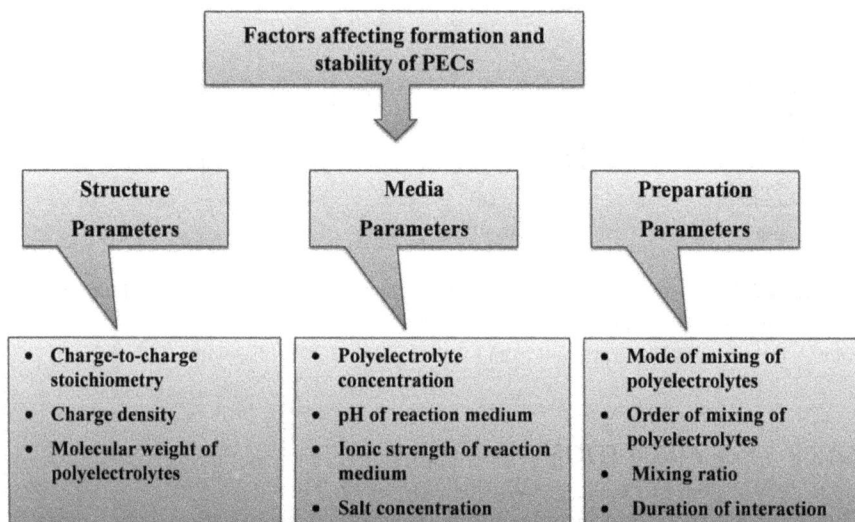

FIGURE 12.5   Illustrative representation of various factors affecting the formation and stability of PECs.

12.6.1   *CHARGE-TO-CHARGE STOICHIOMETRY*

For exploring the complexation in a polyelectrolyte formulation, the positive charge net ratio to the negative charge net ratio (oppositely charged), which is often referred to as *charge ratio*, should be immensely studied. It is represented by 'Z' and is depicted as (+/– or –/+) in subscripted form. The symbol Φ signifies the stoichiometry of the charge-to-charge ratio in the formed PECs. S-PECs (Φ=1) are adequately hydrophobic owing to the reciprocal vetting of the charges and impetuous from the aqueous solution. If the N-PECs (Φ=1) are developed, the overcharging consequences owing to moreover surplus polyanion or polycation can be perceived [11].

12.6.2 CHARGE DENSITY

Dautzenberg and coworkers [22], represented the role of charge density over the acrylamide anionic copolymers and acrylamide cationic copolymers PEC properties. The researchers scrutinized that for equivalent charge density of the polyelectrolyte constituents, the simplex particles assume a compacted organization, whereas in systems with a stalwartly contrary charge density of the polyelectrolyte constituents a slack fluctuating organization exists. Newly, it has been depicted that the contentious observation with anionic poly(styrenesulfonate) (PSS) and cationic methacryloxyethyl trimethylammonium (METAC). At 1:1 stoichiometric ratio, as a decline in charge density is observed, the amount of soluble PECs is obtained as a result of reduced hydrodynamic size (~20 nm) with augmented stability.

12.6.3 MOLECULAR WEIGHT

In recent times, Hu and coworkers [23] presented the possible outcomes of the molecular weight of CHT over the overall dimensions of the carboxymethylpachyman (CMP)/CHT PEC nanoparticles. An enhanced size in the particle (from 135 nm to 279 nm) is reported when the molecular weight is augmented from 12,000 g/mole to 46,000 g/mole. It was concluded by the researchers that positively charged long chains of CHT molecules complexed with large amounts of CMP molecules of negative charge.

12.6.4 POLYELECTROLYTE CONCENTRATION

Schatz et al. [2] reported the augmentation in the dimension of the CHT/DS biopolyelectrolyte complex particles with a rising DS concentration, however, merely at a very high mixing ratio (n^+/n^-). Muller et al. [21] recommended that enhancing the polyelectrolyte concentration and through range dispersive interactions in a primary to secondary PEC particle aggregation model have shown abridged electrostatic revulsion amongst the similarly-charged primary PEC particles which contributed towards superior dispersive attraction. Additionally, an augmentation in the concentration of the polyelectrolyte may moreover result in a huge amount of primary PEC particles per volume, which further leads to the formation of larger secondary PEC particles. Beyond the definite concentration of polyelectrolyte, precipitation may result.

12.6.5   pH

Fukuda and Kikuchi [24] studied the influence of high pH and low pH over the PECs formation between dextran sulfate sodium and CHT [24]. The authors concluded that diverse molecular structures of the complexes were produced under different conditions of pH.

Muller et al. [21] studied the influence of high pH and low pH over the PECs particle size which comprised of poly(acrylic acid) (PAC) and weak polyelectrolytes poly(ethyleneimine) (PEI) at mixing ratio of $X= 1.5$. The investigators found that with a decrease in the values of pH from pH-10, pH-8.5, pH-7, and pH-4 of the PEI solution, the particle size got decreased concurrently from 400 nm to ~160 nm at constant pH of PAC solution. Owing to the mutual electrostatic repulsion, a lesser coagulation propensity of the highly charged PEI/PAC particles was observed at lower pH as compared to the low charged particles at higher pH owing to the electrostatic attractive forces.

12.6.6   IONIC STRENGTH

The dimensions of the final PEC formulations depend immensely on the polyelectrolytes' ionic strength. A lessening in the average diameter of the PEC is observed with the enhanced ionic strength due to the amplification in the chain flexibility [16]. The complexation can result exclusively at the particular pH values in the environs of the *p*Ka interval between the two polyelectrolytes. The polyelectrolytes during the complexation process led to the formation of a less compact hydrogel or coacervate. Precipitation may result when the ionic strength is excessively strong [25].

12.6.7   MODE OF MIXING POLYELECTROLYTE SOLUTIONS

The mixing protocol, the mixing type, and the application of the device largely influence the PECs formation. Ankerfors and coworkers [26], highlighted the role of the mixing procedure in the complexation of PAC with poly(allylamine) (PAH) and further compared with the jet mixing technique employed for the colloids. The study revealed the appearance of small PECs at short mixing times for low molecular weight polyelectrolytes whereas initial dwindle in the PEC size is perceived with a reduction in the mixing time when high molecular weight polyelectrolytes are used, which further starts to augment as a result of adequately rapid formation of diffusion-controlled stable *pre-complexes*. Although, aggregation of non-equilibrium pre-complexes tends to occur when larger polyelectrolytes are employed. It was concluded that colloid titration gave larger PECs whereas jet mixing offered smaller PECs and thereby allowed sufficient mixing time to effectually maintain the PEC size [26]. Sæther et al. [18] detected that the application of high mixing speed through Ultra-Turrax procedure leads to shrinkage in the average particle size of CHT-alginate PECs [18].

12.6.8 ORDER OF ADDITION

The polyelectrolytes addition order may affect the final formulation and many researchers studied the slow mixing of polyelectrolyte solutions with one another [27]. Schatz et al. [2] studied the effect of dropwise slow mixing and compared it with the one-shot rapid mixing in the preparation of CHT-DS PECs. The PECs produced from one-shot rapid mixing was much smaller in terms of diameter as compared to the dropwise slow mixing. The mixing order was critical while adding the solution of the titrant carefully dropwise into the solution of the starting content. Even to avoid the formation of aggregates, the polymer must be added in excess. On the contrary, the order of addition requirement for the one-shot titrant solution addition technique is insensible and a kinetically-driven process takes place in the particle formation [2].

12.6.9 MIXING RATIO

The effect of mixing ratio (X) over the PEC particle size and molecular weight was studied by Dautzenberg [28] employing PSS and poly (diallyldimethylammonium chloride) (PDADMAC). The researchers suggested that when the mixing ratio is increased under saltless condition, a considerable reduction in the particle size from 400 nm ($X = 0.1$) to 200 nm ($X=1.0$) was observed along with an insignificant lessening in the molecular weight. The coiling of the mutual charge-compensated chains might be the reason for the above influence at 1:1 stoichiometry owing to enhancement in the structural density. In contrast to it, under-salted system, lower aggregation characteristics are seen along with an augmentation in the particle size from 50 nm ($X = 0.1$) to about 120 nm ($X = 1.0$) [28].

12.6.10   SALT CONCENTRATION

The properties of the PECs are chiefly affected by the concentration of salt and can be studied truly at complexation levels or after complexation levels.

Dautzenberg [28] studied the influence of 0.01 M and 0.1 M of salt (NaCl) concentration in the formation of PDADMAC (0.0005 M)/PSS (0.00025 M) PEC particles. In the absence of the salt, the average particle size of the PEC around 300 nm, formed at mixing ratio $X = 0.1$, drastically falls to 130 nm at mixing ratio $X = 0.95$. On the contrary, in the presence of NaCl (0.01 M concentration), the size of PECs of about 40 nm is observed at mixing ratio range $X = 0.1$–0.9 while increasing the salt concentration to 0.1 M, the average particle size of the PECs was 50 nm at mixing ratio $X = 0.1$ which augmented concurrently to 120 nm at mixing ratio $X = 0.95$. The author concluded that larger secondary PECs were formed from the primary PECs under the influence of salt concentration which favored the coagulation process; also, the polyelectrolyte shells shrink to a lesser one in the case of ultimately shaped PEC aggregates [28].

Dautzenberg and Kriz [1] studied the influence of various salts such as NaCl, LiCl, and KCl over the PEC size formed from polymethacrylate-complexed acrylamide and PDADMAC at a constant mixing ratio of $X = 0.6$. At $C_{NaCl} = 0$, the average PEC size was found to be 70 nm which further augments to 370 nm size at $C_{NaCl} = \sim 0.5$ M, and interestingly the size of PECs again falls to 80 nm at $C_{NaCl} > 0.5$ M. At salt concentrations of 0–0.5 M, a salt-induced aggregation of the small soluble complexes was dominantly seen. A parallel tendency was detected for the other salt forms, which lead to solubilization of small soluble complexes into the polyelectrolyte components [1].

12.7   APPLICATIONS OF PECS

The PEC forming potentials of some imperative synthetic polymers and natural polymers is depicted in Table 12.1.

12.7.1   APPLICATIONS OF PECS IN DRUG DELIVERY

A wide number of applications of PECs have been reported such as chemotherapeutics [29–31], retroviral [22, 32], various gastric conditions (ulcers) [34], anti-bacterial perspectives (infections related to *Staphylococci*) [35], and anti-fungal perspectives (infections related to *Candida*) [36]. Table 12.2 represented the diverse polyanions and polycations, diseases targeted, and therapeutic agents loaded in particular PECs.

TABLE 12.1   List of Natural and Synthetic Polymers Having PEC Forming Potential

Polymer Category	Cationic	Anionic
Natural	Chitosan, poly(L-lysine), dextran, starch, cellulose	Alginate, carrageenan, carboxymethyl cellulose, gelatin, gellan gum, gum kondagogu, hyaluronic acid, pectin, xanthan gum, xyloglucan, g-poly(glutamic acid), maleic starch, polybetaine, heparin, chodroitin sulfate, poly(l-glutamic acid)
Synthetic	Poly(vinylbenzyl trialkyl ammonium), poly(4-vinyl-N-alkyl-pyridimiun), poly(acryloyl-oxyalkyl-trialkyl ammonium), poly(acryamidoalkyl-trialkyl ammonium), poly(diallydimethyl-ammonium), *N,N,N*-trimethyl chitosan	Dextran sulfate, cross-linked-poly(acrylic acid), eudragit (poly(acrylic or methacrylic acid), polyalkylenoxide-maleic acid, poly-(l-aspartic acid), sodium cellulose sulfate, poly(styrenesulfonic acid), poly(vinylsulfonic acid), poly(itaconic acid)

12.7.2   APPLICATIONS OF PECS IN GENE DELIVERY

For the effectual *in vivo* therapeutic genes loaded delivery of non-viral vectors, biocompatible PECs play a critical role in gene therapy. In gene delivery applications, DNA condensation takes place by acting with polycations, which is referred to as polyplexes. This is considered as an effective approach; however, the effectiveness and safety profile of non-viral vectors still remains a major challenge [37]. Table 12.3 depicted the particular PEC systems employed as gene delivery carriers [38–44].

12.7.3   APPLICATIONS OF PECS IN PROTEIN AND PEPTIDE DELIVERY

PECs have shown the possibilities for the therapeutic delivery of proteins or peptides in a laboratory scale. Based on the principle of non-covalent interactions (majorly, hydrophobic interactions and electrostatic interactions) between the protein/peptide (negatively-charged or positively-charged) and

TABLE 12.2   Applications of PECs as Drug Delivery Carriers

Polycation	Polyanion	Drug	Formulation	Target Disease	References
Chitosan	Dextran sulfate	Curcumin	PEC nanoparticles	Cancer	[29]
TMC	Alginate	Curcumin	PEC	Cancer	[30]
Chitosan	Poly(l-malic acid-co-D,L-lactic acid)	Doxorubicin	PEC nanoparticles	Cancer	[31]
Chitosan	Dextran sulfate, heparin	Adenosine 5'-monophosphate monohydrate	PEC nanoparticles	HIV/AIDS	[32]
Chitosan	Dextran sulfate	Tenofovir	PEC nanoparticles	HIV/AIDS	[33]
Chitosan	Carrageenan	NS	PEC	Gastric ulcer	[34]
Chitosan	Neem gum, Hupu gum	Vancomycin	PEC nanoparticles	*Staphylococci* infections	[35]
Eudragit RL 30D	Carboxymethyl kappa carrageenan	Miconazole	Bioadhesive matrix tablets	Fungal infections	[36]

Note: NS: Not specified; TMC: N,N,N-trimethyl chitosan.

TABLE 12.3 Selected Examples of PECs in Gene Delivery Applications

Polycation	Polyanion	Formulation	Therapeutic Outcomes	References
Chitosan	pDNA	Nanocomplex	Nanocomplexes exhibited high pDNA transfection efficiencies in HEK293 cells *in vitro*	[38]
Chitosan	pDNA	Nanocomplexes	ELISA assay revealed an efficient expression of PDGF-BB and FGF-2 with specific antibodies in mice sera	[39]
Polyethylenimine	pDNA	Nanoparticles	Nanoparticles exhibited high transfection efficiency with the gene encoding human urokinase plasminogen activator (Hu-uPA)	[40]
Chitosan	DNA	Chitoplexes	High binding affinity of chitosan to DNA was obtained at pH 5.4 At high charge ratio, the spherical nanocomplexes were formed, without free DNA	[41]
PEI-PEG-PCP	siRNA	Polyplexes	Polyplexes exhibited high VEGF inhibition efficiency in human prostate carcinoma (PC-3) cells	[42]
PEI	siRNA	Polyplexes	High uptake of siRNA by HeLa cells at higher concentration of copolymer used to modify the surface of polyplexes	[43]
PEI-DA	siRNA	Polyplexes	The polyplexes showed high stability against heparin exchange reaction and improved gene silencing efficacy	[19]
PFNBr	siRNA	Nanocomplexes	Nanocomplexes showed enhanced cellular uptake in PANC-1 cells	[44]

Abbreviations: pDNA: Plasmid DNA; PDGFBB: Platelet-derived growth factor-bb; FGF-2: Fibroblast growth factor-2; VEGF: Vascular endothelial growth factor; PEI-PEG-PCP: Prostate cancer-binding peptide (PCP) conjugated with polyethylenimine (PEI) *via* poly(ethylene glycol) (PEG) linker; PEI-DA: Polyethylenimine-modified by deoxycholic acid; PFNBr: Brush-like conjugated polyelectrolyte nanoparticles.

polymers, these PECs are formed [45]. Few reported PECs for the effective delivery of peptide and protein are depicted in Table 12.4 [46–54].

12.7.4   APPLICATIONS OF PECS IN VACCINE DELIVERY

For the delivery of antigenic molecules in the human body, nanoparticulate formulations or microparticulate formulations are recognized as superior carriers that provide better transport of the antigen, superior protection, long-lasting residence at the required location, and also proffer additional effectual antigen recognition by the immune cells [55, 56].

Lately, Verheul et al. [57] formulated ovalbumin-loaded thiolated hyaluronic acid (HA-SH) and thiolated trimethyl chitosan (TMC-SH)-based polyelectrolyte nanocomplexes stabilized covalently for their applications as intradermal vaccine delivery system or nasal delivery system. This stabilized particulate system demonstrated superior immunogenicity as well as adjuvanticity as compared to the non-stabilized system after the intradermal vaccination. The PEGylation process eliminated the valuable effects of the stabilization characteristics after the nasal vaccination while retaining the comparable immunogenicity as the stabilized particles after the intradermal vaccination [57].

12.7.5   APPLICATIONS OF PECS IN TISSUE ENGINEERING

For the effectual delivery of the therapeutically privileged compounds, biocompatible or biodegradable components are employed as support matrices for facilitating the 3D tissue reconstructions [58] such as engineering of bone tissue [59], engineering of cartilage tissue [60], engineering of cardiac tissue [61], and engineering of dental tissue [62, 63].

12.7.6   DIAGNOSTIC AND IMAGING APPLICATIONS OF PECS

Huang et al. [64] highlighted the gadolinium (Gd) based PECs capable of diagnosis through MRI contrast enhancement. The PECs of 300 nm diameter were formed by complex coacervation process employing CHT with dextran sulfate through diethylenetriaminepentaacetic acid (DTPA) chelation. A noteworthy *in vivo* contrast enhancement of PECs combining grafted Gd-DTPA has been observed which showed mass accumulation in the rat kidneys. These modified PECs offered a great enhancement of MRI

TABLE 12.4 Applications of PECs in Protein and Peptide Delivery

Polycation	Polyanion	Therapeutic Protein/Peptide	Formulation	References
Chitosan	Dextran sulfate and alginate	Insulin	PEC nanoparticles	[46]
Chitosan, Polyethylenimine, Poly-L-lysine	Dextran sulfate	VEGF	PEC nanoparticles	[47]
APEG	PMMA	BSA	PEC nanoparticles	[48]
Chitosan, polyethylenimine, Poly-L-lysine	Dextran sulfate	Repifermin®	PEC nanoparticles	[49]
Chitosan	Alginate	bFGF	Scaffolds	[50]
Chitosan	Hyaluronate	Insulin or Vancomycin	Nasal insert	[51]
Chitosan	Alginate	Ovalbumin	Nanocomplex	[52]
Chitosan	Poly(γ-glutamic acid)	SDF-1	Multilayer films	[53]
Chitosan	NaCS and PPS	Lactoferrin	PEC capsules	[54]

Abbreviations: VEGF: Vascular endothelial growth factor; PMMA: Poly(methacrylic acid); APEG: Bis-(2-aminopropyl)poly(ethylene glycol); bFGF: Basic fibroblast growth factor; SDF-1: Stromal-derived factor-1; BSA: Bovine serum albumin; NaCS: Sodium cellulose sulfate, PPS: Sodium polyphosphate.

contrast through delivery vehicles and find possibilities for quantifying drug biodistribution and drug pharmacokinetics [64].

12.7.7   *NUTRACEUTICAL APPLICATIONS OF PECS*

For endorsing the wellbeing of the human population, nutraceuticals enrichment with staple foods presents a promising strategy. For staying fit, reduction of fats in the regular diet is essential, but the required amount of polyunsaturated fatty acids (PUFA), fat-soluble vitamins, anti-oxidants, and hydrophobic nutraceuticals is seldom required. For stabilizing, solubilizing, and protecting the hydrophobic nutraceuticals in aqueous food or stable clear aqueous drinks, novel technologies for the conservation must be taken to incorporate oil-soluble materials. For an ideal vehicle, transparency needs to be maintained through nano-sized (preferably <100 nm) components, comprised of GRAS, natural inexpensive food materials, competent enough in solubilizing and protecting the components in the aqueous media, promoting higher bioavailability, and preserving sensory features. Limited solutions are yet known for overcoming these challenging requirements; however, no system overall satisfies the requirements [65].

To conquer this drawback, Ron and co-workers developed β-lactoglobuline-polysaccharide complexes as nanovehicles for HN (vitamin D_2) in non-fat foods and clear beverages. It has been found that the nanocomplexes provided better protection to the vitamin against degradation than β-lactoglobuline alone, and stability was significantly better than that of unprotected vitamin dispersed in water.

It has been reported that milk protein-based nanoparticles offer great potential for nanoencapsulation of nutraceuticals [66], as many of the milk proteins have naturally evolved to deliver nutrients from mother to neonate. It has also been found that the core-shell nanoparticles of CHT-coated with β-lactoglobuline were proposed for delivery of nutraceuticals [67].

12.8   CONCLUSIONS AND FUTURE PERSPECTIVES

PECs, being stable, biodegradable ad biocompatible formulations, are capable of merging the unique properties of different polymers without losing their inherent characteristics. The particle formation process can be considered as an environmentally friendly, energy-efficient production process utilizing only aqueous solvents and can be carried out at ambient temperature conditions.

Because of their versatility and above-mentioned merits, PECs find utility as a subject of keen interest for the researchers. A pharmaceutical formulation if, along with academic researchers, well accepted by the pharmaceutical industries for commercialization and clinical applications, would be considered as an effective therapeutic formulation. Since, PECs have already been proven their potential in pharmaceutical, biomedical, and other allied fields; they must engage a sizeable place in the nutraceutical market too. It has been observed that the applicability of PECs in nutraceutical delivery is in the preliminary phase, however, it looked positively by the researchers and health professionals, the promising outcomes will definitely bring the PECs-based nutraceutical formulations on the commercial market very soon.

KEYWORDS

- **active pharmaceutical ingredient**
- **adenosine triphosphate**
- **controlled release solid dispersion**
- **foods for special health use**
- **gastrointestinal tract**
- **hydroxypropyl methylcellulose**
- **polyethylene oxide**
- **gadolinium**
- **anions**
- **biomedical applications**
- **cations**
- **electrostatic interactions**
- **nutraceuticals**
- **polyelectrolyte complex**
- **polyions**

REFERENCES

1. Dautzenberg, H., & Kriz, J., (2003). Response of polyelectrolyte complexes to subsequent addition of salts with different cations. *Langmuir, 19,* 5204–5211.

2. Schatz, C., Lucas, J., Viton, C., Domard, A., Pichot, C., & Delair, T., (2004). Formation and Properties of positively charged colloids based on polyelectrolyte complexes of biopolymers. *Langmuir, 20*, 7766–7778.

3. Wu, D., & Delair, T., (2015). Stabilization of chitosan/hyaluronan colloidal polyelectrolyte complexes in physiological conditions. *Carbohydr. Polym., 119*, 149–158.

4. Mao, S., Bakowsky, U., Jintapattanakit, A., & Kissel, T., (2006). Self-assembled polyelectrolyte nanocomplexes between chitosan derivatives and insulin. *J. Pharm. Sci., 95*, 1035–1048.

5. Sun, W., Mao, S., Mei, D., & Kissel, T., (2008). Self-assembled polyelectrolyte nanocomplexes between chitosan derivatives and enoxaparin. *Eur. J. Pharm. Biopharm., 69*, 417–425.

6. Lankalapalli, S., & Kolapalli, V. R. M., (2009). Polyelectrolyte complexes: A review of their applicability in drug delivery technology. *Indian J. Pharm. Sci., 5*, 481–487.

7. Koetz, J., & Kosmella, S., (2007). *Polyelectrolytes and Nanoparticles*. Springer, Berlin.

8. Boeris, V., Farruggia, B., Nerlia, B., Romanini, D., & Pico, G., (2007). Protein-flexible chain polymer interactions to explain protein partition in aqueous two-phase systems and the protein-polyelectrolyte complex formation. *Int. J. Biol. Macromol., 41*, 286–294.

9. Robertis, S. D., Bonferoni, M. C., Elviri, L., Sandri, G., Caramella, C., & Bettini, R., (2015). Advances in oral controlled drug delivery: The role of drug-polymer and interpolymer non-covalent interactions. *Expert Opin. Drug Deliv., 12*, 441–453.

10. Michaels, A. S., & Miekka, R. G., (1961). Polycation-polyanion complexes: Preparation and properties of poly-(vinylbenzyltrimethylammonium) poly-(styrenesulfonate). *J. Phys. Chem., 65*, 1765–1773.

11. Pergushov, D. V., Muller, A. H. E., & Schacher, F. H., (2012). Micellar interpolyelectrolyte complexes. *Chem. Soc. Rev., 41*, 6888–6901.

12. Philipp, B., Dautzenberg, H., Linow, K. J., Kotz, J., & Dawydoff, W., (1989). Polyelectrolyte complexes - recent developments and open problems. *Prog. Polym. Sci., 14*, 91–172.

13. Kabanov, A. V., & Zezin, A. B., (1984). Soluble interpolymeric complexes as a new class of synthetic polyelectrolytes. *Pure Appl. Chem., 56*, 343–354.

14. Tsuchida, E., (1994). Formation of polyelectrolyte complexes and their structures. *J. Macromol. Sci., Pure Appl. Chem., 31*, 1–15.

15. Zezin, A. B., & Kabanov, V. A., (1982). A new class of complex water-soluble polyelectrolytes. *Russ. Chem. Rev., 51*, 833–855.

16. Delair, T., (2011). Colloidal polyelectrolyte complexes of chitosan and dextran sulfate towards versatile nanocarriers of bioactive molecules. *Eur. J. Pharm. Biopharm., 78*, 10–18.

17. Gucht, J., Spruijt, E., Lemmers, M., & Stuart, M. A. C., (2011). Polyelectrolyte complexes: Bulk phases and colloidal systems. *J. Colloid Interface Sci., 361*, 407–422.

18. Sæther, H. V., Holme, H. K., Maurstad, G., Smidsrod, O., & Stokke, B. T., (2008). Polyelectrolyte complex formation using alginate and chitosan. *Carbohydr. Polym., 74*, 813–821.

19. Lee, D., Kim, D., Mok, H., Jeong, J. H., Choi, D., & Kim, S. H., (2012). Bioreducible crosslinked polyelectrolyte complexes for MMP-2 siRNA delivery into human vascular smooth muscle cells. *Pharm. Res., 29*, 2213–2224.

20. Schatz, C., Domard, A., Viton, C., Pichot, C., & Delair, T., (2004). Versatile and efficient formation of colloids of biopolymer-based polyelectrolyte complexes. *Biomacromol., 5*, 1882–1892.

21. Muller, M., Keßler, B., Frohlich, J., Poeschla, S., & Torgeret, B., (2011). Polyelctrolyte complex nanoparticles of poly(ethyleneimine) and poly(acrylic acid): Preparation and applications. *Polymers, 3*, 762–778.

22. Dautzenberg, H., Linow, K. J., & Philipp, B., (1982). Anionic to form water-soluble polysalts (symplexes) and cationic copolymers of acrylamide. *Acta Polymerica, 33*, 619–623.

23. Hu, Y., Yang, T., & Hu, X., (2012). Novel polysaccharides-based nanoparticle carriers prepared by polyelectrolyte complexation for protein drug delivery. *Polym. Bull., 68*, 1183–1199.

24. Fukuda, H., & Kikuchi, Y., (1977). Polyelectrolyte complexes of sodium dextran sulfate with chitosan. *Macromol. Chem. Phys., 178*, 2895.

25. Berger, J., Reist, M., Mayer, J. M., Felt, O., & Gurny, R., (2004). Structure and interactions in chitosan hydrogels formed by complexation or aggregation for biomedical applications. *Eur. J. Pharm. Biopharm., 57*, 35–52.

26. Ankerfors, C., Ondaral, S., Wagberg, L., & Odberg, L., (2010). Using jet mixing to prepare polyelectrolyte complexes: Complex properties and their interaction with silicon oxide surfaces. *J. Colloid Interface Sci., 351*, 88–95.

27. Mende, M., Buchhammer, H. M., Schwarz, S., Petzold, G., & Jaeger, W., (2004). The stability of polyelectrolyte complex systems of PDADMAC with different polyanions. *Macromol. Symp., 211*, 121–133.

28. Dautzenberg, H., (1997). Polyelectrolyte complex formation in highly aggregating systems. 1. Effect of salt: Polyelectrolyte complex formation in the presence of NaCl. *Macromolecules, 30*, 7810–7815.

29. Anitha, A., Deepagan, V. G., Divya, R. V. V., Menon, D., Nair, S. V., & Jayakumar, R., (2011). Preparation, characterization, *in vitro* drug release and biological studies of curcumin loaded dextran sulphate-chitosan nanoparticles. *Carbohydr. Polym., 84*, 1158–1164.

30. Martins, A. F., Bueno, P. V. A., Almeida, E. A. M. S., Rodrigues, F. H. A., Rubira, A. F., & Muniz, E. C., (2013). Characterization of N-trimethyl chitosan/alginate complexes and curcumin release. *Int. J. Biol. Macromol., 57*, 174–184.

31. Wang, J., Ni, C., Zhang, Y., Zhang, M., Li, W., Yao, B., et al., (2014). Preparation and pH-controlled release of polyelectrolyte complex of poly(l-malic acid-co-d,l-lactic acid) and chitosan. *Colloids Surf. B Biointerfaces, 115*, 275–279.

32. Costalat, M., Alcouffe, P., David, L., & Delair, T., (2014). Controlling the complexation of polysaccharides into multi-functional colloidal assemblies for nanomedicine. *J. Colloid Interface Sci., 430*, 147–156.

33. Polexe, R. C., Terrat, C., Verrier, B., Cuvilier, A., Champier, G., & Delair, T., (2013). Elaboration of targeted nanodelivery systems based on colloidal polyelectrolyte complexes (PEC) of chitosan (CH)-dextran sulphate (DS). *Eur. J. Nanomed., 5*, 39–49.

34. Volodko, A. V., Davydova, V. N., Chusovitin, E. A., Sorokina, I. V., Dolgikh, M. P., Tolstikova, T. G., et al., (2013). Soluble chitosan-carrageenan polyelectrolyte complexes and their gastroprotective activity. *Carbohydr. Polym., 101*, 1087–1093.

35. Kulkarni, A. D., Vanjari, Y. H., Sancheti, K. H., Patel, H. M., Belgamwar, V. S., & Surana, S. J., (2016). Polyelectrolyte complexes: Mechanisms, critical experimental aspects, and applications. *Art Cells Nanomed. Biotechnol., 44*, 1615–1625.

36. Lefnaoui, S., & Moulai-Mostefa, N., (2015). Polyelectrolyte complex based on carboxymethyl-kappa-carrageenan and Eudragit RL 30D as prospective carriers for sustained drug delivery. *Chem. Eng. Res. Des., 97*, 165–174.

37. Amaduzzi, F., Bomboi, F., Bonincontro, A., Bordi, F., Casciardi, S., Chronopoulou, L., et al., (2014). Chitosan–DNA complexes: Charge inversion and DNA condensation. *Colloids Surf. B Biointerfaces, 114*, 1–10.

38. Cifani, N., Chronopoulou, L., Pompili, B., Martino, A. D., Bordi, F., Sennato, S., et al., (2015). Improved stability and efficacy of chitosan/pDNA complexes for gene delivery. *Biotechnol. Lett., 37*, 557–565.

39. Jean, M., Smaoui, F., Lavertu, M., Methot, S., Bouhdoud, L., Buschmann, M. D., et al., (2009). Chitosan-plasmid nanoparticle formulations for IM and SC delivery of recombine FGF-2 and PDGF-BB or generation of antibodies. *Gene Ther., 16*, 1097–1110.

40. Zaitsev, S., Cartier, R., Vyborov, O., Sukhorukov, G., Paulke, B. R., Haberland, A., et al., (2004). Polyelectrolyte nanoparticles mediate vascular gene delivery. *Pharm. Res., 21*, 1656–1661.

41. Liu, W., Sun, S., Cao, Z., Zhang, X., Yao, K., Lu, W. W., et al., (2005). An investigation on the physicochemical properties of chitosan/DNA polyelectrolyte complexes. *Biomaterials, 26*, 2705–2711.

42. Kim, S. H., Lee, S. H., Tian, H., Chen, X., & Park, T. G., (2009). Prostate cancer cell-specific VEGF siRNA delivery system using cell-targeting peptide conjugated polyplexes. *J. Drug Target, 17*, 311–317.

43. Bui, L., Abbou, S., Ibarboure, E., Guidolin, N., Staedel, C., Toulme, J. J., et al., (2012). Encapsidation of RNApolyelectrolyte complexes with amphiphilic block copolymers: Toward a new self-assembly route. *J. Am. Chem. Soc., 134*, 20189–20196.

44. Jiang, R., Lu, X., Yang, M., Deng, W., Fan, Q., & Huang, W., (2013). Monodispersed brush-like conjugated polyelectrolyte nanoparticles with efficient and visualized siRNA delivery for gene silencing. *Biomacromolecules, 14*, 3643–3652.

45. Cheng, W. P., Thompson, C., Ryan, S. M., Aguirre, T., Tetley, L., & Brayden, D. J., (2010). *In vitro* and *in vivo* characterization of a novel peptide delivery system: Amphiphilic polyelectrolyte-salmon calcitonin nanocomplexes. *J. Control Release, 147*, 289–297.

46. Sarmento, B., Ribeiro, A., Veiga, F., & Ferreira, D., (2006). Development and characterization of new insulin-containing polysaccharide nanoparticles. *Coll. Surf. B Biointerfaces, 53*, 193–202.

47. Huang, M., Vitharana, S. N., Peek, L. J., Coop, T., & Berkland, C., (2007). Polyelectrolyte complexes stabilize and controllably release vascular endothelial growth factor. *Biomacromolecules, 8*, 1607–1614.

48. Sajeesh, S., & Sharma, C. P. (2007). Novel polyelectrolyte complexes based on poly(methacrylic acid)-bis(2-aminopropyl)poly(ethylene glycol) for oral protein delivery. *J. Biomater. Sci. Polym. Ed., 18*, 1125–1139.

49. Huang, M., & Berkland, C., (2008). Controlled release of repifermin from polyelectrolyte complexes stimulates endothelial cell proliferation. *J. Pharm. Sci., 98*, 268–280.

50. Ho, Y. C., Mi, F. L., Sung, H. W., & Kuo, P. L., (2009). Heparin-functionalized chitosan-alginate scaffolds for controlled release of growth factor. *Int. J. Pharm., 376*, 69–75.

51. Luppi, B., Bigucci, F., Mercolini, L., Musenga, A., Sorrenti, M., Catenacci, L., et al., (2009). Novel mucoadhesive nasal inserts based on chitosan/hyaluronate polyelectrolyte complexes for peptide and protein delivery. *J. Pharm. Pharmacol., 61*, 151–157.

52. Cegnar, M., Miklavzin, A., & Kerc, J., (2011). Freeze-drying and release characteristics of polyelectrolyte nanocarriers for the mucosal delivery of ovalbumin. *Acta Chim. Slov., 58*, 241–250.

53. Goncalves, R. M., Antunes, J. C., & Barbosa, M. A., (2012). Mesenchymal stem cell recruitment by Stromal derived factor-1-delivery systems based on chitosan/poly(γ-glutamic acid) polyelectrolyte complexes. *Eur. Cell Mater., 23,* 249–261.
54. Wu, Q. X., Zhang, Q. L., Lin, D. Q., & Yao, S. J., (2013). Characterization of novel lactoferrin loaded capsules prepared with polyelectrolyte complexes. *Int. J. Pharm., 455,* 124–131.
55. Csaba, N., Garcia-Fuentes, M., & Alonso, M. J., (2009). Nanoparticles for nasal vaccination. *Adv. Drug Deliv. Rev., 61,* 140–157.
56. Xiang, S. D., Scholzen, A., Minigo, G., David, C., Apostolopoulos, V., Mottram, P. L., et al. (2006). Pathogen recognition and development of particulate vaccines: Does size matter? *Methods, 40,* 1–9.
57. Verheul, R. J., Slutter, B., Bal, S. M., Bouwstra, J. A., Jiskoot, W., & Hennink, W. E., (2011). Covalently stabilized trimethyl chitosan-hyaluronic acid nanoparticles for nasal and intradermal vaccination. *J. Control Release, 156,* 46–52.
58. Liu, C., Xia, Z., & Czernuszka, J. T., (2007). Design and development of three-dimensional scaffolds for tissue engineering. *Chem. Eng. Res. Des., 85,* 1051–1064.
59. Coimbra, P., Ferreira, P., De Sousa, H. C., Batista, P., Rodrigues, M. A., Correia, I. J., et al., (2011). Preparation and chemical and biological characterization of a pectin/chitosan polyelectrolyte complex scaffold for possible bone tissue engineering applications. *Int. J. Biol. Macromol., 48,* 112–118.
60. Whu, S. W., Hung, K. C., Hsieh, K. H., Chen, C. H., Tsai, C. L., & Hsu, S. H., (2013). *In vitro* and *in vivo* evaluation of chitosan-gelatin scaffolds for cartilage tissue engineering. *Mater. Sci. Eng. C Mater. Biol. Appl., 33,* 2855–2863.
61. Ceccaldi, C., Bushkalova, R., Alfarano, C., Lairez, O., Calise, D., Bourin, P., et al., (2014). Evaluation of polyelectrolyte complex-based scaffolds for mesenchymal stem cell therapy in cardiac ischemia treatment. *Acta Biomater., 10,* 901–911.
62. Coimbra, P., Alves, P., Valente, T. A., Santos, R., Correia, I. J., & Ferreira, P., (2011). Sodium hyaluronate/chitosan polyelectrolyte complex scaffolds for dental pulp regeneration: Synthesis and characterization. *Int. J. Biol. Macromol., 49,* 573–579.
63. Chang, H. H., Wang, Y. L., Chiang, Y. C., Chen, Y. L., Chuang, Y. H., Tsai, S. J., et al., (2014). A novel chitosan-γPGA polyelectrolyte complex hydrogel promotes early new bone formation in the alveolar socket following tooth extraction. *PLoS One, 9,* e92362.
64. Huang, M., Huang, Z. L., Bilgen, M., & Berkland, C., (2008). Magnetic resonance imaging of contrast-enhanced polyelectrolyte complexes. *Nanomedicine, 4,* 30–40.
65. Ron, N., Zimet, P., Bargarum, J., & Livney, Y. D., (2010). Beta-lactoglobuline polysaccharide complexes as nanovehicles for hydrophobic nutraceuticals in non-fat foods and clear beverages. *Int. Dairy Journal, 20,* 686–693.
66. Semo, E., Kesselman, E., Danino, D., & Livney, Y. D., (2007). Casein micelle as a natural nano-capsular vehicle for nutraceuticals. *Food Hydrocolloids, 21,* 936–942.
67. Chen, L., & Subirade, M., (2005). Chitosan/β-lactoglobulin core-shell nanoparticles as nutraceutical carriers. *Biomaterials, 26,* 6041–6053.

PART VI
Miscellaneous Nutraceutical Delivery Systems

CHAPTER 13

Micelles: An Insight for Nutraceuticals and Regulatory Status

PANKAJ PADMAKAR NERKAR

Associate Professor, Department of Quality Assurance, R.C. Patel Institute of Pharmaceutical Education and Research, Shirpur, Maharashtra, India, Mobile: +919420151343, E-mail: nerkarpankaj@rediffmail.com

ABSTRACT

Nutraceutical is a collective type of nutritional term related to pharmaceuticals. Creating a pharmaceutical commodity (tablets, powders, capsules, suppositories, etc.), which includes nutraceutical is simple for a formulator, but it is very difficult to obtain an acceptable nutraceutical bioavailability. Nutraceutical bioavailability is often poor due to a lower solubility, lower stability, and lower permeability. For all these problems related to nutraceuticals absorption, micelles can be suitably applied. Detailed discussion on the micelles is given in this section. The information includes the description of the methods for assessing essential micellar concentration, the method for preparing micelles, and various types of micelles recorded in the literature. The information includes the narrative of the critical micellar concentration determination methods, method of preparation of micelles, and diverse types of micelles which are reported in the literature. The description of the electrochemical methods for the assessment of critical micelle concentration (CMC) is given. A variety of factors affecting critical micellar concentration and the micelle size are reported. Micelles can be used for passive targeting against tumors, so various different approaches for the targeting of micelles are also described. Various examples of nutraceuticals that are loaded in different polymeric micelles showing enhanced anticancer activity in comparison to original nutraceuticals are described. Regulatory guidelines for nutraceuticals in India and in the US are described.

13.1 INTRODUCTION

Nutraceuticals product finds its source from food or fortified food that supplements the diet and assists in treating or preventing disease. Nutraceuticals are not tried and controlled to the level of drugs. Nutraceutical is a collective form of the terms as nutrition and related to pharmaceuticals [1, 2].

Creating a pharmaceutical product (tablets, powders, capsules, suppositories, etc.), containing nutraceutical is simple for a formulator, but it is very difficult to obtain a suitable nutraceutical bioavailability. The bioavailability of nutraceuticals is often low due to problems like the little solubility, low stability and permeability and lack of specificity of the bioactive. Colloidal nanocarriers (nanoparticles, micelles, and liposome) are the drug delivery system which satisfies the criteria of increased solubility, increased permeability and stability and site explicitness and targeting. Polymeric Micelles are colloidal nano-particulate carriers formed in an aqueous medium by self-assembly. They consist of amphiphilic polymeric molecules with lyophilic along with lyophobic blocks on a single molecule chain [3]. Polymeric micelles possess a particle size in the range of 10–100 nm. Polymeric micelles for various cancers and other diseases should possess ideal properties such as high encapsulation, prolonged circulation and amassing in the required pathological sites and should be safe. Surfactants assume a significant job in both fundamental and applied science. In aqueous medium surfactants at a specific concentration construct colloidal-sized clusters, which are termed as micelles, and the concentration of the surfactant above which micelles are formed is termed as critical micelle concentration (CMC). As micelles are produced from surfactants, they possess particular significance of potential to improve the solubility of less soluble drugs [4].

Micelles are made up of amphiphiles and surfactants with a hydrophilic head part and a hydrophobic tail component in the second. The radius of a spherical micelle shaped is the same as that of the surfactant monomer's size, which is commonly about 1–3 nm. By aggregating numerous monomers, micelles are generated by non-covalent bonds and are therefore unstable colloidal clusters. Based on its size, there are different forms of micelles such as circular, planar, and cylindrical. The shape of the micelles and also the size depend on different external conditions such as temperature, surfactant structure, surfactant concentration, ionic strength, and pH. By picking the proper size, charge, and surface properties of the micelles, the formulator is free to target specific sites. All these qualities can be achieved in micelles by adding different ingredients to the surfactants before preparation of micelles and by modifying the preparation methods of micelles. The free energy of the process is diminished, and the lyophobic fragments are eliminated from the aqueous atmosphere by creating micelles whose center is stabilized with the lyophobic section when fluid exists [5].

Most nutraceuticals have little solubility in physiological fluids that limit their use, and by loading in micelles, nutraceuticals solubility can be improved. The solubilized nutraceutical will have increased absorption in the body and thus enhanced bioavailability. The nanosize of the micelles also favors in accumulation in leaky vasculature area and to circulate long period in body.

Micelles formation takes place in the surfactant solution is due to the fact that system tries to achieve a low free energy state also there is increase of entropy when the hydrophobic regions of the surfactants are removed from water and the surrounding water molecule structure is lost.

The micellar structure formed by ionic surfactants consists of:

- The micellar core is hydrophobic and consists of long surfactant hydrocarbon chains surfactant;
- A layer of hydrophilic head groups in the company of (1-N) counterions surrounding the hydrophobic center, where N is the aggregation number;
- The hydrophilic layer is encircled by an electrical double layer. The solution's ionic concentration is responsible for the double layer's thickness.

The size of the micelles formed by the nonionic surface-active agents is comparatively more than that of ionic surface-active agents. The shape of micelles may be enlarged to an ellipsoid or rod as in which the center may be hydrophobic shaped by the surface-active agents' hydrocarbon chains. The center of the micelle is surrounded by the surface-active agents' oxyethylene chains.

The micelles formed in a non-aqueous solution may be reversed or inverted as the hydrophilic group containing the core and are surrounded by hydrocarbon chains of the active agents of the ground.

13.2 CRITICAL MICELLE CONCENTRATION (CMC) DETERMINATION

There is a sudden transition in various physical properties of surfactant solution when micelles formation takes place.

The properties include conductivity, surface tension and refractive index, etc. This transition in the physical properties described above is the foundation of CMC determination.

13.2.1   METHODS FOR CMC DETERMINATION [6, 7]

There are various methods which are applied for the CMC determination. These methods are roughly divided into two classes as:

1. **Direct Measurements:** In this technique, there are some properties of solution of polymer which get increased with respective to the concentration of added polymer. The correlation between the value of the property and the concentration of polymer is discontinued when the micelles are produced in the solution. The concentration above CMC is used to prepare micelles.

    Direct CMC measurements methods include physical property measurements method (such as surface tension, electrical conductivity, osmotic pressure, refractive index, and viscosity).

2. **Indirect Measurements:** In this technique of CMC determination, the change of a property of different probe substance which is present in micelle forming polymer solution also changes with respect to concentration of the surfactant solution is observed. UV spectrophotometric method and voltammetric methods are used for indirect measurement of the CMC.

    The CMC is an important property of a surfactant or a polymer. It is the value where the molecule's solution property displays an abrupt change. In aqueous solution surface-active agents' ions or molecules or monomers unite to form larger units at this concentration. These groups of ions or molecules or monomers of active surface agents are called micelles. The CMC determination study of the polymer or surfactant is carried out using the following methods:

    i.   Surface tension method (Stalagmometer-drop count method);
    ii. Iodine UV spectroscopy method;
    iii. Dynamic light scattering method.

13.2.1.1   SURFACE TENSION METHOD (STALAGMOMETER-DROP COUNT METHOD)

CMC is measured by determining surface tension. This is a very common method for measuring surface tension. The theory is to calculate the weight of the drops of the liquid falling from the capillary glass tube and then estimate the fluid's surface tension. Stalagmometer is a glass tool used for surface tension determination. It is also referred to as a stactometer or stalagmometer. The glass apparatus consists of a capillary glass tube whose center section is widened. The bottom piece of the apparatus is lessened to let the fluid fall down from the tube in the shape of a drop. In the experiments, the drops are falling little by little from the tube in a vertical direction. When the size of the drop becomes the highest, the hanging drop starts to fall from the base of the stalagmometer. The volume required to fall from the bottom of the stalagmometer is the distinguishing property of the solution. At this instant, the mass of the drops is in an equilibrium state with the surface tension (Figure 13.1).

$$\text{Surface Tension} = \frac{\text{No of drop of water} \times \text{Density of water}}{\text{No of drop of sample} \times \text{density of sample}} \tag{1}$$

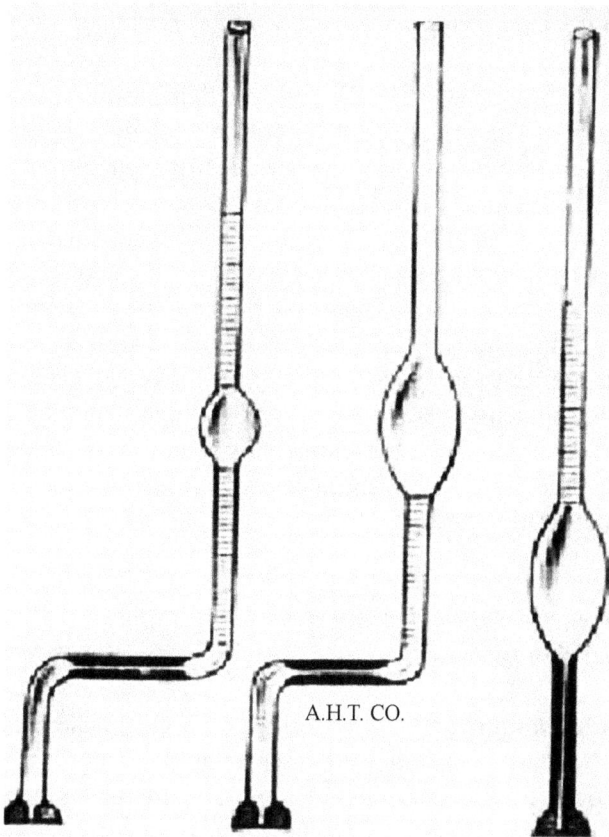

A.H.T. CO.

FIGURE 13.1 Stalagmometer.

13.2.1.2   IODINE UV SPECTROSCOPY METHOD

This is a very simple method to determine the CMC of the polymer in deionized (DI) water. In this method KI/I_2 standard solution is prepared by solubilizing (0.5 g) of I_2 and (1 g) of KI in 50 ml DI water. Various samples of polymer solutions of diverse concentrations are prepared. To each of the sample solutions, equal volume standard preparation is added. Before measurement the solutions are incubated for overnight in a dark. The UV absorbance value of all-polymer concentrations is measured using a UV-Vis spectrometer at 366 nm. The absorption intensity is plotted Vs the polymer concentration. The concentration of the polymer at which there is a sharp rise in absorbance, the concentration is known as its CMC.

13.2.1.3   DYNAMIC LIGHT SCATTERING (DLS) METHOD

CMC values are also detected by the dynamic light scattering method (DLS) using a Zetasizer. The principle of the present technique is as follows if a biphasic dispersion in which particles are in Brownian motion is irradiated with a beam laser, a Doppler Shift is caused when the light strikes the particles, varying the wavelength of the arriving light at different intensities. Analysis of these intensity fluctuations yields the velocity of the Brownian motion and hence the particle size and diffusion coefficient using the Stokes-Einstein relationship. In this method, samples are diluted in various concentrations, and the measurements are carried out using polystyrene Cell at 25°C. The changes in light intensity are reported, and a graph is plotted between the changes in light intensity and the related polymeric solutions concentrations. An increase in the scattering intensity supports micelle formation and polymer concentration as CMC.

13.2.1.4   ELECTROCHEMICAL METHODS FOR THE CMC DETERMINATION [8]

1. **Conductometry:** It is a frequently used electrochemical technique for CMC determination. With increasing concentration of polymeric solution, the conductivity of solution also changes with respect to concentration and at CMC, there is a notable change in the conductivity is observed at CMC. This technique is very simple and economical. In this method, the graph of specific conductivity (k)

against the compound concentration is obtained as two straight lines whose intersection is termed as CMC of the polymeric solution. The equation corresponding to each straight line can be used to determine the CMC analytically. The data obtained can also be reproduced in the molar conductivity and CMC is obtained graphically.

2. **Potentiometry:** In the present method, the ion-selective electrodes are used as these can be selective to the counterion or ion-selective electrodes to the organic fraction of the polymeric solution whose CMC to be determined. In this method, the correlation between ion-selective electrode potential and concentration of micelle forming compound is disrupted at the CMC.

3. **Voltammetric Methods:** In the present process, the changes in the diffusion coefficient of the electrolyte take place at the CMC which lead to limiting the current of the electrolyte. The potential of the species is also affected by the micelle formation. In this method, the presence of strong electrolyte species other than the polymeric compound is necessary for the accurate determination of CMC.

   The CMC value is determined by change of slope of the plot of changes in potential of added electrolyte vs concentration of micelle forming polymer. The addition of strong electrolyte for determination of CMC may alter the value.

4. **Electrophoresis:** It is also called as Electromigration method. By using electrophoresis phenomenon, the CMC can be estimated by following different methods. The starting method involves the plotting of graph of capacity factor vs concentration of micelle forming compound. The CMC value is estimated by extrapolating the graph to k'=0. In the next method plot of electrophoretic mobility of a probe vs concentration of polymeric compound forming micelles is obtained. There is quick transformation in the slope value at the CMC is observed. In the third method, the CMC is obtained by a break on the current vs concentration plot is observed. In this technique, the measurements of electric current of micellar electrolyte solutions as a function of concentration of micelle forming compound at a given applied voltage is plotted.

13.2.2 FACTORS AFFECTING THE CMC AND MICELLAR SIZE

1. **Structure of the Hydrophobic Group:** There is an inverse correlation observed in the chain length of hydrocarbon and CMC, and direct correlation is observed with micellar size.

2.   **Nature of the Hydrophilic Group:** CMC values of non-ionic surface-active agents are very low, but aggregation number is high than that of ionic surface-active agents. As ethylene oxide chain length increases, the CMC of the nonionic surface-active agents also increases.

3.   **Type of Counterion:** For cationic surface-active agents micelles size is observed to be increased as per the series of the counterions $Cl^- < Br^- < I^-$, and for anionic surface-active agents as per the series of the counterions $Na+ < K+ < Cs+$.

4.   **Addition of Electrolytes:** The addition of electrolyte to the solutions of ionic surface-active agents lessens the CMC and enlarges the micellar size. This change is observed as the added electrolyte decrease the forces of repulsion among the charged head groups and the micelle surface, thus the increase in micelle size. If the addition of electrolyte is continued, then the micelles of ionic surface-active agents may be converted into non-spherical shape.

5.   **Effect of Temperature:** Temperature has very less effect on the CMC of the ionic surface-active agents whereas in nonionic surface-active agents, there is an increase in micellar size up to cloud point and a decrease in CMC. Cloud point is the characteristic temperature at which nonionic surface-active agent's aqueous solution becomes turbid.

13.2.3   IDEAL PROPERTIES OF POLYMERIC MICELLES

1.   Should be nano sized structures having size from extents from 10–400 nm so that it can penetrate into tissue.
2.   Should have stealth property against mononuclear phagocyte system (MPS) for a sufficient time to permit build up in target tissue.
3.   Should be eliminated from the body either after degradation or by dissolution.
4.   Should locate and interact with the target cells.
5.   Should have considerable stability.
6.   Should be responsible for the improvement of pharmacokinetic (pk) profile of the encapsulated drug.

13.2.4   VARIOUS ADVANTAGES OF POLYMERIC MICELLES

Following are some advantages of micelles as nanocarriers to improve the solubility and other parameters:

1. Low-molecular-weight drugs are speedily eliminated by excretory organs such as the liver and or kidneys. By encapsulating them in polymeric micelles their bioavailability considerably increases.

2. Due to the small size, nanosized drug carriers are targeted to the tumors by the enhanced permeability and retention effect, leading to the tumor site and decreased toxicity compared to the systemic administration of drug without micellar encapsulation.

3. Intravenous administration of hydrophobic drugs is only possible after the addition of suitable cosolvent which is always have toxic side effects. When such drugs are administered in micelles, solubility will increase, and targeting is also possible.

4. Aqueous concentration of active drug can be increased after micellar encapsulation and which will improve drug circulation.

5. High stability both *in vitro* and *in vivo* and improved biocompatibility is observed in polymeric micelles.

6. Prolonged and extended circulation time for better therapeutic action.

7. Modifying the structure of the amphiphilic copolymers, properties such as the size and morphology of the resulting polymeric micelles can be easily controlled.

8. Polymeric micelles are significantly more stable in case of dilution than surfactant-based micelles and hence shows minimal cytotoxicity as compared to surfactant-based micelles upon dilution triggering lysis of cell membranes.

13.2.5   DISADVANTAGES OF POLYMERIC MICELLES

1. Drugs with a short half-life and low stability cannot be encapsulated in micelles as polymeric micelles in blood may lead to adverse hypersensitivity reactions, albeit these formulations often demonstrate safety *in vitro*.

2. As drugs are physically entrapped in the core of micelles, then upon dilution with blood after intravenous injection, they can easily disassemble, which can result in a quick release of the loaded drug.

3. Polymeric micelles with particle sizes more than 200 nm are easily cleared from blood by macrophages and are mostly distributed in the liver, lungs, and spleen.

13.3 POLYMERIC MICELLE STRUCTURES

Following are examples of structures of micelles. These are mainly three types as:

- self-assembled micelles;
- unimolecular micelles; and
- cross-linked micelles.

13.3.1 SELF-ASSEMBLED MICELLES

Amphiphilic polymers produce this type of micelles which are impulsively form aggregates of nanosize dissolved in water above the CMC. Polymers which are having low water solubility can be solubilized in a volatile organic solvent and dialyzed in suitable buffer containing water. For drug delivery reasons, the polymer should be biodegradable and should have low molecular weight so that it can be excreted through the kidney and can be avoided the buildup in the body. The most developed amphiphilic block copolymers gather into spherical core-shell micelles having size less than 200 nm. The core of such micelles is hydrophobic, and drugs can be loaded in the core. A hydrophilic shell covers the core and act as a hurdle for micelles aggregation and opsonization when administered systemically. Formation of the self-assembled micelles is a thermodynamic and reversible process and is become stable by solvent interactions with the hydrophilic shell.

13.3.2 UNIMOLECULAR MICELLES

These are observed in copolymers with star like polymer molecules in which amphiphile chains are linked covalently. Copolymers which are having dendritic structure can aggregate to produce multimolecular micelles and if its structure and composition is optimized can be successfully used to prepare unimolecular micelles. Dendrimers, due to their highly branched structure, globular shape and surface functionality are generally used to prepare unimolecular micelles. By coupling different generations of dendritic hypercores with PEO chains, this type of micelles can be prepared.

13.3.3 CROSS-LINKED MICELLES

The micelles structure can be resistant by formation of cross-links between the polymer chains. These resulting cross-linked micelles are in essence single molecules of nanoscale size that are stable upon dilution, shear forces, and environmental variations. There are several reports on the stabilization of the polymer micelles by cross-linking either within the core domain or throughout the shell layer.

13.3.4 PREPARATION OF MICELLES

Some methods for the preparation of micelles are discussed in subsections.

13.3.4.1 DIRECT DISSOLUTION METHOD

It consists of direct dissolution of the bulk sample in a specifically chosen solvent for one of the blocks. It should be noted that this method is generally suitable for block copolymers with relatively low molecular weight, and rather short length of the insoluble block. The solubility can be improved by a subsequent annealing process of the solution such as standing, prolonged stirring, thermal or ultrasound treatments. The main disadvantage of this technique is that depending on the block copolymer system, an equilibrium situation is not necessarily reached, especially when the insoluble, core-forming block is characterized by a high glass transition temperature (Tg). The features of these micelles usually depend on the two-phase morphology of the bulk block copolymer sample, and also on the interactions of the selective solvent and the polymer microphases.

13.3.4.2 DISSOLUTION IN NON-SELECTIVE SOLVENT SYSTEM

This method is based on the dissolution of the copolymer in a common good solvent for both blocks, thus forming molecularly dissolved chains. To initiate micelle formation, the properties of the solvent are then changed, either by stepwise addition of a selective solvent for one block and precipitant for the other or by changing the temperature or pH of the solution. The initial common solvent can be further eliminated or gradually replaced by the selective solvent via a dialysis process. This technique is the preferred method of preparation for micellar systems in aqueous solutions. Large aggregates are prevented and micelles from block copolymer with large insoluble block is possible.

13.3.4.3   DIALYSIS METHOD

In this method of micelles preparation solutions of the drug and that of polymer in organic solvent are placed in the dialysis bag, and the solvent is diffused with water by immersing bag into water, inducing micelle assembly. After carrying successful dialysis for 36–48 hours, the solution is lyophilized. By redispersing the freeze-dried product in the correct vehicle drug-loaded polymeric micelles are then prepared.

13.3.4.4   THIN FILM HYDRATION METHOD OR SOLVENT EVAPORATION METHOD

In solvent evaporation or solution-casting technique, a volatile organic solvent is used to dissolve the copolymer and the drug. A thin film of copolymer and drug is obtained after the solvent is removed by evaporation. Drug-loaded polymeric micelles are obtained by reconstitution of film with water or an aqueous phase.

13.4   TARGETING MICELLES [9]

Targeting by polymeric micelles can be achieved by both approaches as passive and active also following are some approaches for targeting such as by enhancing the permeability and retention of micelle, by preparing stimuli-sensitive micelles, complexing micelles surface with particular targeting ligand, and by pairing monoclonal antibodies to the micelle.

13.4.1   STIMULI-SENSITIVITY

During the prolonged circulation of micelles, there should not be release of encapsulated drug, and it should take place at the target site only by a triggering mechanism. Passive triggering mechanism may consist of tumor microenvironment pH, specific enzyme, etc., whereas active triggering mechanism may include temperature, light, magnetic field, ultrasound, etc. After start of the triggering mechanism, the disruption of the micelle structure may be observed, which result in the drug release at a specific target site. The phenomenon in which the disruption of micelles is occurring and which leads to drug release due to the stimulation either by active or by passive triggering mechanism, it is termed as stimuli-sensitivity of the micelles.

13.4.2   ACID-SENSITIVE POLYMERIC MICELLES

Different pH conditions exist in normal and diseased state in our body. The changes in the pH can be used as acid sensitive polymeric micelles for drug targeting to specific site. There are various polymers which are having pH dependent solubility which can be explored for pH sensitive micelle preparation. The tumor microenvironment and inflammatory tissue is observed to possess somewhat acidic pH. This can act as a triggering mechanism for acidic pH sensitive polymeric micelles. The pH of the above-mentioned microenvironment is about 6.8 as compare to that of blood and healthy tissue as about 7.4. The micelles being in nanosize can be getting absorbed in the cells by the process of endocytosis and can enter various cell organelles. There is a marked difference in the pH values which range from 5.5–6.5.

pH-sensitive copolymer can be synthesized by adding groups such as amines, carboxylic acids into the copolymer backbone. This copolymer will lead to alteration of the solubility property of polymer by protonation. This will result in disruption of micellar structure and drug release.

13.4.3   THERMOSENSITIVE POLYMERIC MICELLES

This type of polymeric micelles shows structural changes in response to the rise in temperature, which result in easier absorption by cells. Some polymers show critical solution temperature at which they show a change in volume with a sudden change in the solvation state. Polymers which get solubilized upon heating possess an upper critical solution temperature and solution having lower consulate temperature solubilized at lower temperature. By using thermosensitivity of the polymer, it can be explored by heating the targeted tissue using nearby applied ultrasound. This is also known as the passive way of drug targeting.

13.4.4   COMPLEXING TARGETING LIGAND MOLECULES TO MICELLES

Cell-specific ligand can be attached to the surface of the micelle, which can enhance the internalization of polymeric micelles at targeted tissue. The attachment with ligands includes various ligands such as peptides, folic acid, hyaluronic acids and sugar and some monoclonal antibodies which are covalently attached. For tumor-targeting peptides are having more specificity, and these can be easily derivatized and engineered to achieve better targeting *in vivo*.

13.4.5   TARGETING BY IMMUNOMICELLES

Antibodies are very specific with respect to the receptors so they can be attached to the micelle surface and active targeting can be achieved for cancer tumors.

13.4.6   APPLICATIONS OF MICELLES FOR NUTRACEUTICALS

Following are some reported articles in which nutraceuticals are encapsulated in the micelles and are reported to have enhanced the stability and pharmacokinetic characteristics (Table 13.1):

> ➢ Elham et al. [10] prepared and evaluated polymeric micelles of pluronic F68 containing naringin. In this study, the authors studied the antitumor activity of polymeric micelles containing naringin against cell lines such as HepG2, MCF-7, and Caco2. Naringin, a nutraceutical is present in grape and citrus fruits. Grapefruit juice consists of up to a concentration of 800 mg/L of naringin. It is having activities such as antioxidant, antiulcer, antiallergic, anticancer, and blood lipid-lowering activities. Naringin get degraded in the gastrointestinal tract (GIT) due to harsh pH and enzymatic degradation also it is having very less bioavailability of about 8%. Authors observed an extended-release of naringin up to 48 hrs by the polymeric micelles as compared to free naringin in different pH media with improved antiulcer and anticancer activity.
> ➢ Zhaokun et al. [11] prepared Pluronic F127-stearoyl chloride grafted polyethylenimine copolymer (C18-PEI) based micelles containing ursolic acid for improved internalization. Ursolic acid is chemically

TABLE 13.1 Reported Micelles and Their Activities

SL. No.	Nutraceuticals	Activities	Polymer Used	References
1.	Apigenin	Antioxidative, vasoprotective, anti-inflammatory, hypocholesterolemic	Pluronic P123 and Solutol HS 15	[15]
2.	Naringin	Antioxidative, vasoprotective, anti-inflammatory, hypocholesterolemic	Pluronic F68	[10, 16]
3.	Ursolic acid	Vasoprotective, anti-inflammatory, hypocholesterolemic	Pluronic F127-stearoyl chloride grafted polyethylenimine copolymer	[11]
4.	Hesperidin	Antioxidative, antimicrobial, anti-inflammatory	Cetyl trimethylammonium bromide (CTAB)	[17]
5.	Piperine	Vasoprotective, anti-inflammatory	Poloxamer 407 and D-α-tocopheryl polyethylene glycol 1000 succinate (TPGS)	[18]
6.	Curcumin	Gastroprotective, anti-inflammatory, antioxidative, hepatoprotective	Soluplus and D-α-tocopheryl polyethylene glycol 1000 succinate	[12]
7.	Eugenol	Antioxidative, anti-inflammatory, anticarcinogenic	Non-ionic surfactant Surfynol 485W	[19, 20]
8.	Diallyl sulfide	Antioxidative, anti-inflammatory, anticarcinogenic	Propylene glycol, alcohol, Tween 80	[13]
9.	Gingerol	Antioxidative, anti-inflammatory, anticarcinogenic	D-α-Tocopheryl polyethylene glycol 1000 succinate (TPGS) and poly(ethylene glycol)-poly(ε-caprolactone) (PEG-PCL)	[21]
10.	Thymoquinone	Antioxidative, anti-inflammatory, cardioprotective, antimicrobial	PLGA	[22]
11.	Capsaicin	Antioxidative, anti-inflammatory, anticarcinogenic	Polyvinylpyrrolidone (PVP)-sodium cholate-phospholipid	[23]
12.	Honokiol	Antioxidant, anti-inflammatory, and anticancer activities	Vitamin E-D-α-tocopheryl polyethylene glycol succinate	[14]

pentacyclic triterpenoid obtained from *Hedyotis diffusa Willd.* Ursolic acid is reported to have anticancer activity against different cancers cells such as colon cancer, endometrial cancer, and melanoma. Ursolic acid is having poor bioavailability due to less solubility and hence less efficacy. Authors reported the improved internalization of ursolic acid in the micellar form, which in turn increased the efficacy of it.

➢ Ji et al. [12] developed a mixed micelle based on Soluplus and D-α-tocopheryl polyethylene glycol 1,000 succinate (TPGS) containing curcumin for oral administration. Curcumin is obtained from *Curcuma longa* L., turmeric. Curcumin is reported to possess anticancer and anti-inflammatory action. It also reported to possess low bioavailability due to low solubility and low stability in alkaline pH. The prepared micelles were evaluated for sustained release and *in vitro* anticancer activity by MTT assay. The results of these evaluations were observed to be promising for internalization and anticancer activity for curcumin.

➢ Ju et al. [13] prepared and evaluated self-assembled diallyl trisulfide micelles injection based on propylene glycol, alcohol, Tween 80, and water. Diallyl trisulfide, diallyl sulfide, and diallyl disulfide are reported to be water-insoluble thioether compound possessed anti-thrombotic and anticancer properties. These thioether compounds are extracted from garlic *Allium sativum*.

➢ Godugu et al. [14] formulated and evaluated a Vitamin E-D-α-tocopheryl polyethylene glycol succinate-based Honokiol containing nanomicellar formulation for the treatment of orthotopic triple-negative breast cancer in mouse models. Honokiol is a lignan isolated from Magnolia plant. It is reported to possess different pharmacological activities such as antioxidant, anti-inflammatory, and anticancer activities. It is having low solubility and thus low bioavailability. The authors concluded the study as improved solubility as well as bioavailability after converting Honokiol into micelles form.

13.5 REGULATORY GUIDELINES FOR NUTRACEUTICALS

13.5.1 REQUIREMENTS FOR THE INDIAN MARKET [24, 25]

Currently, not a specific guideline is there for nutraceuticals in India however Food Safety and Standards Authority of India (FSSAI), which is the food regulatory body of India consider Nutraceuticals "Foods for special dietary uses."

The FSSAI were established in India under the Food Safety and Standards Act, 2006. These fuses various acts in different ministries and departments to carry food-related issues.

The purpose of the creation of FSSAI is to establish science-based minimum requirements for food items and to standardize their manufacture, storage, distribution, sale, and import to secure the availability of healthy and safe food for human consumption in multiple ministries and departments. It therefore includes products such as nutraceuticals and dietary supplements (DS). Different central acts such as Prevention of Food Adulteration Act-1954, Fruit Products Order-1955, Meat Food Products Order-1973, Vegetable Oil Products (Control) Order-1947, Edible Oils Packaging (Regulation) Order-1988, Solvent Extracted Oil, De-Oiled Meal and Edible Flour (Control) Order-1967, Milk, and Milk Products Order-1992, etc., have been revoked following commencing of FSS Act-2006.

Under the new regulations given by FSSAI claims to simplify the licensing and registration procedure for nutraceuticals, but the real process differs significantly. For registration a product in India, various licenses are needed which depends on actual product status like which requires many documents to report to the government officer by the person who imports they also need to interlink the dossiers of the product with the licensing procedures:

- Import;
- License for manufacture;
- License for marketing;
- Other state and national level clearances/licenses required from the regulatory side, which need to be taken care of before launching these products in India.

13.5.1.1   HEALTH CLAIMS AND LABEL CLAIMS

It is very important to know the regulatory frames of nutraceuticals which are totally different from the other countries. All the health as well as label claims should be notified and followed carefully [26]. Following are some points to be considered for the registration of product to India:

- India has its specific packaging as well as labeling requirements;
- Packaging also needs to show up their components of the consignment along with same need of the sample product to get it packed according to Indian specification;

- Content which has to be included in the claim;
- Structure claim;
- Functional claim.

13.5.2   REGISTRATION OF DIETARY SUPPLEMENT IN INDIA

FSSAI authority registration for dietary supplement is required to enter the Indian market. There are different procedures provided by the FSSAI to register in India as a dietary supplement. It is becoming very difficult for businesses to get their dietary supplement approved because of the strict rules and regulations. But for the proper public safety, it is required to follow all the guidelines and regulations of registration procedures. Two forms like FORM A and B are required to be filled and get approved to place their product in the market. There are various rules given by the FSSAI to be followed for the registration and licensing of food products like DS and nutraceuticals. It also has given various claims regarding the label and packaging and various standards and their limits of additives are also mentioned. Hence all the standards have to be maintained to get their product approved. Hence there are various departments from the production to distributors. FSS regulations, 2011, mandatory that:

1. The registration form A/B for manufacturing in India must be filled out in accordance with sch-1.
2. If staff needs an import license, it must be issued by the Central Licensing Authority. Following documents are needed for the approval:
   i.   Form A:
       a.   Declaration form which has to be self-attested;
       b.   Manufacturing/import license.
   ii. Form B and C:
       a.   Declaration form which has to be self-attested and the below document copies Documents to be enclosed with new application for license/import license to State/Central Licensing Authority.
   iii. Form-A, B, and C:
       a.   Blueprint can be submitted for the design of the manufacturing system. Processing unit 2 blueprint/layout plan;
       b.   List of directors;
       c.   List of machines used with its name in the manufacture;

       d.   Photo ID with address proof;

       e.   List of the type of food to be made;

       f.   Authority letter with responsible person's name and address;

       g.   NOC and manufacturer's license copy;

       h.   Program and certification for the Food Safety Management System (if any);

       i.   Source of milk or milk supply project like milk collection centers;

       j.   Source of raw material;

       k.   Water residue study;

       l.   Recall plan.

    iv. Form IX:

       a.   Certificate given by the Ministry of Tourism 2;

       b.   Supporting proof for transporters.

13.5.2.1   THE REGULATION OF DIETARY SUPPLEMENTS (DS) IN US

The U.S. Food and Drug Administration (FDA) is in charge of regulating DS in the U.S. and is supervised by the USFDA through its various food industry centers. Food and drug cosmetic act subsequently governed or amended as DSHEA, the 1994 Dietary Supplement Health Education Act. And this DSHEA has provided several expectations that the dietary supplement must meet. USFDA has taken care of the safety of the DS, but their approval by USFDA is not necessary. Prior to producing or selling the products, Dietary supplement manufacturers do not need to register with FDA, or obtain FDA approval:

- Prior to marketing a product, manufacturers are responsible for ensuring that a dietary supplement (or a new ingredient) is safe before it is marketed. FDA has the authority to take action against unsafe dietary supplement products.
- Manufacturers must ensure that their product label information is truthful and not misleading.

13.5.2.2   REGISTRATION OF DIETARY SUPPLEMENTS (DS) IN US

The DS must be according to the definition given in Dietary Supplement Health Education Act-1994, for registration as DS. The active component should follow the regulation given under 21 CFR 190 which is related to DS. At the registration, it should be noted whether it is active ingredient or inactive ingredient and whether it is old or new dietary supplement.

Center for food safety and applied nutrition (CFSAN) perform the pre-market surveillance for the safety of the product in the US market related to the products of New Dietary.

The documents required are as follows:

- Applicants name and address;
- Product name even the botanical name can be included;
- Statement of whether it is a dietary supplement type ODI or NDI;
- Evidence of security measures, if any.

KEYWORDS

- **critical micelle concentration**
- **deionized**
- **dietary supplements**
- **dynamic light scattering**
- **Food Safety and Standards Authority of India**
- **micelle**
- **nutraceuticals**
- **regulatory guidelines**

REFERENCES

1. Kalra, E. K., (2003). Nutraceutical-definition and introduction. *AAPS Pharmsci., 5*(3), 27, 28.
2. Andrew, R., & Izzo, A. A., (2017). Principles of pharmacological research of nutraceuticals. *British Journal of Pharmacology, 174*(11), 1177.
3. Alexander, A., Patel, R. J., Saraf, S., & Saraf, S., (2016). Recent expansion of pharmaceutical nanotechnologies and targeting strategies in the field of phytopharmaceuticals for the delivery of herbal extracts and bioactives. *Journal of Controlled Release, 241*, 110–124.
4. Batrakova, E. V., Bronich, T. K., Vetro, J. A., & Kabanov, A. V., (2006). Polymer micelles as drug carriers. *Nano particulates as Drug Carriers*, 57–93.
5. Jampilek, J., Kos, J., & Kralova, K., (2019). Potential of nanomaterial applications in dietary supplements and foods for special medical purposes. *Nanomaterials, 9*(2), 296.

6. Chidi, O., & Adebayo, I. V., (2018). Determination of critical micelle concentration and thermodynamic evaluations of micellization of GMS. *Mod. Chem. Appl., 6*(251), 2.

7. Mandavi, R., Sar, S. K., & Rathore, N., (2008). Critical micelle concentration of surfactant, mixed-surfactant and polymer by different methods at room temperature and its importance. *Orient. J. Chem., 24*(2), 559–564.

8. Nesměrák, K., & Němcová, I., (2006). Determination of critical micelle concentration by electrochemical means. *Analytical Letters, 39*(6), 1023–1040.

9. Mourya, V. K., Inamdar, N., Nawale, R. B., & Kulthe, S. S., (2011). Polymeric micelles: General considerations and their applications. *Indian J. Pharm. Educ. Res., 45*(2), 128–138.

10. Elham, A. M., Irhan, I. A. H., Rehab, M. Y., Ahmed, A. A. S., Ahmed, R. E., Mohammad, F. H., & Farid, A. E. B., (2018). Polymeric micelles for potentiated antiulcer and anticancer activities of naringin. *International Journal of Nanomedicine, 13,* 1009–1027.

11. Zhaokun, Y., Qingtang, W., Xiaolong, L., Jun, P., Qin, L., Ming, W., & Jiumao, L., (2018). Cationic nanomicelles derived from Pluronic F127 as delivery vehicles of Chinese herbal medicine active components of ursolic acid for colorectal cancer treatment, *RSC Adv., 8,* 15906–15914.

12. Ji, S., Lin, X., Yu, E., Dian, C., Yan, X., Li, L., Zhang, M., Zhao, W., & Dian, L., (2018). Curcumin-loaded mixed micelles: Preparation, characterization, and *in vitro* antitumor activity. *Journal of Nanotechnology, 2018.*

13. Ju, X., Zhang, S., Wang, Q., Li, X., & Yang, P., (2010). Preparation and stability of diallyl trisulfide self-assembled micellar injection. *PDA Journal of Pharmaceutical Science and Technology, 64*(2), 92–96.

14. Godugu, C., Doddapaneni, R., & Singh, M., (2017). Honokiol nanomicellar formulation produced increased oral bioavailability and anticancer effects in triple-negative breast cancer (TNBC). *Colloids and Surfaces B: Biointerfaces, 153,* 208–219.

15. Zhai, Y., Guo, S., Liu, C., Yang, C., Dou, J., Li, L., & Zhai, G., (2013). Preparation and *in vitro* evaluation of apigenin-loaded polymeric micelles. *Colloids and Surfaces A: Physicochemical and Engineering Aspects, 429,* 24–30.

16. El-Desoky, A. H., Abdel -Rahman, R. F., Ahmed, O. K., El-Beltagi, H. S., & Hattori, M., (2018). Anti-inflammatory and antioxidant activities of naringin isolated from *Carissa carandas* L: *In vitro* and *In vivo* evidence. *Phytomedicine, 42,* 126–134.

17. Morteza, J., & Azam, J., (2016). DPPH Radical-scavenging activity and kinetics of antioxidant agent hesperidin in pure aqueous micellar solutions. *Bulletin of the Chemical Society of Japan, 89*(8), 869–875.

18. Jadhav, P., Bothiraja, C., & Pawar, A., (2016). Resveratrol-piperine loaded mixed micelles: Formulation, characterization, bioavailability, safety and *in vitro* anticancer activity. *RSC Advances, 6*(114), 112795–112805.

19. Gaysinsky, S., Davidson, P. M., Bruce, B. D., & Weiss, J., (2005). Stability and antimicrobial efficiency of eugenol encapsulated in surfactant micelles as affected by temperature and pH. *Journal of Food Protection, 68*(7), 1359–1366.

20. Tolen, T., Ruengvisesh, S., & Taylor, T., (2017). Application of surfactant micelle-entrapped eugenol for prevention of growth of the Shiga toxin-producing Escherichia coli in ground beef. *Foods, 6*(8), 69.

21. Zhen, L., Wei, Q., Wang, Q., Zhang, H., Adu-Frimpong, M., Firempong, C. K., Xu, X., & Yu, J., (2018). Preparation and *in vitro/in vivo* evaluation of 6-gingerol TPGS/ PEG-PCL polymeric micelles. *Pharmaceutical Development and Technology,* 1–30.

22. Ganea, G. M., Fakayode, S. O., Losso, J. N., Van, N. C. F., Sabliov, C. M., & Warner, I. M., (2010). Delivery of phytochemical thymoquinone using molecular micelle modified poly (D, L lactide-co-glycolide)(PLGA) nanoparticles. *Nanotechnology, 21*(28), 285104.
23. Zhu, Y., Peng, W., Zhang, J., Wang, M., Firempong, C. K., Feng, C., Liu, H., Xu, X., & Yu, J., (2014). Enhanced oral bioavailability of capsaicin in mixed polymeric micelles: Preparation, *in vitro* and *in vivo* evaluation. *Journal of Functional Foods, 8*, 358–366.
24. Dhar, J., & Puranik, S. B., (2018). Regulatory requirements for registration of biosimilar products and imports in India: A recent scenario. *Research & Reviews: A Journal of Drug Formulation, Development and Production, 4*(2), 32–39.
25. Santini, A., Cammarata, S. M., Capone, G., Ianaro, A., Tenore, G. C., Pani, L., & Novellino, E., (2018). Nutraceuticals: Opening the debate for a regulatory framework. *British Journal of Clinical Pharmacology, 84*(4), 659–672.
26. Singh, M. C., & Gujar, K. N., (2013). Nutraceuticals: Uses, risks and regulatory scenario. *International Journal of Pharmacy and Pharmaceutical Sciences, 5*(Suppl 3), 23–26.

CHAPTER 14

Insights into the Latest Taste Masking Techniques for Nutraceutical Products and Functional Foods

PARAG A. KULKARNI,[1] AMIT B. PAGE,[1] and
DEBARSHI KAR MAHAPATRA[2]

[1]SVKM's NMIMS, School of Pharmacy and Technology Management,
Shirpur Campus, Shirpur, Dhule, Maharashtra, India

[2]Department of Pharmaceutical Chemistry, Dadasaheb Balpande College
of Pharmacy, Nagpur–440037, Maharashtra, India,
E-mail: mahapatradebarshi@gmail.com

ABSTRACT

Taste matters a lot to every individual in this globe. Although patients of any age group may be forced to take the daily medicine requirements but when it comes to nutraceutical products and functional foods, avoidance or skipping tendency dominates, which may have negative results over an individual. This interesting book chapter comprehensively discusses the most prevalent taste-masking techniques for bitter nutraceutical products and functional foods such as flavoring approach, sweeteners approach, amino acids approach, polymer coating, inclusion complexes approach, ion exchange resin complexes, solid dispersion approach, liposomes approach, microencapsulation approach, multiple emulsions approach, lipophilic components approach, adsorption approach, gelation approach, pH modifiers approach, prodrug method, salt formation approach, rheological modification, freeze-drying process (FDP), wet spherical agglomeration (WSA) technique, and continuous multipurpose melt (CMT) technology, etc. The chapter will provide imperative information to the global health researchers regarding ways to overcome this problem and improve individual compliance.

14.1 INTRODUCTION

Till now, learners have understood that nutraceutical is a pharmaceutical product of one or more than one nutritional ingredient prepared to be consumed orally (mostly) for the purpose of prevention of a disease or disorder or for the management of dietary deficiency of certain nutritional compound. A nutraceutical may be of plant, animal, or mineral origin, either in a form of whole extract of fraction of the extract, or even a blend of them. They may be bitter or unpalatable in taste or in some cases they may cause nausea due to obnoxious odor [1].

The taste buds work in harmony with olfactory sensation, therefore for a better acceptance of nutraceuticals; they need to be presented in acceptable taste as well as odor. A simple example can be quoted here for the purpose of understanding; multivitamin multimineral food supplement to be added in milk is flavored in chocolate or vanilla flavor to increase its acceptance in children. Several brands of proteins are presented in the form of flavored powder to be mixed with milk [2].

To increase palatability and acceptance and therefore compliance per say, it is needed that the food supplements or nutraceuticals are either be masked or turned acceptable by converting in tasty, pleasant, and easily palatable forms. In addition to this, the taste improvement is also beneficial for converting the nutraceutical product in the form of chewable or mouth dispersible dosage form for better acceptance [3]. This book chapter will take the readers through basic concepts of taste masking and their applications, particularly in the masking of obnoxious taste or odor of nutraceuticals.

14.2 ANATOMY OF TASTE BUDS AND PHYSIOLOGY OF TASTE

Human has a great sense of taste. Acceptance of any orally consumed substance is determined by its taste. Through around 10,000 taste buds spread over the tongue, humans can sense five major tastes, viz. sweet, sour, salty, hot, and umami (delicious). Sensation of taste is affected by these taste buds, through the taste cells. In certain cases, the taste can be correlated with their chemical nature. E.g., alkaloids mostly tend to be bitter in taste, while, as molecular weights of salts go on reducing the taste tends to get more salty than bitter. There was a concept of having distinct areas of taste sensation for a particular taste, some scientists, however, deny this and suggest of having no such distinction [4].

Taste is a sensory response in reaction to chemical stimulation of taste receptors. Bitter taste perception is considered the most complex modality.

Taste buds are a group of some 50 around columnar cells with sensory nerve endings at its base forming a cluster. These taste buds convert the chemical signal given by a tastant in the generation of neuronal action potential to be transmitted by the through nerve cells to the brain for interpretation. There are three major cranial nerves involved in the sensation of taste or gustation. They include- 7, 9, and part of 10th cranial nerves-the facial, the glossopharyngeal and the vagus nerves, respectively [5].

The salty and sour taste substances activate neurons through ion channel receptors, while sweet, bitter, and umami tastants do it through G protein-coupled receptors. Sweet tastants cause depolarization of gustatory cells leading to the sensation of taste. Bitter tastants even though bind to G-protein coupled receptors (GPCR), due to diversity in chemical nature, behave differently. Some of them produce sensation of taste through depolarization of gustatory cells, while other cause hyperpolarization, some others increase GPCR activation while others can inhibit the activation. The specific response depends on which molecule is binding to the receptor. Further nerves carrying taste information travel to the medulla, then through the thalamus are routed to the primary gustatory cortex, which is responsible for sensations of taste. The nuclei in the medulla can extract some information which may stimulate the hypothalamus and amygdalae causing autonomic reflexes such as nausea, vomiting, or salivation [6].

The primary visual cortex, primary olfactory cortex, and primary gustatory cortex are situated in three different areas of the brain. Each of these primary areas are associated with higher-order secondary areas, which have a communication with each of these (taste, vision, and odor), which further integrate the information and give a specific reaction. This is the reason, when good appearance or smell of food stimulates salivation or chemical with offensive odor tends to taste bitter [7]. This is another reason to have a better appearance and flavor in addition to masking of taste (Table 14.1).

Nutraceuticals obtained from plant, animal, marine as well as mineral sources are claimed to lower the risk of chronic diseases like cancer and cardiovascular disease (CVD), as well as increase immunity and general health. Studies on the mechanisms of these actions are focused on phenols and polyphenols, flavonoids, isoflavones, terpenes, and glucosinolates present in them. Enhancing the phytonutrient content of plant foods through selective breeding or genetic improvement and extraction of active components from them has resulted in an excellent supplement for disease prevention. However, most of these active principles are bitter, acrid, or astringent, which in turn reduce acceptance of them by consumers [8].

TABLE 14.1 Human Threshold Values of Taste and its Masking

Taste	Substance	Threshold for Tasting	Masking Agent
Salty	NaCl	0.01 M	Butterscotch, maple, apricot, peach, vanilla, wintergreen mint
Sour	HCl	0.0009 M	Citrus flavor, licorice, root beer, raspberry
Sweet	Sucrose	0.01 M	Vanilla, fruit, and berry
Bitter	Quinine	0.000008 M	Wild cherry, walnut, chocolate, mint, anise

14.3 TASTE MASKING TECHNIQUES

A discussion is provided for the most prevalent taste-masking techniques for bitter nutraceutical products and functional foods such as flavoring approach, sweeteners approach, amino acids approach, polymer coating, inclusion complexes approach, ion exchange resin complexes, solid dispersion approach, liposomes approach, microencapsulation approach, multiple emulsions approach, lipophilic components approach, adsorption approach, gelation approach, pH modifiers approach, prodrug method, salt formation approach, rheological modification, freeze-drying process (FDP), wet spherical agglomeration (WSA) Technique, and continuous multipurpose melt (CMT) technology, etc. Table 14.2 depicts the list of few common taste-masking agents.

TABLE 14.2 Some Common Taste Masking Agents Examples

Nutraceutical Product	Product Form	Taste Masking Agents
Eucalyptus oil	Solutions	Fenchone, borneol or isoborneol
Thymol	Solutions	Anethole, eucalyptol, and methyl salicylate
Theophylline	Capsules	D-sorbitol, sodium saccharin, sodium glutamate, and vanilla essence
Caffeine	Capsules	Starch, lactose, mannitol
Saponins	Fortified foods	Glycine, alanine
Gymnema Sylvestre	Tablet	Chitosan
Polylactic acid	Fortified foods	Sodium chloride, calcium chloride

14.3.1 TASTE MASKING WITH FLAVORS, SWEETENERS, AND AMINO ACIDS

This is the most common, simplest, and common practiced technique for masking the taste of highly bitter nutraceuticals where amino acids, natural sweeteners (fructose, sucrose, mannitol, glucose, sorbitol, etc.), artificial sweeteners, and flavors (menthol) are employed. These coating materials (often referred to as excipients) are high aqueous (saliva) soluble and effectively coats the taste buds [9].

14.3.2 POLYMER COATING OF THE DRUG

The polymer coating (hydrophilic polymers, hydrophobic polymers, sweeteners, lipids, etc.), is one of the best taste masking technique that represents an effective barrier (physical) for the nutraceutical products by preventing any plausible interaction with the taste buds [10].

14.3.3 FORMATION OF INCLUSION COMPLEXES

For the delivery of low dose bitter nutraceuticals, the inclusion complexes are utilized effectively where Van der Walls type of interaction takes place between the active functional food (termed as guest) and complexing agent (termed as host). The complexing agent (such as cyclodextrin (CD), a sweet cyclic oligosaccharide) compromises the solubility of the guest and restricts the particles to come in contact with the taste buds which lead to masking attributes [11].

14.3.4 ION EXCHANGE RESIN COMPLEXES

The taste masking is achieved even through ion exchange resins where weak anion exchange (tertiary amine substituents, etc.), and weak cation exchange (carboxylic acid moieties, etc.), are employed for exchanging the charged counter ions. The high molecular weight water-insoluble polymers absorb the ions of the groups of nutraceutical material into the polymer matrix [12].

14.3.5 SOLID DISPERSION

Solid dispersions (SDs) are the formulations exclusively recommended for the nutraceuticals for taste masking (by employing sugar or suitable agents) where ingredients are dispersed in an inert polymeric solid carrier (polyethylene glycols, hydroxypropyl methylcellulose (HPMC), urea, ethylcellulose, mannitol, povidone, etc.), formed by the melting-solvent method or kneading method [13].

14.4   MICROENCAPSULATION

The modern technique of microencapsulation offers protection of active nutraceutical components in both liquid form and solid form by employing suitable polymeric material such as hydroxyethylcellulose, gelatin, shellac, carnauba wax acrylics, povidone, ethylcellulose, and beeswax [14]. These microencapsulated components prevent the direct contact of the nutraceutical product with the human tongue and effectively produced the taste masking. This pharmaceutical process may be achieved by one of the subsequent procedures:

- Solvent evaporation;
- Air suspension coating;
- Pan coating;
- Interfacial polymerization;
- Spray drying and spray congealing;
- Multiorifice-centrifugal process;
- Coacervation-phase separation.

14.4.1   MULTIPLE EMULSIONS

Multiple emulsions technique comprising of w/o/w emulsion (nutraceuticals or functional foods are dissolved in internal aqueous phase) or o/w/o emulsion (nutraceuticals or functional foods are dissolved in external aqueous phase) is an impressive approach for the useful masking of the bitter nutraceuticals. The bitter taste masking attributes are best for both the types of multiple emulsions [15].

14.4.2   LIPOSOMES

Liposomes are the lipid carrier comprising of multiple lipid layers which are composed of phosphatidylinositol, soya lecithin, phosphatidic acid, etc. It is quite effective in masking the taste of bitter hydrophobic functional foods by entrapping them within the lipid core [16].

14.4.3   PRODRUG METHOD

This is a rare option for taste masking where a chemically inactive form of the nutraceutical is produced, just like a prodrug. Here, the inactive form of the nutraceutical product is biotransformed into active form by changes in the chemical groups. The degree of the amount of the disagreeable taste receptor-substrate adsorption can be customized [17].

14.4.4   TASTE MASKING WITH LIPOPHILIC COMPONENTS

Polyalcohols, surfactants, oils, and lipids are employed as potential vehicles for effective taste masking. These vehicles owing to the enhanced viscosity, completely coat the taste buds. A large amount of lecithin is sometimes added to makeover the unpleasant taste of the nutraceutical products [18].

14.4.5   FORMATION OF SALT AND DERIVATIVE

The preparation of salts results in an abrupt reduction in the solubility profile of the nutraceutical component which leads to decrease in the horrid taste. The ionized nutraceutical molecules are formed through salt formation by proton removal or addition [19].

14.4.6   TASTE MASKING WITH EFFERVESCENT FORMULATIONS

Nutraceuticals under dissolved form in carbonated water helps overcoming the nasty taste of the product form. The nutraceutical sieved material is mixed uniformly with sodium bicarbonate, an effervescence producing component that releases the carbon dioxide (CO_2) in the presence of water (hence, is termed carbonated water) [20].

14.4.7   RHEOLOGICAL MODIFICATION

This is a brilliant approach for preventing the diffusion of bitter nutraceutical components from the saliva of the buccal cavity to the human taste buds by applying carbohydrates (microcrystalline cellulose, etc.), or gums xanthan gum, etc., as the rheological modifier [21].

14.5   FREEZE DRYING PROCESS (FDP)

This method is used to develop fast-dissolving oral technologies such as Zydis and Lyoc technology. Zydis is a tablet-shaped dosage form that spontaneously disintegrates in the mouth in seconds. This is due to the high porosity produced by the FDP. The Zydis process requires the active ingredient to be dissolved or suspended in an aqueous solution of water-soluble structure formers. The resultant mixture is then poured into the preformed blister pockets of a laminate film and freeze dried. The two most commonly used structural excipients are gelatin and mannitol, although other suitable excipients can be used (e.g., starches, gums, etc.). This process is ideally suited to low solubility drugs as these are more readily freeze-dried. Taste is very important for this type of dosage form, and it is possible to produce palatable formulations by using artificial sweeteners (e.g., aspartame) and conventional flavors. Lyoc differs from Zydis in that the product is frozen on freeze-dryer shelves [22].

14.5.1   TASTE MASKING BY ADSORPTION

This is a well-known taste-masking technique that is recently in application for the bitter nutraceutical substances. These formulations were prepared by initially mixing the nutraceuticals with a powder material (bentonite, silicates, veegum, silica gel, etc.), that is insoluble in water. The insoluble powder absorbs the drug and the solvent is removed concurrently. Further, the powders are dried and then these dried adsorbents are prepared as the final formulation. This adsorbed nutraceutical formulation restricts the solubility of the material in the saliva and therefore makes easy administration of the product [23].

14.6   pH MODIFIERS

Partial taste masking of the nutraceutical products or functional foods can be achieved through synthetic polymers, natural polymers, waxes, and resins. Eudragit L, the enteric polymer which solubilizes beyond pH 5.5 is one of the most widely employed polymers for taste masking as the salivary pH is nearly 5.8. Nutraceuticals coated with Eudragit L are dispersed in the liquid orals that prevent leaching of the content in the buccal cavity [24].

14.6.1 TASTE MASKING BY GELATION

For the effectual taste masking of bitter functional foods containing tablets, water-insoluble gel coating is applied. Usually, this water-insoluble gelation is performed by employing sodium alginate in the presence of bivalent metal (Ca^{2+}, etc.), ions. Sometimes, calcium gluconate overcoating is applied. The tablet remains tasteless and can be administered to all ages with simple water [25].

14.7 WET SPHERICAL AGGLOMERATION (WSA) TECHNIQUE AND CONTINUOUS MULTIPURPOSE MELT (CMT) TECHNOLOGY

Wet spherical agglomeration (WSA) is a combined taste-masking technique with a new microencapsulation approach originally taken into application for the coating of the therapeutically privileged substances and continuous granulation. This novel technique may also be applied for successfully overcoming the bitter taste of functional foods.

14.8 CONCLUSION

The chapter content will provide information to all enthusiastic researchers across the globe regarding the various techniques, approaches, and methods for masking the bitter taste of nutraceutical products and functional foods.

KEYWORDS

- continuous multipurpose melt
- freeze-drying process
- functional foods
- G-protein coupled receptors
- masking
- nutraceutical products

REFERENCES

1. Abraham, A. and Mathew, F., (2014). Taste masking of pediatric formulation: A review on technologies, recent trends and regulatory aspects. *Int. J. Pharm. Pharm. Sci., 6*(1), 12–19.

2. Sharma, S., & Lewis, S., (2010). Taste masking technologies: A review. *International Journal of Pharmacy and Pharmaceutical Sciences, 2*(2), 6–13.

3. Ayenew, Z., Puri, V., Kumar, L., & Bansal, A. K., (2009). Trends in pharmaceutical taste-masking technologies: A patent review. *Recent Patents on Drug Delivery & Formulation, 3*(1), 26–39.

4. Vummaneni, V., & Nagpal, D., (2012). Taste masking technologies: An overview and recent updates. *International Journal of Research in Pharmaceutical and Biomedical Sciences, 3*(2), 510–524.

5. Pein, M., Preis, M., Eckert, C., & Kiene, F. E., (2014). Taste-masking assessment of solid oral dosage forms: A critical review. *International Journal of Pharmaceutics, 465*(1, 2), 239–254.

6. Ahire, S. B., Bankar, V. H., Gayakwad, P. D., & Pawar, S. P., (2012). A review: Taste masking techniques in pharmaceuticals. *Pharma Science Monitor, 3*(3).

7. Sharma, V., & Chopra, H., (2010). Role of taste and taste masking of bitter drugs in pharmaceutical industries an overview. *Int. J. Pharm. Pharm. Sci., 2*(4), 123–125.

8. Douroumis, D., (2007). Practical approaches of taste-masking technologies in oral solid forms. *Expert Opinion on Drug Delivery, 4*(4), 417–426.

9. Wagh, V. D., & Ghadlinge, S. V., (2009). Taste masking methods and techniques in oral pharmaceuticals: Current perspectives. *J. Pharm. Res., 2*(6), 1049–1054.

10. Joshi, S., & Petereit, H. U., (2013). Film coatings for taste masking and moisture protection. *International Journal of Pharmaceutics, 457*(2), 395–406.

11. Mulay, M. S., (2012). Taste masking by inclusion complexation: A review. *International Journal of Pharmaceutical Research and Development, 397,* 3547.

12. Suhagiya, V. K., Goyani, A. N., & Gupta, R. N., (2010). Taste masking by ion-exchange resin and its new applications: A review. *Int. J. Pharm. Sci. Res., 1,* 22–37.

13. Gupta, K., Madaan, S., Dalal, M., Kumar, A., Mishra, N., Singh, K., & Verma, S., (2010). Practical approaches for taste masking of bitter drug: A review. *International Journal of Drug Delivery Technology, 2*(02), 12–22.

14. Dhakane, K., Rajebahadur, M. C., Gorde, P. M., & Gade, S. S., (2011). A novel approach for taste masking techniques and evaluation in pharmaceutical: An updated review. *Asian J. Bio. Pharm. Sci., 1,* 18–25.

15. Jain, M., Pareek, A., Bagdi, G., Aahmad, D., & Ahmd, A., (2010). Taste masking methods for bitter drug: A review. *International Journal of Pharmacy and Life Sciences, 1*(6), 336–339.

16. Thoke, S. B., Gayke, A., Dengale, R., Patil, P., & Sharma, Y., (2012). Review on: Taste masking approaches and evaluation of taste masking. *Int. J. Pharm. Sci., 4*(2), 1895–1907.

17. Amita, N., & Garg, S., (2002). An update on taste-masking technologies for oral pharmaceuticals. *Indian Journal of Pharmaceutical Sciences, 64*(1), 10.

18. Chatap, V. K., Gupta, V. B., Sharma, D. K., & Nandgude, T. D., (2007). *A Review on Taste Masking Methods for Bitter Drug* (Vol. 5, No. 4). Pharmainfo.net.

19. Gandhi, C. K., Patel, M. R., Patel, K. R., & Patel, N. M., (2011). A review: Taste masking in pharmaceutical. *International Journal of Pharmaceutical Research and Development, 3*(3), 19–26.

20. Wadhwa, J., & Puri, S., (2011). Taste masking: A novel approach for bitter and obnoxious drugs. *International Journal of Biopharmaceutical and Toxicological Research, 1*(1), 47–60.

21. Chirag, J. P., Tyagi, S., Dhruv, M., Ishita, M., Gupta, A., Mohammed, U. M. R., & Paswan, S. K., (2013). Pharmaceutical taste-masking technologies of bitter drugs: A concise review. *Journal of Drug Discovery and Therapeutics, 1*(5), 39–46.

22. Deepthi, P. Y., Chowdary, Y. A., Murthy, T. E. G. K., & Seshagiri, B., (2012). Approaches for taste masking of bitter drugs. *ChemInform., 43*(30).

23. Sajal, J. K., Uday, S. R., & Surendra, V., (2008). Taste masking in pharmaceuticals: An update. *Journal of Pharmacy Research, 1*(2), 126–130.

24. Tripathi, A., Parmar, D., Patel, U., Patel, G., Daslaniya, D., & Bhimani, B., (2011). Taste masking: A novel approach for bitter and obnoxious drugs. *JPSBR, 1*(3), 36–142.

25. Kaushik, D., & Dureja, H., (2014). Recent patents and patented technology platforms for pharmaceutical taste masking. *Recent Patents on Drug Delivery & Formulation, 8*(1), 37–45.

Index

H

For Product Safety Concerns and Information please contact our EU
representative GPSR@taylorandfrancis.com
Taylor & Francis Verlag GmbH, Kaufingerstraße 24, 80331 München, Germany

www.ingramcontent.com/pod-product-compliance
Lightning Source LLC
Chambersburg PA
CBHW060749220326
41598CB00022B/2373